Forensic Odontology

Forensic Odontology

Principles and Practice

EDITED BY

Jane A. Taylor

Faculty of Health and Medicine
University of Newcastle
Australia

Jules A. Kieser (Deceased)

Faculty of Dentistry
University of Otago
New Zealand

WILEY Blackwell

Library of Congress Cataloging-in-Publication Data

Forensic odontology (Taylor)
Forensic odontology : principles and practice / edited by Jane Taylor, Jules Kieser.
     p. ; cm.
   Includes bibliographical references and index.
   ISBN 978-1-118-86444-9 (cloth)
I. Taylor, Jane (Jane A.), editor.   II. Kieser, Jules (Jules A.), editor.   III. Title.
   [DNLM: 1. Forensic Dentistry. W 705]
   RA1062
   614′.18–dc23
                              2015029796
A catalogue record for this book is available from the British Library.

Set in 9.5/13pt Meridien by SPi Global, Pondicherry, India

1   2016

Contents

Contributors

Richard Bassed
Victorian Institute of Forensic Medicine, Victoria; and Monash University, Australia

Eleanor Bott
Healthscope Pathology, Australia

Maurice Churton
Oral and Maxillofacial Surgeon (Retired), New Zealand

Gemma Dickson
Victorian Institute of Forensic Medicine, Australia

Denise Donlon
Discipline of Anatomy and Histology, University of Sydney, Australia

Terry Lyn Eberhardt
PestLab, AsureQuality Ltd, New Zealand

Norman Firth
Faculty of Dentistry, University of Otago, New Zealand

Alex Forrest
School of Natural Sciences, Griffith University Nathan Campus and Health Support Queensland, Australia

Jeremy Graham
School of Dentistry and Oral Health, La Trobe University, Australia

Denice Higgins
Forensic Odontology Unit, University of Adelaide, Australia

Erin F. Hutchinson
School of Anatomical Sciences, University of the Witwatersrand, South Africa

Helen James
Forensic Odontology Unit, University of Adelaide, Australia

Zaf Khouri
New Zealand Society of Forensic Odontology, New Zealand

David C. Kieser
Christchurch Hospital, New Zealand

Jules A. Kieser (Deceased)
Faculty of Dentistry, University of Otago, New Zealand

Stephen Knott
Queen Elizabeth Medical Centre and Faculty of Medicine, Dentistry and Health Sciences, University of Western Australia, Australia

Russell Lain
Oral Surgery and Diagnostic Imaging Department, Sydney Dental Hospital, Australia

Mark Leedham
Northern Territory Coroner's Office, Australia

Alain G. Middleton
NSW Forensic Dental Identification Unit, Westmead Hospital, Australia

David L. Ranson
Victorian Institute of Forensic Medicine; and Monash University, Australia

Alistair Soon
Health Support Queensland, Australia

Jane A. Taylor
Faculty of Health and Medicine, University of Newcastle, Australia

Hugh G. Trengrove
New Zealand Society of Forensic Odontology, New Zealand

J. Neil Waddell
Faculty of Dentistry, University of Otago, New Zealand

Dedications

Anthony (Tony) John HILL (2.5.1945–22.12.2013)

Tony was born and educated in New Zealand and eventually settled as a private practitioner in Melbourne, Australia. In 1992 he enrolled in the Diploma of Forensic Odontology course at the University of Melbourne under the tutelage of Professor John Clement, and worked at the Victorian Institute of Forensic Medicine (VIFM) on a volunteer basis for a number of years. In 2004 he retired from general dentistry to take up a position at the VIFM as Senior Forensic Odontologist.

Tony's empathy for those in our society who die with no one to mourn for them or to care for their remains was always evident – he was a man who wore his heart very much on his sleeve. He spent many years working with the Victoria Police long-term missing persons unit attempting to identify the remains of unidentified people who would otherwise be buried in anonymous graves. Tony played a large role in the identification of the remains of Ned Kelly, Colin Ross and Ronald Ryan, all of whom were exhumed from Pentridge Prison in 2009.

The contribution Tony made to the identification of people who died in tragic circumstances in mass fatality incidents has been an enduring testament to his professionalism. He played a major role in the Disaster Victim Identification teams deployed to identify the deceased following the 2002 Bali bombings, the 2004 Boxing Day tsunami in Thailand, and the Black Saturday bush fires in Victoria in 2009. Throughout these physically and emotionally demanding operations Tony always maintained a sense of cheerfulness, generosity and professional empathy that was an example for us all.

The recipient of several awards, including the Australian Federal Police Operations Medal and a Premier's Citation, Tony will be sadly missed by all who had the good fortune to work with him and benefit from the enormous breadth of his knowledge and experience. He was a compassionate and kind person, and despite spending so many years dealing with some of the more difficult aspects of humanity, always maintained his empathy and respect for his fellow man.

Julius (Jules) August KIESER (20.12.1950–10.6.2014)

It takes a noble man to plant a seed for a tree that will someday give shade to people he may never meet.

(Chinese proverb)

Jules was a man with an insatiable appetite for knowledge that he loved to share. He was born in Pretoria, South Africa, and educated at the University of the Witwatersrand in Johannesburg where he completed his BSc in 1971 and qualified as a dentist in 1975. He practised in the outback of South Africa and subsequently in London and Johannesburg. He gained a PhD (Medicine) in 1989 and in 1991 was appointed as reader of craniofacial biology and in 1994 as honorary professor of anatomy.

In 1996 he moved to Dunedin with his wife, Glynny, and their four teenage children, where he assumed the position of chair and head of the department of oral sciences and orthodontics at the University of Otago. Jules was a well-respected and much-loved teacher who was an extraordinary inspiration to all those around him. He had an extensive range of research interests, which led to many exciting PhD theses. Jules assisted in police investigations ranging from child abuse and trauma analysis to disaster victim identification. He played a leading role in the identification of victims of the Boxing Day tsunami in 2004 and the Christchurch earthquake in 2011. For these he was awarded a New Zealand Special Services Medal, a Canterbury Earthquake citation and a fellowship of the Faculty of Maxillofacial Pathology from the Royal College of Pathologists of Australasia.

Jules obtained a DSc from his alma mater in 2001 and in 2004 was awarded an ad hominem fellowship in dental surgery from the Royal College of Surgeons, Edinburgh. In 2006 he was elected a professional fellow of the Forensic Science Society (UK) and in 2009 was appointed as the inaugural director of the Sir John Walsh Research Institute at the University of Otago.

Through all his research and his academic life, and his commitment to forensic sciences, Jules always remained a man for all and one who cared about each and every individual in his life.

Preface

The genesis for this book was the inclusion of forensic odontology as an independent stream in the Faculty of Oral and Maxillofacial Pathology in the Royal College of Pathologists of Australasia. Jules and I thought it would be fantastic to have a dedicated textbook to support the curriculum that had been developed. Our vision was an awareness text rather than a didactic discourse. After John Wiley & Sons kindly supported the initiative, we then set about asking fellows to contribute, and I would like to thank each and every one of them for their efforts and the timeliness of their contributions. I would particularly like to thank David Kieser, Erin Hutchinson, Terry Eberhardt and Gemma Dickson who stepped in for Jules after his passing. A text such as this can only ever be seen as a group project and all authors have willingly given their time and expertise to participate.

Our first sadness came with the passing of our esteemed colleague Tony Hill in December 2013. It was not a hard decision to decide to dedicate this text to Tony as he epitomised everything we love about our profession. Our next sadness was the passing of Jules Kieser in June 2014. While potentially catastrophic for the text, once again the decision was not hard; that Jules would remain as an editor of the book. For me personally Jules was someone I looked up to as a role model and mentor as well as a good friend. His enthusiasm for forensic work, generosity of spirit in sharing knowledge and commitment to teaching the next generation is something I can only dream of emulating. I know that since June I have mentally consulted him frequently about content and progression of the book, so I feel he has well and truly earned his place on the front cover. Some comments about Jules from our authors are presented below.

> Of a legend I write, an infinite intellect, extraordinary mind and insatiable thirst for knowledge. Jules Kieser is best described as a gentle giant whose youthful enthusiasm for everything around him endeared him to both colleague and student alike. He was a phenomenal supervisor, colleague and friend who inspired those around him to strive far beyond their own expectations or self-imposed limitations. (E Hutchinson)

> Jules was one of the great enthusiasts and supporters of forensic medicine. He was a master of his subject and someone who could hold an audience in the palm of his hand and leave them both awed and enthused. Hugely respected by his peers, he was a practitioner, researcher and teacher. As a teacher he truly inspired his students and left them with a desire to push the boundaries and commit to supporting the forensic sciences. (D Ranson)

An outstanding academic with a heart of gold who always put his students and colleagues first. (N Waddell)

I had the pleasure of meeting Jules for the first time in Darwin, when he was keynote speaker at a forensic odontology meeting. He immediately impressed me as a great speaker, researcher and person. I was looking forward to seeing Jules again when I heard of his loss. The scientific community and his family have lost a wonderful man. (M Leedham)

Jules was a true gentleman in every respect. Slow to judge, quick to support, first to honour and lead by example. Those of us who were lucky enough to have worked with him are better people for having known him. (A Forrest)

Jules Kieser contributed mightily to the discipline of dental anthropology. His research into odontometrics was particularly valuable and an example of his great breadth of research, crossing over into palaeoanthropology and forensic anthropology. (D Donlon)

Following the Asian tsunami in Thailand, I fortunately found myself working with a very committed and caring guy called Jules. Since that time our friendship evolved and I became aware of Jules' dedication to his work and his drive to research the unknown. (S Knott)

An inspiration to both students and colleagues alike. (D Kieser)

All that being said, this book would not have been possible without the dedication and ceaseless work of Jules' wife Glynny. She has kept me, and the authors, on the straight and narrow and prodded and poked us to make sure we met deadlines. She has my unending admiration, thanks, gratitude and love.

It is fitting to express our thanks and gratitude to the Office of the Dean (Dentistry) at the University of Otago for editorial funding. Further thanks go to Rachael Ballard and Fiona Seymour who worked on the manuscript during its infancy, Audrie Tan who has been an unfailing support throughout, Jenny Cossham, Janine Maer and all at John Wiley & Sons. Thank you to Caro McPherson for her copyediting and to Sandeep Kumar at SPi Global for overseeing the production of this book.

Jane A. Taylor
2015

CHAPTER 1

Foundation knowledge in forensic odontology

Jules A. Kieser[1,†], Jane A. Taylor[2], Zaf Khouri[3] and Maurice Churton[4]

[1] Faculty of Dentistry, University of Otago, New Zealand
[2] Faculty of Health and Medicine, University of Newcastle, Australia
[3] New Zealand Society of Forensic Odontology, New Zealand
[4] Oral and Maxillofacial Surgeon (Retired), New Zealand

> I'm not young enough to know everything.
>
> J. M. Barrie, *The Admirable Crichton*, Act I (1903).

Introduction

Forensic odontology has been variously described as 'the application of dental science to the administration of the law and the furtherance of justice' [1] and 'that branch of dentistry, which in the interest of the law, deals with the proper handling and examination of dental evidence and the proper evaluation and presentation of such evidence' [2] and 'the overlap between the dental and the legal professions' [3].

The dates of these references show us that forensic odontology has been developing as a specialist discipline for the last 50 or so years. Once the remit of the merely interested or community minded and conscientious, dentists now require rigorous training and commitment to practise within the profession. The discipline is recognised as a speciality of dentistry in a number of countries including Australia, and has a dedicated training stream within the Royal College of Pathologists of Australasia.

To the general community, forensic odontology is most frequently associated with personal identification of the deceased, and gains significant publicity at the time of disasters, natural or manmade, that claim many lives at a single point in time. The actual scope of practice of forensic odontology is considerably broader than this. In addition to human identification forensic odontologists are also involved in the examination and assessment of bite mark injuries, orofacial injuries following assault or trauma and child abuse injuries; age assessment of both living and deceased persons and civil cases involving malpractice and fraud allegations.

†Deceased

Forensic Odontology: Principles and Practice, First Edition. Edited by Jane A. Taylor and Jules A. Kieser.
© 2016 John Wiley & Sons, Ltd. Published 2016 by John Wiley & Sons, Ltd.

Practitioners must also have a sound working knowledge of dental anatomy and pathology; comparative dental anatomy; the natural sciences; legal system law and relevant legislation. An understanding of the activities and interactions of other forensic disciplines is also important in developing an appreciation of the scope and practice of forensic odontology.

On a personal level, forensic odontologists should have broad dental experience, a methodical and analytical approach with considerable patience and attention to detail. Personal honesty and integrity and emotional stability are vital. Good communication and interpersonal skills and the ability to work as part of a team, as well as autonomously, are important, as is the ability to formulate and articulate well-balanced views.

This text will work its way through current best practice in a number of these areas. It aims to support those undertaking training in forensic odontology in the development of their knowledge base, which forms alongside their clinical skills. The text is designed at the awareness level rather than aiming to be an exhaustive discourse. Contemporary excellent references are provided to extend reading beyond the introductory.

Recent reviews into the scope and reliability of all forensic evidence have seen an explosion of research and literature relating to improving the performance and professionalism of practitioners [4–6]. Recent rulings challenging admissibility of specialist evidence, recognition of specialist disciplines and the evidentiary weight of forensic evidence also highlight the need for continued research into aspects of practice and the need to establish and maintain high professional standards [7–9].

A short history of forensic odontology

Although it was reported that forensic odontology was used to identify victims of a fire in the Vienna Opera House in 1878 [10,11], the modern era of forensic odontology is said to have commenced with the identification of the victims of the Bazar de la Charité fire which occurred on 4 May 1897 in Rue Jean-Goujon, Paris. One hundred and twenty-six members of the Parisian aristocracy perished after an ether–oxygen film projector ignited a rapidly destructive fire. All but 30 of the victims were identified visually or by personal effects, mainly jewellery, on the day after the fire.

The honour of being the 'father of forensic odontology' is often bestowed on Oscar Amoedo, a Cuban dentist working in Paris at the time of the fire, but he did not in fact do any of the odontology work at this incident. The author of *L'Art dentaire en Medecine Legale* [12], which was a considerable text on many aspects of the use of teeth for legal purposes, merely reported the outcomes of the work done by other dentists after the fire. The credit for the idea of using dental information to assist the final identifications actually belongs to the

Paraguayan Consul, Mr Albert Haus. With the identification of the last 30 victims seeming almost impossible, Mr Haus suggested consulting the dentists who had treated the remaining missing persons. One of the unidentified victims was the Duchesse d'Alencon, who was a daughter of the Duke of Bavaria and sister of Elisabeth, Empress of Austria and Anne, Queen of Naples. A Dr Isaac B Davenport had provided dental services to the duchess and many of the other victims. He was apparently a trained botanist as well as a dentist and his detailed notes included excellent drawings of the dentition. He examined the majority of the remaining unidentified bodies and was eventually able to identify the duchess via her dentition. Subsequently, a number of other dentists were invited to examine the remains of the deceased, and eventually all but five of the victims were identified. The police accepted these dental identifications and released the bodies to the families [13,14].

Prior to the Bazar de la Charité fire, the most frequently cited examples of the use of teeth and dental work in the identification of the deceased were those of Lollia Paulina by Agrippina using visual recognition of 'distinctive teeth' in AD 49; Charles the Bold in 1477; General Joseph Warren by Paul Revere via a fixed wire silver bridge in 1776; Dr Parkman by Nathan Keep from the fit of dentures on study models in 1849 and Napoleon the IV in 1879 [14,15].

In 1954 Strom [16] reported that the use of teeth to aid identification in the modern understanding had in fact initially been proposed by Godon in 1887, but a report by M'Grath in 1869 [17] described the use of dental characteristics to differentiate between two incinerated females.

After the Bazar de la Charité fire many authors published case studies on the use of forensic odontology in both single and multiple fatality incidents. Rosenbluth [18] described a case in the United States in 1898 where dentistry played a pivotal role in a murder case. Ryan [19] mentioned the identification of US Sailors from an accident in 1927, commenting on the high quality of the dental records kept by the Navy, and Gustafson [11] recounted a fire in Oslo in 1938 where 29 people died. Simpson [20] summarised a number of English cases of the early 20th century. Strom [16] and Gustafson [11] reported on the identification of victims of the Second World War via forensic odontology. Teare [21] discussed the identification of 28 victims of a plane crash in 1950; Frykholm [22] described a Swedish shipping accident in 1950 where 15 were killed and Mercer, Reid and Uttley [23] and Warren [24] a rail accident in New Zealand in 1953 where 151 perished. Bradley and Miller [25] described the use of odontology in the identification of victims of a plane crash in Canada. The odontology aspects of the identification of the 118 victims of a fire aboard the SS Noronic in Toronto Harbour were described in detail by Grant, Prendergast and White [26].

While these reports would appear to indicate that forensic odontology was well recognised as a discipline, Frykholm [22] did comment that both the German and Swedish authorities involved in his case report 'reflected a certain disbelief' about the value of forensic odontology, and that the assisting dentists had no personal experience in forensic odontology prior to this case. It would be reasonable to assume that both appreciation of the value and experience in forensic odontology were varied across the globe, as can be expected with any relatively new and emerging area of knowledge and investigation.

Histories of forensic odontology acknowledge that the next significant publication after Amoedo was that of Gustafson in 1966 [11]. This comprehensive text covered principles of identification in single and multiple death situations, information that can be ascertained from the dentition, the responses of teeth and restorations to various traumas and the investigation of bite mark injuries. Although more than 40 years old, the text remains relevant for contemporary practitioners. Texts by Furuhata and Yamamoto [27], Luntz and Luntz [28], Sopher [29], Cameron and Sims [30] and Harvey [31], and an edition of the *Dental Clinics of North America in 1977* soon followed, marking the arrival of a new specialist discipline within the field of dentistry. Professional associations relating to forensic odontology soon followed, for instance the Canadian Society of Forensic Odontology was formed in 1970 [32], the British Association of Forensic Odontology in 1983, the New Zealand Society of Forensic Dentistry in October 1985 and the Japanese Society of Forensic Odontology in 1988 [33], thereby exposing the discipline to larger numbers of interested dentists.

The American Society of Forensic Odontology formed in 1970 as a group open to any person with an interest in forensic odontology [15]. In 1976 the American Board of Forensic Odontology (ABFO) was incorporated under the auspices of the American Academy of Forensic Sciences to 'establish, enhance and revise qualifications and standards' and has developed a role as a certifying board of forensic odontologists [34]. This is the only international society to take on such a formal role.

The International Association of Forensic Odonto-Stomatology (IOFOS) held its inaugural meeting in Paris in June 1973 [35]. Membership was initially open to any individual with an interest in forensic odontology, and was not limited only to dentists. It has since grown to be a group where membership is country based, having 32 member countries in 2015, and is the organisation representing the majority of forensic odontologists internationally.

The only international journal dedicated to forensic odontology, *The International Journal of Forensic Dentistry*, was published from 1973–1977 and was the forerunner to the *Journal of Forensic Odonto-Stomatology*, which commenced publication in 1982 [35].

In Australia, The Australian and New Zealand Forensic Science Society was formed in 1971 with the aim of bringing together scientists, police, pathologists and members of the legal profession [36]. Dentists were, and still are, members of this group. Dentists with a special interest in forensic odontology formed The Australian Society of Forensic Dentistry, now known as The Australian Society of Forensic Odontology (AuSFO) in 1984.

Forensic odontology in Australia

Pounder and Harding [37] reported that the first autopsies were conducted in Australia in 1790, one on a victim of inanition (starvation) and the other on the governor's gamekeeper who was allegedly murdered by Aborigines. Pounder [38], reporting on death investigations in the early years (1839–1840) of South Australia, indicated that both the coroner and jurors were required to view the body of the victim as part of the inquest procedures. Although the stated purpose was for the examination of marks of violence, it could also be surmised that it was also for the formal identification of the victim. This practice remained until 1907. Cordner, Ranson and Singh [39] indicated that the first lectures on forensic medicine were held in Melbourne in 1866.

It is not really known when forensic odontology was first used in Australia. A report in the New South Wales Police News in 1943 reported the identification in Melbourne, Victoria of a murder victim, Bertha Couphlin, in 1923 and of Norman List in 1924, using dental evidence [40]. This article also mentioned that the identity of three victims of a plane crash in the Dandenong Ranges in 1938 'could only be established by means of the teeth'. Cleland [41] mentioned the identification of a New Zealand citizen in Western Australia in 1930, although this identification appeared to rely more on circumstantial dental evidence than true dental identification.

The most famous identification case from that era occurred in New South Wales in 1934. Colloquially known as the Pyjama Girl Case, the outcome highlights the value of dentistry in identification, but also the pitfalls that can derail the well intentioned but ill prepared, dental practitioners and investigating police officers. It involved a murdered woman who remained unidentified for 10 years, ostensibly due to unreconciled dental information. The badly burned remains of the victim were discovered by a farmer in a road culvert near Albury in September 1934. The body was clothed only in pyjama remnants and revealed little other identifying information. A post-mortem was carried out and a local dentist, Dr Francis Jackson, was asked to complete a dental autopsy. His unorthodox procedures can best be explained by his inexperience in forensic odontology, but mitigated by the fact that few people had any experience at that time. At the subsequent Supreme Court trial he admitted that this was his only experience of forensic odontology and he found the process 'revolting and unnerving' [42, 43].

Dr Jackson's unconventional examination occurred over three visits. On the first he made some observations and extracted two teeth, on the second he extracted an additional four teeth and on the third he took upper and lower impressions of the jaws. The extracted teeth were then mounted into the stone dental models made from the impressions 'in approximately the same position as they were in the mouth'. During the course of these examinations Dr Jackson incorrectly identified one tooth and failed to observe restorations in two other teeth. These inaccuracies proved pivotal in the inability to identify the remains for 10 years. Photographs of the casts with the extracted teeth in situ were distributed to dentists in Australia and New Zealand, and every dentist in metropolitan Melbourne and Sydney was personally contacted by police. Information about this case, including images of the extracted teeth, was also displayed as 'ads' in movie theatres. Unsurprisingly, none of these activities yielded any useful information.

The police relied on public appeals to attempt to identify the victim. Apparently over 500 women who had been reported missing were located in the course of the investigation. Ultimately the remains were preserved in a formalin bath, and it became quite a social outing to visit 'the body in the bath' at Sydney University. Many false identifications were offered to police from these viewings. About nine months after the victim was found, police interviewed a man, Antonio Agostini, whose wife Linda had been reported missing by a family friend. This gentleman indicated that he did not recognise the lady in the bath, but provided police with the details of his wife's dentist.

The information provided by this dentist did not match the post-mortem information provided by Dr Jackson and the investigation continued. Interestingly, the dental information provided by the treating dentist was also somewhat unorthodox. It transpired that he kept no formal clinical records and the information he provided was an amalgamation of personal recollection and ledger entries of fees paid. This information would be legally inadmissible today.

In 1944 new investigating officers decided to review all the information relating to the case and asked another dentist, Dr Magnus, to re-examine the body. Dr Magnus was more thorough in his work, correctly identifying all the teeth and locating previously unobserved restorations. On comparison the new charting matched the ante-mortem dental information of Linda Agostini. Antonio Agostini subsequently admitted to having murdered his wife in 1934 [42, 43].

This case highlights the importance of experience and procedure in forensic odontology, the value of comprehensive clinical records and attention to detail during the collection of post-mortem information. Despite this recognition it still took a number of years before formal services in forensic odontology were established in Australia. Interestingly, this development followed a similar path in most states and territories. From around the early 1960s there was spasmodic use of dentists to assist police in identification procedures. This was generally an informal arrangement with little or no remuneration, which meant that the dentists providing the services frequently had to complete examinations and prepare reports after hours and at weekends. In the vast majority of cases a single practitioner provided the entire service. Limited training in forensic odontology was available to these dental practitioners and it is a credit to their dedication and professionalism that the discipline has developed to the high standard and international reputation it enjoys today.

Dr Gerald (Gerry) Dalitz provided the early forensic odontology services in Victoria from the 1950s. In 1961 he was awarded a Doctor of Dental Science for a thesis entitled 'Some aspects of dental science – Identification of human remains' by the University of Melbourne. While collecting data for his research his expertise came to the attention of the Victoria Police and they slowly began utilising his services. Dr Ross Bastiaan started working with Dr Dalitz in 1979, continuing until 1989. Professor, then Dr, John Clement arrived from the UK in 1989 to take up a position in the dental school at the University of Melbourne. Professor Clement had considerable experience in forensic odontology and had worked on a number of mass fatality incidents including the Free Enterprise at Zeebrugge in 1987. Upon arriving in Melbourne, Professor Clement was instrumental in establishing a broader and more professional forensic odontology service in Victoria, including the introduction of the first graduate training program and the only Chair in Forensic Odontology in Australia [44].

In New South Wales the Chief Dental Officer, Dr Norbert Wright, together with Drs Max Bullus, John Wild, Sydney Levine and Barry Barker provided the odontology services on a similarly informal basis. It was not until 1981, when Associate Professor Griffiths completed a Masters in Public Health relating to Disaster Victim Identification and took up a position at Westmead Hospital, that forensic odontology was formally recognised and funded through the New South Wales Health Service [44].

In South Australia, Dr Kenneth Brown's interest in forensic odontology was sparked in 1961 when he attended a lecture entitled 'Dental aspects of forensic medicine' presented by Professor Gosta Gustafson who was the Professor of Oral Pathology at the University of Lund in Sweden. In 1967 he responded to a request by the South Australian Police Department who were looking for volunteer dentists to provide them with dental expertise. Dr Brown read widely, but as there were no formal training programs in Australia at the time, he used a Churchill Fellowship in 1976 to travel internationally to increase his knowledge and experience in the field of forensic odontology. His honorary work for the South Australian Police continued until a formal post in forensic odontology, the first such position in Australia, was created at the University of Adelaide in 1980. Drs Jane Taylor (2000–03) and Helen James (2004–present) have succeeded Dr Brown as leaders of this unit [44].

Pocock, in his 1979 paper on the provision of a forensic pathology service in Western Australia [45], commented that a part-time forensic odontologist was 'available for consultation in any problem of identification'. This position had been established in the early 1960s and was held by Dr Frank Digwood, and became a formal part-time position in the 1980s. Dr Stephen Knott provided assistance to Dr Digwood from 1991, and succeeded him on his death in 1993 [44].

Dr Kon Romaniuk moved from New Zealand to take up a position in the dental school at the University of Queensland as an oral pathologist in the mid 1960s. As appears typical for most developing services in Australia, he provided an honorary consultation service in forensic odontology, later establishing a more formalised arrangement that provided a modicum of remuneration. Dr Alex

Forrest started working as an assistant to Dr Romaniuk in 1985, and became the consultant forensic odontologist in 1994 after a traffic accident necessitated Romaniuk's retirement [44].

Early forensic odontology services in Tasmania were by Dr Eric Canning MBE, a non-practising dentist who worked in the anatomy department at the University of Tasmania. Dr Paul Taylor has provided these services since 1989 [44].

It is believed that early forensic odontology services in the Northern Territory were provided by Dr T. Paul Boyd who worked part time as an oral surgeon in the public health system. Dr John Plummer had an interest in forensic odontology from his undergraduate years but his first exposure came in the late 1970s when he was the government dentist in Katherine and was asked to help identify a family who had drowned after a flash flood had washed away their homestead. Dr Plummer continued his professional development in forensic odontology by using a Churchill Fellowship, awarded in 1985, to travel extensively and meet and work with a number of forensic odontologists internationally. As a health service employee Dr Plummer continued his involvement in forensic dentistry on an honorary basis until his retirement in 2002, which proved satisfactory as the caseload in the Northern Territory was not large [44].

The Australian Capital Territory was the last of the Australian jurisdictions to establish any regular service in forensic odontology, and this occurred as a consequence of poor identification procedures in a murder that led local dentist Dr David Griffiths to develop an interest, undertake some training and offer his services [44].

Also quite interestingly, all states and territories in Australia have experienced major incidents which required the services of forensic odontology and which served to increase the profile of the emerging discipline across the country.

The Ash Wednesday bushfires of 1983 claimed 47 lives in Victoria: 14 of the 22 (64%) Victorian victims who could not be visually recognised were identified via forensic odontology [46]. Forensic odontology now forms a routine part of single and multiple death investigations in Victoria, including the Kew Cottages Hostel fire in 1996 (nine deceased); the Linton bushfires in 1998 (five deceased); a light plane crash at Myrrhee in 2002 (six deceased); the Mt Hotham plane crash in 2005 (three deceased); a car accident at Donald in 2006 (eight deceased); the Kerang train crash in 2007 (nine deceased); the crash in the Burnely Tunnel in 2007 (three deceased); and in a major national Disaster Victim Identification (DVI) incident, the Black Saturday bushfires of 2009 that claimed the lives of 174 people [44].

The Grafton bus crash in 1989 highlighted the limitations of visual identification and changed identification practices in New South Wales. One of the 21 victims of this accident was initially incorrectly visually identified, so when just over two months later 35 people were killed in a collision between two buses near Kempsey, forensic odontology was used to identify the majority of the victims. Subsequently, forensic odontology has been used as part of the identification repertoire in all mass fatality incidents in New South Wales including the Newcastle earthquake in 1989 (13 deceased), the Thredbo landslide in 1997 (19 deceased), the Glenbrook train accident in 1999 (seven deceased) and the 2003 Waterfall train disaster (seven deceased) [44].

The largest mass fatality incident in the recent history of South Australia was the 'Ash Wednesday' bushfires of 1983. Twenty-eight South Australians lost their lives in fires in the hills surrounding Adelaide and in the south east of the state near Mount Gambier. This incident saw the first activation of the newly written State Disaster Plan. Eight (29%) of the South Australian victims were identified by dental comparison [47]. Subsequent to this South Australia seemed to develop a national reputation as the locale for bizarre murders with the victims of many of these incidents being formally identified by forensic odontology, including the Truro murders in 1978 (seven victims) [48–50], the Family Murders over the period of 1979 to 1983 (five victims) and the Snowtown murders in 1999 (11 victims) [44].

One of the earliest incidents of significance for the recognition of forensic odontology in Australia occurred in Western Australia with the crash of a Viscount aircraft in Port Hedland in 1968. Dental comparisons played a significant role in the identification of the 29 victims. Forensic odontology provided the identification for eight of the 10 victims of the 1982 Merredin bus crash, and seven of the 10 victims of the 1988 Leonora plane crash, and was important in the identification of the victims of the Gracetown Cliff collapse which killed 18 teenagers in 1998 [44].

Significant incidents in Queensland have included the crash of two Blackhawk helicopters near Townsville in 1996 (15 deceased), the Childers Backpackers Hostel fire in June 2000 (15 deceased) and the Lockhart River plane crash in May 2005 (15 deceased) [44].

While the Mt St Canice Boiler explosion in September 1974 (eight deceased) and the Tasman Bridge collapse in January of 1975 (12 deceased) were major incidents for Tasmania, it is the Port Arthur massacre of 1996, where Martin Bryant shot and killed 35 and wounded 19, that stays in the national memory. Three of these victims were subsequently burnt beyond recognition in a fire set by the gunman in a nearby guest house where he had held them hostage overnight. The identification of these three victims was assisted by odontology evidence. The fire was so extensive and intense that almost 30 kilograms of debris was collected during the recovery of the bodies to ensure all possible remains were located. One body was so severely incinerated that only fragments of both jaws and a few teeth were able to be located. Two of the victims wore dentures, one a full upper against some remaining lower natural teeth, the other full upper and lower dentures. One full upper denture survived the conflagration. Dental and medical radiographs of the head area were instrumental in confirming the identification of these victims [44, 51].

Although the Northern Territory has not experienced many mass fatality incidents, one of Australia's largest did occur in Darwin. Cyclone Tracy, which struck on Christmas Eve in 1974, resulted in the death of 71 people. While it is believed that those who were recovered at the time of the cyclone were identified visually, a number of victims who were recovered in later years were identified via forensic odontology. All 13 victims of the collision of two hot air balloons over Alice Springs in 1989 were also identified via dental comparison [44].

Covering a small geographic area, the Australian Capital Territory has not experienced many multiple fatality' incidents. Incidents such as the 1991 plane crash in the Brindabellas (four killed) and the 1993 MIG crash at Canberra airport were coordinated and managed by the Search and Rescue division of the Australian Federal Police ACT with identifications being completed via dental comparison [44].

Dr Anthony Lake of South Australia has completed a comprehensive history of forensic odontology in Australia which can be accessed on the Australian Society of Forensic Odontology website http://www.ausfo.com.au.

Forensic odontology in New Zealand

The contemporary history of forensic odontology (as it is now known) in New Zealand began in 1946 and has been well documented by Churton (Fig. 1.1) [52]. The first recorded use of dental identification of deceased individuals in this country came in 1946, after the end of the Second World War, when Lt Col O.E.L. Rout RNZDC was tasked with the formal identification of the New Zealand war dead. Most of these individuals had perished in battlefields across North Africa, Italy, Europe and the Pacific and many had been buried where they fell. Correct identification of the exhumed remains was important prior to re-interment in official war cemeteries.

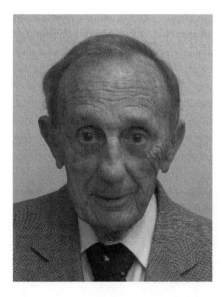

Fig. 1.1 Dr Maurice Churton.

Rout noted that dentists were not always present when bodies were recovered, so he wrote a very detailed document entitled 'Posthumous Dental Identification'. This document was used with great success by the lay personnel of the Graves Registration Units (GRU). Churton remarks that, surprisingly, there is no mention of Rout's work in Brooking's text, *A History of Dentistry in New Zealand* [53].

The Tangiwai Bridge rail disaster on Christmas Eve, 1953 (in which 151 people died) prompted a concerted effort in this country to establish forensic odontology as a permanent, scientific discipline. Some of those killed were recent arrivals to New Zealand who had no relatives and no local medical or dental records to help in their identification. Of the dead, the bodies of 20 were never recovered and may have been washed out to sea [54]. Of the bodies that were found, some were initially misidentified and 21 others were eventually buried unidentified in a common grave at the Karori Cemetery in Wellington [23].

Subsequent disinterment of these remains was undertaken in April 1954 and 16 of these bodies were identified, nine by dental means. The dentists involved were Dr G. McCallum and Dr O.E.L. Rout.

Churton [52] stated that these events were the catalyst for the development of forensic interest by the profession. In particular, Associate Professor Frank Shroff, from the University of Otago School of Dentistry, took up the challenge.

Professor Shroff gave a paper on dental identification at a Christchurch dental conference in the mid 1950s and subsequently produced a 28-page document entitled 'Procedure for the examination of human remains for the purpose of identification' in 1954. The intention was to have police print and distribute this procedure manual to the profession and to selected pathologists. In addition, bulk supplies were to be held at various police centres and made available in the event of a major disaster.

In 1958, negotiations began between the New Zealand Dental Association (NZDA) and various government agencies to print the manual. NZDA members were canvassed to determine which practitioners were interested in being involved in this field of practice.

Despite the continued endeavours of Professor Shroff, a plan for printing and distribution of the manual and the establishment of a national forensic dental practitioner group did not progress until the procedure manual was eventually published as a hard-backed booklet in 1968. The manual was printed and distributed to a number of police districts.

In 1963 another incident rekindled interest in forensic dentistry. On 3 July 1963, a DC3 passenger aircraft with 23 people on board crashed into a vertical rock face in the Kaimai Ranges near Matamata, while on a flight from Auckland to Tauranga in poor weather. All on board died and four of the bodies were never recovered.

Of the 19 bodies recovered from the crash site, 13 were identified on the basis of dental evidence [55]. The forensic dental examinations of the recovered bodies were undertaken by Dr Colin Powell and Dr Edward Blair, both from Hamilton. This disaster helped cement forensic odontology in the consciousness of the New Zealand Police.

During the mid 1960s, the national discussion revolved around the labelling of dentures and the desirability for dental practitioners to retain radiographs for extended periods of time.

In 1966, two homicides in Auckland (the Soutter and Harvey killings) once again galvanised the attention of the profession and police. In both cases, an extended post-mortem interval made it difficult to identify the victims by what were considered to be conventional means at the time. The dentists involved were Professor Shroff, Dr Euan Moore and Dr Robert Max. For the first time in this country forensic odontology became a significant player in criminal investigations.

Meanwhile, discussions and correspondence between the police and the dental profession continued on two levels.

On the one hand, while the NZDA was communicating with police hierarchy, concurrent private correspondences were being conducted between individual members of both organisations. This resulted in confusion and stalled progress.

Professor Shroff advanced his strongly held view that one practitioner, specifically trained in forensic odontology, should be appointed for each island to assist police with such matters as homicides and accidents. He also foresaw the need for a larger group of dentists to deal with disaster situations.

On the other hand, Dr Moore supported the appointment of one or two dentists in each major centre, who would act as a 'link' between the profession and police.

Churton [52] observed that the entire thrust of discussions became focused on one aspect of forensic odontology – namely, the identification of the dead. That such should be the case is perhaps understandable, but even so it was unfortunate, because it imposed limitations on the role of dentistry and denied the police, and through them the community, the full range of expertise potentially available through the profession. This narrow perception of forensic odontology persists today, even among some who are involved in the provision of these services.

It was eventually decided by the NZDA that each of its various branches would be asked to put forward recommendations of those 'interested in forensic dentistry' for subsequent appointment to a nation-wide team. Those nominated were to have 10 years' experience in practice. The proposal outlined was that this group would be trained in court and police procedures and receive basic training in post-mortem methods, forensic medicine and certain relevant laboratory skills. In addition, each appointed dentist would be required to report annually to the NZDA, at which time the appointments would be re-affirmed.

This course of action was approved by the NZDA in 1967. In 1968 a panel of 19 interested practitioners (one for each police district) was appointed, chaired by Dr Moore. The stated intention was not only to train this group for their roles in their individual communities, but also for their secondary, but no less important, role as a national dental forensic team capable of dealing with major disasters.

Unfortunately, few of the proposals regarding education, training and reporting came to fruition. A seminar involving Auckland members, police and medical personnel was held in 1969, but this appears to have been the only one of its type. Literature was not circulated and no formal educational seminars were held. Indeed, only one was proposed – to be given by Professor Shroff in Dunedin; but this had to be cancelled due to a lack of support. The only formal education included as part of the dental undergraduate course at the time was delivered by Professor Shroff as part of the oral pathology curriculum. This ceased when he retired from the School of Dentistry in 1974.

From 1969 until the Erebus disaster in 1979, the national panel barely functioned. At a local level, some panel members were involved with police while others were not. It would appear that the level of activity depended not so much on the expertise of the individual practitioner, but more on the whims of the constabulary as often the practitioner of the victim would be called rather than the nominated panel member. A further problem revealed by the passage of time was the cyclic transfer of senior police contacts. This often broke the invaluable personal contact and the dental panel member would be repeatedly faced with re-establishing his credibility and acceptability to the police replacements. Finally, in some areas, another trend began to emerge. With increasing frequency, full-time hospital-based dental officers became involved in identifications at the request of the police. Whilst this may have given a degree of flexibility to the police, it was certainly not looked upon as an encouraging development by those members of the profession outside the hospital dental service who over the years (often at significant personal sacrifice) had been involved in police matters. Throughout this period, although individual practitioners, panel members and others were involved with homicide investigations, aircraft crashes, fires, drownings, and the like, the emphasis was always on post-mortem dental identification rather than forensic odontology.

The result of this lack of organised activity, together with piecemeal utilisation of panel members and a dearth of formal education in forensic odontology, was inevitable – the panel ceased to exist as a functional entity. The fact that some of its members continued their involvement was a tribute to their professional dedication and personal motivation rather than a reflection of any encouragement received. This situation continued unaltered until the Erebus disaster in 1979.

On 28 November 1979, an Air New Zealand DC10 aircraft crashed on Mount Erebus in Antarctica with the loss of 257 passengers and crew. At the time of writing, this disaster ranks as the worst disaster the country has ever suffered.

The weeks that followed saw the recovery of bodies from Antarctica, their transportation to Auckland and the successful identification of 213 victims. The dental team consisted largely of Auckland practitioners with no experience in DVI. The result achieved by the 10 dentists involved had a major impact on the overall success of this DVI operation with identification by dental means accounting for approximately 60% of all of the identifications achieved.

The Erebus debrief, to which not all who had been involved in the dental DVI team were invited, should have provided an opportunity to propel forensic odontology into a new era in the 1980s. Unfortunately, this opportunity was missed and the school of thought that carried the day was that the coordination of future operations of this type should be left to senior clinicians in the hospital dental service. The reasoning for this was that it was better to have an 'office' rather than an individual as the first point of contact for police. Furthermore, Auckland was proposed as the obvious place to deal with large numbers of disaster victims. To support this view, it was suggested that private dental practitioners could not be expected to be involved in major disaster victim identification operations because of the attendant financial losses and disruption to their practices.

This decision was made despite the fact that the majority of those involved in Erebus and the prior DVI operations were in private practice (either part time or full time) – a state of affairs that has continued to apply through to the present day.

These proposals and others were discussed with a senior police officer and as a result a report was presented to the Council of the NZDA. In line with these proposals, a plan agreed to by both the police and the dental profession was put in place to deal with future disaster situations. By 1983, the wheel had turned a full circle as the NZDA once again requested the names of those wishing to be involved in forensic work.

Churton concluded his history (to 1983) by lamenting the fact that forensic odontology had not become firmly established in New Zealand. He proposed five reasons for this failure.

1 The profession and the police had failed to appreciate the real meaning of forensic odontology. Rather, the term had become synonymous with the identification of the dead by dental means. While this latter skill had been, and will always remain, an important aspect of the subject, it must be fully appreciated that it is only a part and not the whole.
2 Despite several resurgences of interest due to large-scale or high-profile events, the groundswell of enthusiasm had not been capitalised on prior to 1983. The result was a loss of interest and enthusiasm.
3 The profession failed to heed and properly utilise great teachers such as Frank Shroff and R.M.S. Taylor.
4 A flawed decision-making process whereby, over the years, decisions of ever-increasing importance have been made without full and free discussion and without the involvement of many of those with a proven interest in, and knowledge of, this topic.
5 A flawed method of appointments. It is a fundamental tenet that all professional appointments in clinical fields should be made as a result of properly described and advertised job descriptions. It is unacceptable that a particular individual is *ipso facto* the most suitable person for a position simply because he or she holds an unrelated appointment.

Table 1.1 NZSFO president and secretary/treasurer, by year.

Year	President	Secretary/treasurer
1984	Maurice Churton	John Gilhooly
1987	Maurice Churton	John Gilhooly
1991	Maurice Churton	John Gilhooly
1994	Don Adams	Mike Bain
1997	Denis Beale	Mike Bain
2000	Kerry Sullivan	Mike Bain
2002	Howard Mace	Mike Bain
2004	Wayne Laing	Hugh Trengrove
2006	Bruce Murdoch	Hugh Trengrove
2008	Zaf Khouri	David Antunovic
2010	Jules Kieser	David Antunovic
2012	Craig Campbell	David Antunovic
2014	James Hannah	David Antunovic

In December 1983, a request was made by Dr Churton to form a special Society of Forensic Dentistry under the aegis of the NZDA. Approval was immediately forthcoming. On 22 June 1984, the first meeting of the New Zealand Society of Forensic Dentistry (NZSFD) was held in the Conference Room of the Freyberg Building at Wellington. For the first time, all those with an interest or involvement in forensic matters had the opportunity to participate in a formal society for mutual benefit and advancement of knowledge. The previously conflicting approaches of Shroff and Moore were finally reconciled.

The new society began with an enthusiastic membership of 16 and elected the inaugural president – Dr Maurice Churton (Fig. 1.1), who was subsequently re-elected for a further two terms. Dr Churton is regarded as the 'father of the NZSFO'. A list of presidents and secretary/treasurers is given in Table 1.1.

The constitution of the Society refers to its objectives as to:

a) Foster and coordinate and advance forensic odontology howsoever and to inter alia hold conferences of high scientific merit.

b) Seek and maintain association with the International Organisation of Forensic Odonto-Stomatology (IOFOS) and the New Zealand Dental Association Incorporated.

c) Pursue and advance the recognition and acceptance of the practice of forensic odontology within the fields of forensic science and odontology, and to establish high professional and clinical standards for the practice of forensic odontology.

d) Stimulate interest in forensic odontology generally, and to establish liaison with organisations with kindred interests.

e) Raise money.

f) Publish literature.

g) Enlist support of government and any other appropriate organisation or group.

h) Give advice on matters related to forensic odontology.

i) Do all such things as are incidental or conducive to any of these objectives and, as such, are necessary or desirable to encourage, directly or indirectly, the attainment thereof.

The NZSFD became the vehicle for a forensic voice of the dental profession and a motivator for its members. A conscious decision was made at the outset to bring acknowledged overseas experts in forensic dentistry to its meetings – a decision which proved invaluable. Annual conferences have been held every year, and attendance numbers have steadily increased.

In the 30 years of its existence, the membership of the society has grown to a present day number of 89, as per Table 1.2. This healthy membership arises as a result of a collegial spirit of support and the free sharing of knowledge and experience.

While society membership was initially comprised exclusively of dentists and dental specialists with no formal qualifications in forensic odontology, interest was such that, in 1990, two members sought training overseas and both Drs Denis Beale and Zaf Khouri returned with Graduate Diplomas in Forensic Odontology – the first practitioners in New Zealand to have formal training in the discipline. They have since been joined by several others with similar qualifications and yet others who have undergone other forensic training.

In 1991, after discussions between the NZSFD and the New Zealand Police and subsequent advertising for applicants, the New Zealand police appointed six regional advisors on forensic dentistry. This system worked well for a few years, but suffered the same fate as the previous attempts at formalised police involvement in the 1960s, 1970s and early 1980s, and for the same reasons. A national advisory panel to police was then convened, but this also failed in short order.

The 1990s ticked along unremarkably, with a good representation of casework being reported at the NZSFD annual meeting each year. During this period, the society appointed seven regional coordinators to act as first contact points for police and anyone else who wished to access the services that society members could offer.

In 1996, Professor Jules Kieser was appointed to the Chair and Head of the Department of Oral Sciences and Orthodontics at the University of Otago in Dunedin.

Table 1.2 Membership of the NZSFO.

Year	Status	Number
1984	Full members	16
2014	Full members	56
	Associate members	22
	Overseas members	5
	Honorary members	6

He promptly joined the NZSFD in 1997 and was elected onto the Executive of the Society in 2000, subsequently becoming president in 2008. Professor Kieser was instrumental in bringing to the profession all that Professor Shroff before him had aspired to achieve – scientific rigour touched with human kindness.

Formal teaching in forensic odontology became part of the undergraduate curriculum again, and through his enthusiasm and engagement with students, Professor Kieser lifted the forensic consciousness of the dental academic community to new highs. In 2009 he was appointed as the inaugural director of the Sir John Walsh Research Institute and continued to inspire and lead undergraduate students and postgraduate research. Through his research, his teaching, his comradeship and his leadership, Professor Kieser contributed much to the knowledge, training and promotion of forensic odontology in New Zealand. He remained an active, contributing and highly respected member of the Executive of the NZSFO until he passed away on 10 June 2014.

In 2005, the National Forensic Pathology Service was launched. This service employs seven full-time and experienced forensic pathologists based in Auckland, Palmerston North, Wellington and Christchurch, who provide 24/7 national coverage for all suspicious deaths and homicides as well as regional coverage for routine coronial deaths. They also provide a support service to coronial pathologists (laboratory-based anatomical pathologists) for all complicated and infectious cases [56].

The net effect of this on forensic odontology was profound and immediate. Casework in the 'regional centres' dropped dramatically (because the forensic pathology was no longer being carried out in the regional hospitals), while casework in the main centres increased.

Through the NZSFO, this situation was addressed by way of an internal understanding whereby practitioners in the main centres, upon receiving forensic cases from other areas, agreed to offer these cases back to the Regional Coordinator for the geographic area of origin. In this way, an equitable distribution of casework was ensured so that all members could remain actively involved in forensic odontology and continue to develop their knowledge and experience.

On 29 August 2006, the new Coroners Act 2006 received royal assent and came into effect on 1 July 2007, repealing and replacing the previous Coroners Act 1988. This established the office of a chief coroner and a series of full-time coroners and saw the end of an ad-hoc coronial service with many part-time coroners spread all over the country.

The main function of the chief coroner is to 'ensure the integrity and effectiveness of the coronial service provided for by the Act with the objective of raising the professionalism of the coronial service and to promote consistency of the coronial practice throughout the country in a timely and efficient way whilst respecting the rights and interests of the bereaved'.

District Court Judge Neil MacLean was appointed the first chief coroner of New Zealand and took up his new position in February 2007. He soon became closely associated with the NZSFD and has attended and spoken at several annual meetings. The chief coroner has had valuable input into the development of this society and some of its core policies.

The relationship with New Zealand Police on a national level is strong, thanks mostly to the tireless work of Drs Warren Bell and Hugh Trengrove. The National DVI team includes a permanent NZSFO representative. The society now has an agreed range of fees for identification cases, odontology opinions and bite mark analysis and this is reviewed by the society from time to time. There are brief descriptions of selected forensic odontology procedures in the Police Manual and also key contacts for advice. There are contacts on the police intranet available for police officers nationwide to access at any time. The society website (www.nzsfo.org.nz) also has a list of regional advisors and their contact details that is freely available to anyone wishing to contact us. At the time of the 2004 Asian Ttsunami, the society negotiated an overseas deployment contract with police. This document is currently being re-negotiated.

In 2009, on its 25th anniversary, the society changed its name to the New Zealand Society of Forensic Odontology (NZSFO) – to better reflect the nature of the discipline and to remain in step with international practice.

In 2011, after several years' hard work, much consultation and many drafts, a credentialing [57] framework was put into place, authored principally by Dr Hugh Trengrove. Credentialing relates to an individual's competence to work in a particular subject area (scope of practice). This provided a mechanism for the NZSFO to provide governance and oversight for forensic odontology activities in New Zealand, in the absence of Dental Council recognition of forensic odontology as a dental speciality. The purpose of credentialing is to provide assurance concerning the competence of personnel performing forensic odontology activities. Currently, the defined scopes of practice include General Forensic Odontology, Forensic Odontology Extended Scope – Bite Marks, Forensic Odontology Extended Scope – Disaster Victim Identification, General Forensic Odontology Scope of Practice – Allied Practitioner and Forensic Odontology Extended Scope – Forensic Auxiliary Procedures.

Credentialing has had a significant impact on how forensic odontology is perceived by police and coronial users of our services. This has resulted in increased confidence in members who are credentialed and a better understanding of why a mechanism to monitor competence is important.

The early 21st century has seen New Zealand forensic odontologists contribute to the identification efforts following a number of significant disasters (as well as the steady stream of sporadic casework). Teams were deployed to Phuket, Thailand after the Boxing Day 2004 Asian tsunami, to assist our Australian colleagues after the Victorian 'Black Saturday' bushfires of February 2009 and after the Christchurch earthquake in February 2011. It is fair to say that, due to education and training, largely through the NZSFO, New Zealand is internationally regarded as a leader in disaster victim identification.

Despite the healthy state of membership of the society, it is interesting to observe that, while many things have changed, much remains the same. In the 1950s and 1960s, Professor Shroff lamented the lack of understanding about what forensic odontology can offer – both within organised dentistry and in police circles. He was a firm believer in formal training and education and, on a number of occasions, stated that a simple interest in forensic odontology was unacceptable as a qualification to undertake the work. Dr Churton was of the same view, and this was a major factor in his drive to establish the NZSFD. Dr Churton noted that police seem to be singularly interested in identification of the dead while disregarding, out of ignorance, the wealth of other assistance available to them. He also remarked on the cyclic frustration of 'educated' senior police moving on and leaving behind a vacuum of knowledge and experience so that forensic odontologists have to start all over again with building relationships.

The recurrent wax and wane of topics such as retention of records, denture marking and universal baseline dental charting in general dental practice continues. Other perennial subjects of discussion are our relationships with police, pathologists and coroners. All these will need to be addressed through our society if progress is to be made.

Where to from here? The future of forensic odontology in this country lies with the NZSFO. This organisation is firmly established as the authoritative voice of the discipline in this country. It is critical, however, if the frustrations of the past are to be avoided in the future, that the society takes a proactive approach to advancement. This will involve recognition by our members that forensic odontology is not merely identification of the dead by dental means. It will require a continued commitment to (and investment in) training and, for some, the pursuit of formal postgraduate qualifications. It will necessitate continued engagement with police, coroners and other healthcare professionals and building increasing awareness and closer relationships with them. It will involve the collegial sharing of information and knowledge among ourselves and with these other groups. Contentiously, it will also mean the establishment of formalised professional standards and a mechanism for policing those standards while maintaining the supportive, inclusive and enabling principles upon which the Society was founded and its credentialing process enshrines.

Working as an odontologist

One important aspect of forensic work is the physical and emotional toll it can take on an individual. This is as much the case for those contemplating a career in the forensic area as it is for those already involved. Exposure to the deceased, either in routine forensic casework or in the disaster situation, is an understandably stressful experience. In addition, much of the casework of the odontologist is often the result of traumatic circumstances, which seem to amplify the less desirable side of human nature. The work environment can be physically challenging. Practitioners need to be aware of the potential impact on their health and actively check in on their mental and physical wellbeing at regular intervals.

Jones [58] surveyed 225 US Air Force personnel who were involved in body movement and identification subsequent to the Jonestown mass suicide in 1978: 32% of respondents reported feeling anxious and depressed immediately after the mission, and for 21% these symptoms continued long term. Those most severely affected were reported to be younger (less than 25 years of age), African American and had a higher level of direct exposure to the remains of victims. Ursano and colleagues [59] reported that identifying with the deceased, particularly as a friend, increased the risk of Post Traumatic Stress Disorder (PTSD) amongst the disaster workers.

McCarrol and colleagues [60] looked at the post traumatic stress experienced by forensic odontologists after the Waco, Texas siege in 1993, where 85 Branch Davidian sect members were incinerated. They found that higher levels of stress were directly related to longer periods of exposure, younger age, less previous disaster experience and the level of personal support. Epstein, Fullerton and Ursano [61] reviewed 355 workers for an 18-month period after their involvement in the air crash at the Ramstein Airshow in 1988. The crash killed 70 and injured many more. They found that lower levels of education, personal exposure to those affected by gross burns, a feeling of numbness and stressful personal circumstances in the six months following the accident were useful indictors for PTSD. Brannon and Kessler [62] commented that stress experienced by DVI practitioners is frequently not reported as it tends to be covert or silent. They concluded from their personal experiences in 10 disasters, that stress was less of a problem for older, more experienced practitioners. These comments were reinforced by Perrin and colleagues [63] who reported that PTSD in workers at the World Trade Centre disaster in 2001 was more likely to occur in those with no or limited prior experience or training. PTSD experienced among disaster rescue workers is 10–20% in the first year after the disaster [64]. This is perhaps reasonably logical, but of little comfort for the new and enthusiastic to forensic odontology.

References

1 Taylor DV. (1963) The law and the dentist. *British Dental Journal* **114**, 389–392.
2 Keiser-Nielsen S. (1970) Forensic Odontology – Cases and comments. In: Wecht CH (ed.) *Legal Medicine Annual*. Appleton Century Crofts, New York.
3 Pretty IA, Sweet D. (2001) A look at forensic dentistry – Part 1: The role of teeth in the determination of human identity. *British Dental Journal* **190**, 359–366.
4 Saks MJ, Koehler JJ. (2005) The coming paradigm shift in forensic identification science. *Science* **309**, 892–895.
5 Pyrek KM. (2007) *Forensic Science Under Siege*. Elsevier Academic Press, Burlington.
6 National Research Council. (2009) *Strengthening Forensic Science in the United States: A Path Forward*. National Academies Press, Washington.

7 Rule of Law Institute of Australia. (2014) *Honeysett v The Queen* HCA 29.
8 Supreme Court of South Australia. (2013) *R v Sumner; R v Fitzgerald SASCFC* 82.
9 LIAC Crime Library. (2008) *R v Tang HCA* 39.
10 Strom F. (1954) Dental aspects of forensic medicine. *International Dental Journal* **4**, 527–538.
11 Gustafson G. (1966) *Forensic Odontology*. Staples Press, London.
12 Amoedo O. (1898) *L'Art Dentaire en Medicine Legale*. Masson et Cie, Paris.
13 Amoedo O. (1897) The role of the dentists in the identification of the victims of the catastrophe of the 'Bazar de la Charité', Paris, 4 May,1897. *The Dental Cosmos* **39**, 905–912.
14 Hill IR, Keiser-Nielsen S, Vermylen Y et al. (1984) *Forensic Odontology – Its Scope and History*. Ian R Hill, Bicester.
15 Luntz LL. (1977) History of forensic dentistry. *Dental Clinics of North America* **21**, 7–17.
16 Strom F. (1954) Dental aspects of forensic medicine. *International Dental Journal* **4**, 527–538.
17 M'Grath JM. (1869) Identification of human remains by the teeth. *Dental Cosmos* **11**, 77–78.
18 Rosenbluth ES. (1902) A legal identification. *Dental Cosmos* **44**, 1029–1034.
19 Ryan EJ. (1937) Identification through dental records. *Journal of Criminal Law and Criminology* **28**, 253–260.
20 Simpson K. (1951) Dental data in crime investigation. *International Criminal Police Review* **6**, 312–317.
21 Teare D. (1951) Post–mortem examinations on air–crash victims. *British Medical Journal* **2**, 707–708.
22 Frykholm KO. (1956) Identification in the Ormen Friske disaster. *Acta Odontologica Scandinavia* **14**, 11–22.
23 Mercer JO, Reid JD, Uttley KFM. (1954) The identification of exhumed bodies. A brief report of the exhumation of the unidentified dead after the Tangiwai railway accident. *New Zealand Medical Journal* **53**, 329–334.
24 Warren JLeB. (1955) The identification of bodies in mass accidents. *New Zealand Dental Journal* **51**, 22–23.
25 Bradley TP, Miller LW. (1955) Suggestions for guidance of dentists establishing identity of disaster victims. *Oral Hygiene* **45**, 452–455.
26 Grant EA, Prendergast WK, White EA. (1952) Dental identification in the Noronic disaster. *Journal of the Canadian Dental Association* **18**, 3–18.
27 Furuhata T, Yamamoto K. (1967) *Forensic Odontology*. Ishiyaku Publishers, Tokyo.
28 Luntz LL, Luntz P. (1973) *Handbook for Dental Identification. Techniques in Forensic Odontology*. JB Lippincott Co., Philadelphia.
29 Sopher IM. (1976) *Forensic Dentistry*. Charles C Thomas, Springfield.
30 Cameron JM, Sims BG. (1974) *Forensic Dentistry*. Churchill Livingstone, London.
31 Harvey W. (1976) *Dental Identification and Forensic Odontology*. Henry Kimpton Publishers, London.
32 Burgman GE. (1987) A history of forensic odontology in Canada. *American Journal of Forensic Medicine and Pathology* **8**, 39–41.
33 Suzuki K. (1996) The history of forensic odontology in Japan. *Forensic Science International* **80**, 33–38.
34 Dorion RB. (1990) Disasters big and small. *Journal of the Canadian Dental Association* **56**, 593–598.
35 Rotzscher K. (1992) The origins and development of FDI, INTERPOL and IOFOS: International co-operation in identification. *Journal of Forensic Odontostomatology* **10**, 58–63.
36 Payne–James J, Byard RW, Corey TS et al. (eds) (2005) *Encyclopedia of Forensic and Legal Medicine*. Elsevier Academic Press, Oxford.
37 Pounder DJ, Harding HWJ. (1984) Forensic services in Australia. *American Journal of Forensic Medicine and Pathology* **5**, 269–278.
38 Pounder DJ. (1984) Death investigation in early colonial South Australia, 1839–1840. *Medicine, Science and the Law* **24**, 273–282.

39 Cordner SM, Ranson DL, Singh B. (1992) The practice of forensic medicine in Australasia: a review. *Australian and New Zealand Journal of Medicine* **22**, 477–486.

40 Anonymous. (1943) Identification by teeth. *New South Wales Police News*, March **1**, 10–12.

41 Cleland JB. (1944) *Teeth and bites in history, literature, forensic medicine and otherwise. Australian* Journal of Dentistry September, 107–123.

42 Coleman R. (1978) *The Pyjama Girl*. Hawthorn Press, Melbourne.

43 Brown KA. (1982) The identification of Linda Agostini. The significance of dental evidence in the Albury 'Pyjama Girl' case. A case report. *Forensic Science International* **20**, 81–86.

44 Taylor J. (2009) A brief history of forensic odontology and disaster victim identification practices in Australia. *Journal of Forensic Odontostomatology* **27**, 64–74.

45 Pocock DA. (1979) Forensic pathology service in Western Australia. *Forensic Science International* **12**, 207–209.

46 Bastiaan RJ. (1984) Dental identification of the Victorian bushfire victims. *Australian Dental Journal* **29**, 105–110.

47 Pounder DJ. (1985) The 1983 South Australian bushfire disaster. *American Journal of Forensic Medicine and Pathology* **6**, 77–92.

48 Brown KA. (1983) Developments in cranio-facial superimposition for identification. *Journal of Forensic Odontostomatology* **1**, 57–64.

49 Brown KA. (1993) The Truro murders in retrospect: A historical review of the identification of the victims. *Annals of the Academy of Medicine* **22**, 103–106.

50 Auslebrook WA, Iscan MY, Slabbert JH et al. (1995) Superimposition and reconstruction of forensic facial identification: a survey. *Forensic Science International* **75**, 101–120.

51 Taylor PTG, Wilson ME, Lyons TJ. (2002) Forensic odontology lessons: multishooting incident at Port Arthur, Tasmania. *Forensic Science International* **130**, 174–182.

52 Churton MC. (1984) New Zealand. In: Hill IR, Keiser-Nielsen S, Vermylen Y, Free E, de Valck E, Tormans E (eds) *Forensic Odontology: Its Scope and History*. Ian R Hill, Bicester, pp. 174–184.

53 Brooking TWH. (1980) *A History of Dentistry in New Zealand*. New Zealand Dental Association Inc, New Zealand.

54 'Search and rescue – Tangiwai disaster' URL: http://www.nzhistory.net.nz/culture/responding–to–tragedy/tangiwai–1953 (Ministry for Culture and Heritage), updated 6 January 1914.

55 Blair E. (1964) Identification of casualties from the Kaimai Air Disaster. *New Zealand Dental Journal* **60**, 151–159.

56 Stables S. (2014) *Clinical Director, National Forensic Pathology Service of New* Zealand. Personal Communication.

57 Credentialing in Forensic Odontology. (2005) New Zealand Society of Forensic Odontology.

58 Jones DR. (1985) Secondary disaster victims: The emotional effects of recovering and identifying human remains. *American Journal of Psychiatry* **142**, 303–307.

59 Ursano RJ, Fullerton CS, Vance K et al. (1999) Posttraumatic stress disorder and identification in disaster workers. *American Journal of Psychiatry* **156**, 353–359.

60 McCarroll JE, Fullerton CS, Ursan et al. (1996) Posttraumatic stress symptoms following forensic dental identification: Mt Carmel, Waco, Texas. *American Journal of Psychiatry* **153**, 778–782.

61 Epstein RS, Fullerton CS, Ursano RJ. (1998) Posttraumatic stress disorder following an air disaster: A prospective study. *American Journal of Psychiatry* **155**, 934–938.

62 Brannon RB, Kessler HP. (1999) Problems in mass–disaster dental identification: A retrospective review. *Journal of Forensic Science* **44**, 123–127.

63 Perrin MA, DiGrande L, Wheeler K et al. (2007) Differences in PTSD prevalence and associated risk factors among World Trade Centre disaster rescue and recovery workers. *American Journal of Psychiatry* **164**, 1385–1394.

64 Galea S, Nandi A, Vlahov D. (2005) The epidemiology of post–traumatic stress disorder after disasters. *Epidemiologic Reviews* **27**, 78–91.

CHAPTER 2

Jurisprudence and forensic practice

David L. Ranson

Victorian Institute of Forensic Medicine; and Monash University, Australia

Legal systems and the healthcare community

The legal aspects of their work often confront healthcare practitioners who frequently complain about the effect that the legal rules regulating healthcare practice have on their work. They may express the view that this represents a form of outside interference with their professional freedom and this is often coupled with a viewpoint that suggests that the healthcare professional always knows best. Such views, of course, are a direct confrontation to the notion of patient autonomy and the right of the community to decide how it wants its healthcare services provided.

When asked why law matters, the response from many healthcare practitioners is 'because you will get sued if something happens to your patient'. Such a narrow view of the law is understandable as medical law education was not included in undergraduate medical curricula or postgraduate specialist training courses until relatively recently.

In reality the legal system supports healthcare professionals more than it restricts them. As a group of professionals, healthcare practitioners probably have an easier time with regard to civil litigation than many other professional groups. If an architect or civil engineer designs a wall and the wall falls over, it will be far more difficult to defend them against an allegation of negligence as compared to a surgeon who carries out a surgical procedure that is complicated by a post-operative wound infection.

Understanding medical law is not about how to avoid being sued. Rather, the primary objective of medical law systems is to ensure better patient outcomes by increasing knowledge and understanding of both the healthcare professionals' obligations and responsibilities and those of patients and their families. In order to understand how legal rules influence and benefit medical care, it is important to understand the way in which law contributes more generally to society. In particular, how it facilitates the maintenance of a safe and nurturing environment, in which a community can grow in size and complexity, develop new

Forensic Odontology: Principles and Practice, First Edition. Edited by Jane A. Taylor and Jules A. Kieser.
© 2016 John Wiley & Sons, Ltd. Published 2016 by John Wiley & Sons, Ltd.

services for personal health and welfare and be inclusive in the way rules are developed and social decisions made.

For the forensic practitioner who supports the civil, administrative and criminal legal processes, an understanding of their own role within the legal system as well as the purpose of a legal system in modern society can make their job easier and better focused on their clients' needs.

The question 'Why law?' has challenged legal theorists over the centuries. The general public usually understands the concept of law in a personal sense, although there are individuals in most communities who appear to have great difficulty in comprehending why they should obey such rules! It is not enough to just examine the philosophical issues surrounding why we have rules, because to come to an understanding of what the law is about we must also examine the procedural mechanisms by which laws are created and enforced. Healthcare professionals can become involved in both of these processes, and indeed it is essential that those engaged in healthcare industries ensure that their expertise is called upon and directly influences the creation of laws and the operation of relevant parts of the legal system.

All human communities and societies have laws and legal systems. This appears to be true even of so-called primitive societies. While a citizen in a modern, sophisticated society might have difficulties recognising formal laws in primitive communities, the fact that the community operates in such a way that its individuals know what is expected of them and how they should behave with respect to others indicates the existence of customary rules or laws. Perhaps the simplest expression of this can be seen in everyday phrases such as 'the law of the jungle' where the term law is used loosely to refer to behaviour typical of animals. Perhaps it is going too far to suggest that groups of animals have laws or legal systems. However, animal behaviourists have been able to demonstrate the existence of repetitive forms of behaviour that appear to regulate the conduct of animals within their social grouping and that seem to provide the group with a distinct survival advantage.

Perhaps this is the origin of the law in human communities. If human survival and growth are based on people acting together in coordinated groups, then the existence of a system of behaviour modifying rules which can be enforced, could enhance the survival of such communities.

When we examine human societies and groups, whether we are looking at a single-parent family or a complex federal system of government, we can see that rules and behaviour-controlling systems are in place. The breakdown of such systems is associated with dysfunction within the community, and it can result in economic loss, physical harm and death. Not all of these rules are, of course, laws in the strict sense. But whether the rule is made by a parliament seeking to prevent drink-driving in the community, or by parents seeking to regulate their child's television watching in the home, the existence of these rules has a particular meaning for the relevant social group. Such rules impose obligations on members of the particular community or group whose behaviour the rule seeks to address. Thus, in the case of family rules, the children are made aware of the rule and, although they may dislike it and decide to break it, in most cases they understand the consequences of disobedience. Similarly, a rule promulgated by government places an obligation upon members of the community who, even if they dislike the rule, are made aware of the consequences of breaking it.

Most individuals in the community accept the vast majority of rules and laws. Even if there is dissatisfaction with certain laws, usually in advanced societies the opposition is restrained rather than violent. Of course, at times rules and laws emerge which a community finds completely unacceptable. Such rules may arise as a result of dictatorial power being established or because of political pressure from minority groups. It is interesting to note that if widespread community opposition to a law exists, the legislation rarely survives for long. The prohibition laws relating to alcohol in the United States of America in the early twentieth century are a good example of this. Civil disobedience of law, if persistent and widespread, brings the law into disrepute; as a result, despite all enforcement attempts, the majority of prohibition laws were eventually relaxed.

Why then, should we obey rules and laws, and why are most people within a community happy to accept the laws we live under? To the behaviourist, the animal models are clear. Troop, pack and herd animals survive better in groups and this survival is enhanced in well-ordered groups. Similarly, human communities grow, develop and live in better conditions where the activities of the individuals within the community are coordinated. Laws and rules help in developing and maintaining social cohesion. The safety and security that this provides for individuals within a community are very powerful attractions for individuals who wish to join or stay within it.

Not all rules or laws have obvious advantages. Sometimes a law has both advantages and disadvantages for the community. Patent law dealing with the protection of inventions and ideas in the commercial world is a good example. The law purports to defend the intellectual property or ideas of an inventor and to prevent others from capitalising on those ideas by making profits at the expense of the originating inventor. At first glance this appears to present a great restriction upon the growth of a community by preventing individuals from developing their own wealth. But it has long been argued that if inventors invest their own money in the development of ideas and products that will assist society, they must have some assurance that having spent their money and their time on the project they will reap some financial benefit. The absence of patent laws restricting the freedom of individuals in the community to copy the work of others would in fact inhibit the development of inventions and new products. Without patent law, inventors and investors would be unlikely to put their money into developing new ideas, because they would have no assurance that they would receive adequate financial reward for their effort. Thus, whilst rules dealing with patents and copyright appear to be oppressive from one viewpoint, they are in fact designed to assist in the advancement of society.

The existence of laws and rules, therefore, appears to be necessary for social cohesion. Humans, as complex social animals, require high levels of coordination and cohesion within their community groups in order to be successful. In this way, law is the oil that lubricates the machinery of society and provides one of the elements required for social cohesion.

While the purpose of law, when viewed from a community perspective, can be seen as supporting and maintaining of social cohesion, there is nevertheless an individual or personal basis to law that exists alongside the broad community interest. There is value for the community in the law being focused on individuals. Society prospers where individuals are valued in their own right and their interests are supported by the community as a whole. Personal rights and personal obligations are of direct legal interest to the whole community and lie at the heart of the everyday operation of the law. Just as everyday dealings between individuals in a society require each person to behave fairly with respect to the other, the same is true for legal dealings. Indeed these basic principles of fair play are reinforced by the way in which the law regulates and reviews dealings between individuals. In simple terms, it is this concept of fair play in a broad social sense that underpins the concept of justice in society.

For legal rules to be effective in regulating and controlling social order, it is not enough for there to be a mechanism for enforcing the law. What is required is for the community at large to accept laws, not just because of a fear of retribution if legal rules are not followed, but by virtue of agreeing with the principles that the law seeks to regulate and enforce. In other words, it seems important that the community as a whole appreciates that the operation of the law and the legal rules that regulate everyday actions are right and proper, and meet the needs of individuals as members of the community.

For legal processes to be fair requires a set of general values that underpins their operation. In our legal system these are often referred to as principles of natural justice. With regard to the criminal law, it is for the courts to be sure that an individual who is charged with having broken the law is treated fairly with regard to these principles. In this way an accused person must be told what crime they have been charged with as well as being given the right to defend themselves in a manner that allows them to be freely heard. Critically for the forensic practitioner these fairness rules include provisions that include provision that ensure that a conviction must be based on real evidence rather than supposition and that any bias or risk of conflict of interest is eliminated.

Justice therefore comprises the way in which legal rules are acted upon and enforced as well as the content of the legal rules themselves. Criticism of justice systems often includes comments addressing the way in which the legal rules are put into practice. Indeed, enforcement of the law is also often subject to criticism. In some cases, the particular ways in which normally considered just laws are enforced, can be perceived by some sections of society as unjust. Put more simply, a rule can be correct in a general sense but in a particular instance, for a particular individual, the enforcement of the rule can be unfair and as a consequence unjust. For such situations to be handled appropriately, machinery must be in place to allow the application of laws to individuals to be examined and reviewed. The machinery of justice, comprising the law courts and associated tribunals, plays a major part in this area. With regard to the criminal law, it is for the courts to be sure that an individual who is charged with having broken the law is treated fairly with regard to the principles of natural justice. In this way an accused person must be told what crime they have been charged with as well as being given the right to defend themselves in a manner that allows them to be freely heard.

The concept of justice, however, extends beyond the rights of a person who has been accused of a criminal offence. What are the rights of the family of an individual who has been killed? What about the rights of a child who has been abused, or the rights of a spouse during divorce proceedings? Just like the ramifications of medical treatment legal actions have the capacity to affect the lives of many individuals. Traditionally the law has taken a narrow approach with regard to individuals who are affected by its operation. In many cases courts have confined themselves to dealing with the issues between the particular parties appearing in court. Thus, in a criminal matter, the issues are between the person charged with the crime and the prosecution which is to bring the action before the court. The rights of a victim such as an abused child, or of the family of a victim such as a murdered man's wife, traditionally were not part of the court proceedings and therefore were not taken into account by the legal process. However, this narrow view of the law has changed. Victim impact statements are used in criminal cases, and courts may consider the psychological and emotional injuries suffered by the family of an individual as a result of negligent acts.

For the courts, it can be difficult to balance the competing interests of individuals who are directly or indirectly involved in a case. In child-care proceedings, the wellbeing of the child is usually considered paramount. But what about the rights of the biological parents, the step-parents, the grandparents and other close members of the family? Competing interests often arise, and the concept of justice requires that these interests be balanced to arrive at what the community will accept as a just solution. Conflicts arise in many situations. Even in death it is not uncommon for various groups and factions within a family to compete for possession of the body and to seek to have control over the funeral. Families are in many ways a microcosm of the community. In a family, there may be no easy answer to a complex problem that has many emotional overtones; the range and complexity of problems is increased manyfold when we look at the issues that disturb whole communities. Arguments about what is just and right and proper create the concept of justice, and such principles apply to the community as a whole as well as to the individuals within it.

Forensic practitioners will often encounter potential conflicts between the rights of a victim of crime to receive confidential medical services, and the need of investigators to obtain forensic medical evidence. Where a victim of crime refuses to be examined, or to have their examination results communicated to investigators, potential evidence that could be used to prosecute an offender is lost. The loss of such a prosecution, which has the potential to prevent an offender from causing further damage to the community, is a legitimate concern for governments, the community and law enforcement agencies alike. Balancing an individual's right to self-determination with regard to medical treatment and medical examination with the community's desire for safety from the risk of personal injury caused by criminal activity, is an important task for law makers and the courts that apply the rules.

A similar issue can arise with regard to potential offenders. An accused person has a right not to be assaulted, and in many legal jurisdictions has a right to remain silent when questioned regarding the crime of which they are suspected. The medical examination of such an individual for the purpose of obtaining evidence for a subsequent prosecution may become problematic. New legislation in some jurisdictions permits force to be used to examine such individuals and obtain medical and scientific forensic samples from them. Such legislation has been widely criticised on medical, legal, civil libertarian and human rights grounds. In recent times the increased risk of acts of terrorism taking place in our community and the need to detect the preparation of such activities has resulted in legal amendment that some people might see as a breach of civil liberty principles. Yet the political and social imperatives that have led to such legislation appear to express real community concerns regarding the need to prevent these crimes. Given the availability of modern scientific forensic techniques, such as molecular biology technology (DNA) for the purpose of identifying offenders, criminal justice systems can claim scientific justification/benefit for seeking powers to take compulsory samples from a range of individuals in the community. The potential for conflict between individual human rights and the need for safeguarding the community has already been demonstrated by the concern that some of this legislation has caused.

Forensic medical practitioners can also become involved in human rights issues that have an international perspective. Human rights abuses identified by the international community include the infliction of trauma upon individuals. The forensic interpretation of the resulting injuries plays an important part in identifying and monitoring such abuse. For this reason, the independence of any forensic medical service should be paramount.

Types of law

Laws are established as a result of various needs and pressures that arise within society. As we have seen, rules governing human behaviour and relationships appear to be a constant feature of human society. Whether or not formal laws are present and enforced, customary behaviour and attitudes within a society regulate the ways in which groups and individuals operate in relation to each other. Such traditions and customs in both primitive and advanced communities may operate as extremely persuasive and powerful rules that amount to formal laws. Much of the formal law we have today arose out of these customary practices of our ancestors. If historical custom within human societies forms one of the basic sources of law in modern societies, it is important to understand these traditions in order to truly appreciate our current law and legal processes.

An example of this is the early English coroner system that originally operated simply to raise taxation and revenue for the Crown. For example, when the Normans invaded England in 1066 they developed a system whereby, if a person were found dead, the body was assumed to be Norman. (Presentment of Englishry.) Unless the local inhabitants could prove that the body was Anglo-Saxon, they had to pay a heavy fine. In this way the community of Norman invaders was able to protect itself. Today the coroners' jurisdiction is focused on death investigation for the purposes of prevention of avoidable deaths and is a far cry from its taxation origins.

Each country or state has its own legislation and legal rules. The physical, political, legal and social grouping within which people live is referred to as a jurisdiction, and it forms the arena within which a given set of legal rules applies. Within this grouping there are a number of smaller legal jurisdictions where a particular court or tribunal has the power to consider matters of a particular type. Such local jurisdictions have particular judges or legal officers who have specific powers to act in particular ways. Differences between the various local jurisdictions within a state have to do with the areas of law covered, the types of legal procedure employed, and the level of penalties and awards that can be made. Most states form their own jurisdiction within which their rules apply. Despite the fact that there is a wide range of human societies in the world, many of the legal rules by which they live are remarkably similar. However, differences do exist and these can create difficulties in international disputes. The field of international law is a broad one, and despite the existence of international courts, legal disputes between citizens of different countries may not be easy to resolve. Formal diplomatic arrangements as well as international treaties can clear the way for solutions to be found to such international legal conflicts.

Matters of international law are rarely of concern to the forensic practitioner. However, issues may arise in relation to international forensic practice, particularly in situations involving disaster victim identification (DVI), where a doctor or dentist has to work overseas within different legal jurisdictions. It is essential in such a situation that they accurately inform themselves of the legal rules and procedures within the foreign jurisdiction so that their work in determining identity is legally valid.

The creation of laws today follows a growing trend to codify and collate the rules by which society operates, resulting in substantial formal documents that can be stored, referenced and recorded. Within Anglo-Australian jurisdictions, such documents are usually developed by a legislative assembly such as a parliament. By a variety of constitutional procedures they are declared to be a part of the formal law. Such documents – acts of parliament or statutes – may represent completely new rules but often they reflect customary provisions, traditions and local rules that have ordered the society in the past and adapt them to the changes in attitude and structure that the society has undergone over recent years. In some cases these new or amended laws reflect the influence brought to bear on the previous law by the judiciary when the judges interpret the law to meet modern needs. Such codification of recent judicial decisions allows the parliament to recognise the work of the courts in attempting to interpret older statutes with, in many cases, parliament adopting the modern judicial interpretations of the old law and so bringing legislation up to date. As a result of the incorporation of all these influences, the parliament arrives at a statement of the law that is relevant to the present structure of the society. Such statements are direct legislation; they set the legal rules or laws that the legislators wish to have operating in their jurisdiction.

In addition to this direct form of legislation, there are other ways in which elected lawmakers can formulate legal rules. One of these is through the use of so-called delegated legislation. It would be far too onerous for a parliament or similar body to make the rules that regulate every facet of a complex modern society. For this reason, parliaments often formulate legislation that sets out the general principles of law that should apply in an area, and then lists, specifically, who should be permitted to make the precise legal rules that shall apply and how they should be made. Such legislation nominates a specific individual (often a government minister) or organisation to be responsible for the 'nitty-gritty' of the actual law in the designated area. These laws therefore specifically delegate to an individual the responsibility for making the detailed rules, and because the power has been delegated to them by parliament in the relevant legislation, the rules made by the individual have the same force as if they had been made by parliament directly.

In fact there are many activities within society that do not require parliamentary debate on the details of their regulations. For example, in order to assure the safety of the public with respect to buildings, regulations need to be in force regarding the composition of building materials. It would not be appropriate for parliament itself to debate the issues surrounding the composition of concrete. Indeed, a high level of technical knowledge is required to specify accurately how concrete should be made in different construction settings. A parliament therefore might pass legislation that specifically delegates a minister or an executive agency to make the rules regarding the composition of different types of concrete and the circumstances in which they should be used.

At first glance it may seem dangerous for a parliament to give an individual or an outside organisation the power to make the actual laws. But in practice, the details of this delegated legislation are reviewed by parliament. The delegated legislation is tabled, that is, set before parliament, so that the parliament has the opportunity to examine the rules that have been made. The courts also can review the way in which delegated legislation was made, and have the power to rule that delegated rules made outside parliament are invalid in certain circumstances. To take the previous example, suppose parliament has enacted that a particular minister 'may make regulations regarding the composition of house bricks, after consulting with representatives of the building industry', and the minister does not consult with the building industry before making the regulations; the courts may declare those regulations invalid because the minister did not formulate the rules according to the manner which parliament determined. Similarly, if a minister made rules that were outside the area of responsibility delegated by parliament, then the courts could hold that these rules were invalid because the minister had exceeded their powers under the legislation enabling the delegated power.

Whether laws are made by direct or delegated legislation, the complexity of human interactions means that situations are bound to arise that fall outside the specific provisions of the law as stated in the statutes. Similarly, given the inventiveness of the human mind, legislation that defines legal rules in formal words is capable of a variety of interpretations, each of which could amount to a substantial difference in the meaning of the law. While language is the best means we have for conveying ideas, it can be an inexact medium. A piece of writing may mean different things to different people.

Society relies on certainty in the law in order that members of society can plan their activities in a way that will not cause a conflict with the law. Such planning, for example, may result in a commercial contract. In such a situation, both parties to the contract need to have faith and belief in the certainty of the law relating to that contract in order for them to risk their money and goods. Similarly, the trust that develops between a purchaser and a vendor relating to the sale of property is based on the fact that both parties are complying with a stable and comprehensible set of legal rules relating to contracts of sale. Where a dispute arises, it is often based on the meaning of the law of contract in relation to the particular sale. In many cases, even the most clearly worded legislation proves to be ambiguous in relation to a specific section or phrase that deals with the issue in dispute. In order to resolve such difficulties, specialist legal advice has to be sought as to the probable meaning of the legislation in this area, and if agreement is still not reached then recourse to a formal hearing of the matter before a court may be required. Each party argues their own interpretation of the law before a judge or other legal arbiter; the parties agree to be bound by the verdict of the arbiter as to the meaning of the words in the legislation, regardless of the effect this has on the business relationship between them.

As a result of analysing legislation during disputes regarding the relevant law, judges and legal arbiters enlarge and expand upon the legislation by interpreting the statutes on a case-by-case basis. These judicial decisions regarding interpretation of statutes also form part of the substantive law of the jurisdiction and they can be referred to by individuals as additional legal rules that apply when a dispute arises. Such judge-made rules form part of what is termed the common law. Although not enshrined in legislation, the additional rules are recorded, documented and referenced as case law so that the rules can be proved to exist and can be referenced in later legal disputes.

The power of judges in this area is considerable. If no legislation exists dealing specifically with the issue in dispute and no judge has considered the matter before, then effectively the judge can seem to be 'making new law' regarding the issue. As far as the legal system is concerned, the judge is not making new law, but is merely declaring what the law has always been on this point (even though a dispute has never arisen before). Occasionally a judge's modification of legislation alters the thrust of the legislation. In the past some governments have had to repeal judicially interpreted legislation and create new legislation in order to remove ambiguity and restore the law to their original intent. However, as commented above, there are situations where judges have personally developed the law in a particular area with such skill that a government has taken the judge's rules and formulated specific legislation to incorporate those rules. Whilst judges cannot alter a rule clearly set out in legislation, they can interpret the legislative rules and give them practical meaning in relation to disputes between individuals. In such a way judges are able to define and modify the meaning of legislation so it can be applied to the situation of a particular dispute.

The coronial system

All death investigation takes place in a medical, scientific, administrative and legal environment that is specific to that type of community and legal jurisdiction within which the death occurred. The differences among jurisdictions arise from a variety of interrelated factors including social, religious, political and legal influences, as well as the development of the medical profession and its specialities. At the most mechanical level, systems are in place to ensure that records are generated and retained about who has died. In the vast majority of deaths it is the treating medical practitioner who knows the patient best and is charged with providing a cause of death based on their knowledge of the patient's recent illness and medical history. This cause of death is recorded within a registry office inside government bureaucracy, generally by recording on a death register the cause of death given in the report or certificate of the treating doctor.

The maintenance of a death register and a birth register has important social implications. A community needs to know information regarding those who make up its population. From a practical perspective this is needed in order to ensure that community services are appropriate to the size and make up of the population. However, at a deeper level our concerns about threats to our safety generate a desire to find out more about deaths that occur in our community and to understand their causes and what has brought them about so that we can feel less threatened. Community and personal grief involve important emotions that can have deep effects on the functioning of individuals, families and in some cases the whole community. In this environment a society's ability to independently investigate critical deaths from a perspective that is focused beyond that of any individual professional group, such as scientists, the medical profession or the police, is important.

Different jurisdictions have solved the problem of the need for independent death investigation in a variety of ways. Jurisdictions based on the English legal system have tended to employ 'coroners' as the independent death investigators. Over time individual coroners have developed from being unqualified individuals of some general standing in the community to being judicial legal officers, although in some jurisdictions independent medical practitioners still have a role to play. Today in Australia and New Zealand coroners are full-time judicial officers appointed by the Crown and chief coroners are often judges of intermediate level courts.

The need for death investigation systems that are independent of treating medical practitioners, the police and other aspects of government requires both medical and legal practitioners to operate as independent investigators who can respond to community concerns regarding certain death types.

Our community has a need to process a range of deaths to understand why they happened and to put the risk of these deaths occurring again into a social context. Sometimes it seems that the media drives this demand in a manner that may be considered by some to be salacious. News reports often contain the details and profiles of both victims and perpetrators of homicide, lethal error and catastrophe. Cases involving the discovery of hidden bodies, terrorist attacks, pandemics, tsunamis, uncontrolled bushfires, homicidal medical practitioners, toxic spillages, gangland killings and dangerous workplaces are just some of the deaths that particularly concern the community and as a result receive the particular attention of the public media. This focus places medical and legal death investigators directly in the public eye, and for many this is a radical departure from their traditional quiet and confidential medical or legal role.

Not all deaths investigated by a coroner are subject to such public concern or scrutiny. With some deaths the treating medical practitioner cannot explain what happened or provide a cause of death. For example: the deceased person may not have seen their treating medical practitioner for some time, there may be multiple factors or aetiologies that could have caused the death, the death may have happened unexpectedly or in suspicious or unnatural circumstances, it may have occurred while or shortly after the deceased underwent a medical procedure in a hospital. In other situations the environment of the death is a critical factor; the death may have happened while travelling on public transport, in the course of an aeroplane flight or while the person was on board a boat, the death may have occurred during confinement in prison or police custody or in the course of an involuntary in-patient admission at a psychiatric hospital. All such circumstances require further information because abuse or neglect may have needlessly endangered the life of the person who was, or should have been recognised as vulnerable.

Balanced perspectives in assessing causes of death can be difficult. It is not easy to come to terms with the fact that sometimes people simply pass away – that deaths just happen. It is very tempting to expect or insist upon there being someone to blame when a loved one passes away. This is so whether they are young or of advanced years. Could not something have been done? If someone had intervened would not the person still be alive? If more care had been taken, would not the likelihood of their death have been reduced? Lives lost in such a manner call for explanation and there is the temptation to find someone to blame.

Grief can readily lead to guilt, frequently unwarranted but nonetheless burdensome to survivors and to carers left behind. This means that there is a constant pressure for investigation into circumstances of death and a need to evaluate whether conduct that brought about death should not have occurred. The other aspect of independent death investigation is the consideration of what needs to be done to avoid its repetition. Sometimes there are ready answers, such as criminal prosecutions of the homicidally culpable. Sometimes there are complex, systemic responses that might reduce the potential for other fatalities.

Those involved in death investigation should never lose sight of the social importance of the work they undertake. It is all too easy to become involved in the technical and scientific aspects of solving the death puzzle and as a result fail to be aware of the personal, family and community loss. Similarly it is easy to become enmeshed in the often complex administrative and bureaucratic processes that surround death investigation with the result that the human aspects of grief and loss become invisible.

Commonly, death investigation systems involve a combination of medical, legal and administrative structures. The differences among jurisdictions arise from a variety of interrelated factors including social, religious, political and legal influences, as well as the development of the medical profession and its specialties.

The continental European and Scandinavian systems, as well as a number of medical examiner systems, focus upon whether criminal behaviour has brought about a death. By contrast, coronial death investigations in the Anglo-Australian jurisdictions take a broader and more public health perspective, inquiring in a wide variety of circumstances whether the conduct that gave rise to a death could or should have been different and whether alternative processes might in the future avoid such deaths. This means that the distinctive systems of coronial investigation are focused on both accuracy of the public record about deaths and prophylaxis – learning from deaths so as to minimise the risks of recurrence. This also results in the majority of the coroner's investigations involving non-criminal matters such as deaths in natural and manmade disasters, workplace and transport accidents and unsatisfactory medical treatment events.

From a legal perspective, the coroner functions as an inquisitorial process embedded in the broader adversarial English legal system. In the death investigation court hearing or inquest the coroner functions as both an investigator, assembling the evidence they need, and as a decision maker. This is quite different to the system in place in the criminal and civil courts in the same jurisdiction that operate in an adversarial fashion. In these adversarial hearings the judge sits as an impartial observer and decision maker, but is not involved directly in the management of the investigation process.

In order to be able to investigate the death a coroner must be convinced that a death has occurred and in circumstances that mean that the death is within their legal jurisdiction. For example, where body parts are found the coroner will need to be convinced that the parts of the body recovered mean that the individual is necessarily dead. For example if a hand or arm was discovered it would not be appropriate to necessarily conclude that the individual had died, indeed such limb parts may have been removed as part of a surgical procedure to save the life of the individual. Where the body part identified was of a significant internal organ such as the heart or lungs or substantial portions of the brain, then a coroner could conclude that the loss of such tissue in particular circumstances, such as a plane crash, would inevitably mean that the individual was dead.

Many coroners' jurisdictions permit the coroner to investigate deaths that have occurred outside their state or country. This allows coroners to investigate the deaths of citizens when the death occurs overseas, for example while they are travelling overseas on holiday.

The law in relation to those deaths that must be reported to a coroner differs from jurisdiction to jurisdiction. Reportable deaths must be reported to a coroner, often with legal penalties for those who fail to do so. However, the legislative reporting requirement is often satisfied where the death is reported to the police, who in turn have a duty to inform the coroner and assist in the coroner's investigation. While the whole community has a responsibility to report reportable deaths to the coroner, in some jurisdictions this duty is usually made a specific statutory responsibility of the medical profession and the police. This is for purely practical purposes, in that these two groups are most likely to be present at some stage following a death.

In understanding which deaths must be reported to a coroner, it is important to consider both the legal definitions of reportable death in the legislation of the relevant jurisdiction and the principles of public safety and administration of justice that lie behind the purpose of the coroner's jurisdiction.

Different legal jurisdictions will have different legislative requirements regarding the reporting of particular deaths; however, there are a number of common features that are found in most coroners' jurisdictions. Deaths that are related to unnatural or violent events or that have resulted directly or indirectly from accident or injury are usually reportable to a coroner. It is not always clear what is meant by unnatural or indirect injury. It may well be that a death that has occurred 20 or 30 years after an injury is still reportable to the coroner. For example a spinal injury resulting in bladder dysfunction may lead to ascending urinary tract infections that over many years cause damage to the kidneys with the eventual death decades later from septicaemia associated with pyelonephritis. Although such a death might seem to be natural as a result of an infectious process, it could be considered the indirect result of an injury and might therefore be reportable to a coroner. Similarly a death from lung cancer could occur as a result of a purely natural disease process, but if the lung cancer was caused by industrial exposure to asbestos it might be considered to be a non-natural or unnatural disease process and therefore reportable to the coroner. Things become far less clear in relation to chronic complications of the use of alcohol or smoking tobacco, as it would be possible to consider that diseases such as alcoholic cirrhosis or smoking related lung cancer are in fact unnatural, as they have been caused by an external process.

Another group of deaths that are reportable to a coroner are those occurring in circumstances where the person has been detained or had their freedom constrained by a government agency or as a result of legislation. This means that deaths occurring in prison or in custody of the police as well as individuals who are in the care of local authorities or of government departments are often reportable to a coroner. This is to ensure that the agency responsible for caring for the person had acted appropriately and had not contributed to the death occurring as a result of neglect or inappropriate actions.

Other situations that involve compulsory reporting to the coroner include deaths occurring in a setting of medical treatment where the death was not expected as an outcome of that treatment.

There are other situations which make deaths reportable to a coroner; these include factors such as the absence of a valid death certificate and uncertainty as to the identity of the deceased person. It is interesting to note that the word 'suspicious' is rarely found in the coroner's legislation, while consideration of whether a death is the result of a criminal act is certainly within the coroner's jurisdiction. The majority of coroner's legislation is not structured around the criminal justice process, so-called suspicious deaths being captured by the other provisions regarding reportable deaths.

The endpoint of a coroner's investigation, whether or not an inquest is held, involves the setting out of a finding and, or the delivery of a verdict. The transition from a coroner's verdict to that of a discursive, structured set of findings is a particular feature of the modern development of the coronial jurisdiction as it has moved away from its English origins in Australia, New Zealand and Canada. Traditionally, coroners have to determine who the deceased was, when and where they died, the cause of death and how they died. The identification of individuals who have contributed to a death may also form part of a coroner's finding. Indeed in some jurisdictions the coroner has the power to refer individuals to the Director of Public Prosecutions where the coroner believes a criminal action may have been involved. Historically coroners and or their juries were able to add riders to their verdicts in which they could comment on broader matters surrounding the death including steps that might be taken to prevent such deaths occurring in the future. Modern legislation often permits coroners to make specific recommendations in matters affecting public health and safety and the administration of justice. The power to make a recommendation as part of a finding is not unfettered. Indeed there should be a clear nexus between the comments or recommendations made and the circumstances surrounding the death into which the coroner inquires. In the context of an inquest into the deaths of prisoners in a jail fire in Victoria, in the case of Harmsworth v State Coroner, his Honour Justice Nathan noted the power to make comments and recommendations, but held unequivocally that the power to comment is incidental and subordinate to the mandatory power to make findings related to how the deaths occurred, their causes and the identity of any contributory persons [1]. Although the finding as to how a death occurred or what were the circumstances of death associated with recommendations regarding death prevention is perhaps the most important outcome of a death investigation and inquest, the key administrative outcomes of an inquest, including the determination of the particular items of information required to register the death, remain at an important part of the coroner's function. This information is essential in order for the public record to be made complete and if necessary set straight.

It is in this administrative area that the question of identity is such an important consideration for the coroner. Not only must identity be confirmed even in those cases where there is no particular problem with the identification of the deceased person, such as an individual being found deceased at home or in their car. But it also includes the identification of human remains such as skeletal remains and decomposed individuals found in remote locations.

A particular feature of identification within the coroner's jurisdiction relates to the identification of individuals in settings of mass disaster. Here, although police and other agencies will often apply the standard Interpol DVI criteria and procedures in the Anglo-Australian jurisdiction, it is the coroner who is ultimately responsible for the legal identification of deceased persons and who has the power to control the investigation processes involved.

While standard Interpol procedures for human identification distinguish between primary identifiers such as fingerprints, dental features and molecular biology techniques and secondary identifiers including property such as jewellery, documents or clothing, coroners are not obliged to apply these strict investigative procedures and can determine identity in any manner they see fit. Very occasionally when no primary or secondary identifiers are available coroners will still determine that a person has died as a result of a disaster on broad circumstantial grounds. Despite this, coroners will usually rely on the expert scientific and medical processes in order to obtain a sufficient evidence base to determine identity.

The investigators within the coroner's jurisdiction

General police, namely uniformed police officers, have an important role at death scenes. In many cases it is the uniformed police who are the first investigators on the scene, and in such situations they have the role of ensuring that scene management begins appropriately. They also have the role of initially reporting the death to the coroner. It is at this time that an initial decision is taken as to whether the police and coroner should consider the death suspicious or not. This decision will underpin the remainder of the death investigation. The failure to recognise the suspicious nature of the death may prejudice future criminal issues. Where there is doubt about the nature of the death, the uniformed police will usually involve local detectives or one of the specialist police squads or units that are responsible for investigating particular crimes.

In non-suspicious cases, the uniformed police will collect the basic information required by the coroner and arrange with the coroner's office for the body to be collected. The police will make their own general assessment of the death scene and take statements from appropriate witnesses or friends or relatives of the deceased. In some situations it is possible for the uniformed police at the death scene to obtain formal identification of the deceased person from friends and relatives. This removes the necessity of a formal identification at the mortuary, which would require family or friends to travel to the mortuary at a later time. In the case of apparently natural deaths, the police will make inquiries to determine who was the deceased's local doctor and then contact the doctor to obtain further medical information that could have a bearing on understanding of the cause or manner of death. Following the autopsy and subsequent medical testing, the coroner's office will usually contact the original uniformed police officer involved in the case and request that further statements be taken to assist in compiling a brief of evidence, which the coroner can use in making their finding.

In suspicious cases the primary role of general police is to ensure that the appropriate specialist police units are informed and that the scene is appropriately secured prior to their arrival. This will involve the establishment of crime scene boundaries and the creation of a crime scene log to record all persons who enter the scene and to document their names, the organisations they are from, and the time they entered and left the scene. Some suspicious scenes of death may require security for prolonged periods of time. Major mass death scenes may require such security for days or weeks. Homicide death scenes may require security for several days. In some cases where the circumstances of the death are unclear, it may be necessary to maintain a security guard and log on the death scene even after the body has been removed. This can be an efficient method of handling a suspected suspicious death scene where, prior to requesting any formal examination of the scene by forensic crime scene experts, it is considered appropriate to wait to see what the autopsy reveals. In these situations, if the autopsy determines that the cause of death is natural, then no detailed forensic scientific examination of the scene may be considered necessary and the security log on the scene can be abandoned.

Because of the work structure of uniformed police with regard to shift work and rosters, they are ideally placed to provide long-term logistics support in a death scene investigation. They can provide traffic management to ensure access for emergency service personnel and re-routing of traffic to minimise the impact on the local community. In many situations members of the public will be permitted to enter the outer low-security areas of a crime scene. This may be because these areas include their residence or contain some of their property. In these situations the uniformed police will escort them in and out of the low-security area as required. Manpower issues of policing at a crime scene can also be assisted by local uniformed police taking routine statements from people in nearby premises, thereby relieving the investigating detectives of some of these more routine functions.

Crime scene management and support also contains roles with which the uniformed police can help. These include artificial lighting, catering, media liaison, counselling and debriefing services. The administration of these services is often delegated to uniformed police in order to permit the other death investigators to concentrate on the matter at hand.

There are a number of agencies and individuals that provide the coroner with the specialist investigators essential to the work of the jurisdiction. While the routine aspects of the coroners' investigation are performed by police officers, and forensic pathologists carry out the medical investigations focused around the examination of the deceased person, many death procedures lie outside the knowledge of the police or the pathology profession. Toxicologists deal with issues surrounding the impact of drugs and poisons, dentists, anthropologists and molecular biologists are closely involved with the determination of human identity and entomologists with the determination of the time of death and any post-mortem interference with the body. While the work of these investigators is centred on the body of the deceased person, other issues arise that require an assessment of the circumstances in which the death occurred. These investigations involve a range of disciplines that include a knowledge of engineering, architectural design, military procedures, fire services, maritime matters, accountancy and the wide range of biological and physical forensic sciences that may arise in cases from time to time. It is appropriate that these issues are comprehensively addressed. To this end the coroner may well contract out this part of the investigation by commissioning external experts in the relevant field and providing them with relevant information from the coroner's case file.

Such commissioned expert reports received by the coroner are then added to the case file and evaluated by the coroner as part of the death investigation. In many situations where such experts are used, the case will proceed to inquest, and the experts will be called as witnesses and subjected to questioning by the coroner and interested parties. The coroner is often assisted in the hearings by police officers seconded from other duties who assist in compiling the brief for the coroner and in presenting the evidence at the inquest. In addition, often they act in a liaison/operational role between the coroner and operational police units, including general duty police and detectives. This is a very efficient arrangement in many coroners' investigations. However, where a death involves police operations, such as a death in custody, there is the potential for allegations of conflict of interest. In such cases the coronial service needs to have special procedures in place for the appointment of other investigators, legal counsel, or independent supervisors who can oversee the police investigation. Such cases are a minority within coronial practice and for the most part, the advantages of the close working relationship between coroners and the police outweigh the disadvantages.

In larger coroners' offices the role of the police can be more focused on the inquest, with police personnel assisting the coroner in the hearing by calling witnesses and presenting the evidence contained in the brief to the court. In some cases a police officer attached to the coroner's office will directly act as the leading police investigator. This situation arises when the death is one that demands a level of knowledge in a particular field that the general duty police do not have. Police on general duties have a limited involvement in death investigations, whereas coroners' police assistants deal with the issues on a daily basis. Indeed, coroners' police assistants help in the investigation of many more deaths than a specialist police homicide investigation unit. The investigation of deaths occurring in the setting of medical care as well as transport-related deaths involving aircraft, marine craft and trains is often supervised and managed by coroners' police assistants. Where complex issues in relation to identification of the deceased are concerned, particularly when there has been a multiple fatality event, police will take charge of the DVI process for the coroner.

The most common external medical investigation service used by a coroner is the autopsy service provided by forensic pathologists. Death investigation systems, such as those operated by a coroner, usually have the power to order that an autopsy be carried out to assist in the determination of the manner, circumstances and cause of death. The detail of how this is carried out and incorporated within the coroner's investigation is set out in Chapter 4. It is significant that the autopsy and medical aspects of the death-scene investigation are carried out very early on in the coroner's investigation process. In many jurisdictions the medical death-scene investigation and autopsy are completed within one or two days of the death. The results of these initial medical investigations often shape the nature of subsequent investigations on behalf of the coroner. As a consequence, the professional relationship between pathologists and coroners' staff is usually close.

Although pathologists are the group of medical practitioners most closely involved in the work of coroners, increasingly a range of other medical specialists are being utilised by coroners in death investigations. Deaths occurring in the setting of medical treatment may require investigations to be carried out by non-pathology medical specialists. Experts in anaesthetics, intensive care, radiology pharmacology and accident and emergency services, as well as specialist physicians and surgeons, may have an important role to play in the evaluation of such deaths. Today, the advent of the use of alternative death investigation processes, in addition to or as a replacement for the autopsy, demonstrates the need for a wider range of medical specialists to be engaged by a coroner. Medical investigations incorporating therapeutic management review or post-mortem radiology will clearly be enhanced by the involvement of the appropriate clinical specialist or radiologist, rather than expecting a forensic pathologist to try to cover these medical specialist areas.

Court procedures and the expert medical witness

In the practice of the forensic healthcare disciplines, it is important to recognise that the principal output or endpoint of the work of the forensic practitioner is not to deliver healthcare to a patient, but rather to deliver the results of the medico-legal examination, including the medical opinion and comments, to investigators and to the courts. As a result, forensic medical skills are not confined to the science and art of healthcare, but must include knowledge and skill in the areas of law and technical communication. The forensic healthcare practitioner therefore needs to have a basic understanding of court procedure and advocacy, as well as specialist skills regarding the construction of medico-legal reports and the presentation of oral evidence.

While a coroner may be informed in any way they see fit and does not need to apply the rules of evidence found in criminal and civil courts, the fundamental principles of fairness exemplified by the natural justice provisions are still relevant. The inquisitorial nature of the coroner's enquiry makes it easier for the forensic healthcare practitioner to deliver complex technical evidence in that they only need to satisfy the coroner that there is a sound evidence base for the opinion they express. Such an inquisitorial procedure still allows individuals, involved in the death, to have a lawyer to represent their interests in the inquest and to test the expert's assertions.

In contrast, the court procedure in the Anglo-Australian tradition is principally adversarial. Here each party before the court seeks to advance their case by calling witnesses to present their own version of the facts to the court. At the same time, each party seeks to demonstrate that the other party's case is either not made out, flawed or unbelievable. The adversarial nature of the proceedings within the civil and criminal jurisdictions means that the forensic practitioner is more carefully led through their evidence in such a way that it meets the needs of the party calling them. It also follows that the other party before the court may seek to challenge their evidence and do so in a way that gives the witness very little room to manoeuvre or to independently assert their opinion.

While the courts are established by the state and are operated and administered through the legislation established by the government, the judiciary organises the day-to-day procedure within the court. Therefore in criminal matters, the prosecutor presents the case on behalf of the state, whilst the judge formally presides over the court as an impartial umpire supervising the proceedings and dealing with matters of law and procedure including the admissibility of evidence. It follows, therefore, that in a criminal matter it is up to the prosecutor to inform the court about those facts of the case that the prosecutor believes support the charge against the accused person. The prosecutor need not lay all the facts before the court, and can leave out pieces of information that are not thought to be relevant to their case. While prosecutors must not deliberately hide information that is relevant to the issue before the court, they are not usually obliged to lay before the court all the information that they know. Modification of legislation in Anglo-Australian legal systems has developed the law further on this point, so that in many jurisdictions the prosecution is obliged to make the defence aware of all information that it has prior to trial. In recent years in Australia the defence has similarly been under an obligation to make expert evidence upon which they seek to rely available to the prosecution prior to the commencement of the trial. Of course this only relates to expert opinion that they seek to directly admit into evidence. It is entirely open to the defence to obtain an expert opinion in relation to the evidence and then use the information contained in that opinion to cross-examine the prosecution's expert witness on the relevant points. If they do not call their own expert to give evidence then they are not obliged to make that expert's opinion available to the prosecution in advance.

The task of the defence in the adversarial system is to demonstrate to the court that the prosecution has not made out a satisfactory case, so that there is no case for the accused to answer; or to demonstrate the weaknesses and errors in the prosecution case, so as to show that the matters alleged cannot be believed to have occurred beyond all reasonable doubt. A wide range of defences is open to accused persons, a defence barrister may rely on one or several of these. As the prosecution relies on the oral testimony of witnesses giving evidence from the witness box, the defence, in some cases, tries to discredit the reliability of the prosecution witnesses or to demonstrate that what the witnesses say is incorrect or capable of another interpretation. It follows that it is legitimate for the defence to attack the credibility and truthfulness of prosecution witnesses. In the same way it is open for the prosecution to attack the credibility and truthfulness of any witnesses that are subsequently called to give evidence by the defence.

The adversarial process in a criminal matter comprises the examination of witnesses alternately by the prosecution and defence lawyers. The judge plays little or no part in this process, although on occasions a judge intervenes to ask questions or to clarify a point that has been raised.

The procedure for examining witnesses is straightforward. The person or party calling the witness asks questions first, and elicits from the witness the information that they require in order to prove their case. This process is referred to as examination-in-chief. The prosecution evidence elicited during examination-in-chief is fundamental to the process of any criminal trial because it must set out all of the evidence that the prosecution requires to prove its case. Leading questions, that is questions that imply the nature and content of the answer, are not usually permitted in examination-in-chief. So a forensic medical witness would not be asked a question 'Did you observe a fresh bruise over the right side of the man's forehead and underlying facial fractures in keeping with him being struck by a clenched fist?' Instead they would be asked 'What did you observe on examination of the face and skull?' and then 'How might such an injury have been caused?' Despite this rule, in practice it is not uncommon for prosecution forensic medical witnesses to be asked less controversial leading questions during examination-in-chief, provided that the prosecutor has first obtained express consent to do this from the other party's barrister and the judge.

If a forensic practitioner is to give expert opinion as well as factual evidence during examination-in-chief, it is the task of the party calling them to set out the nature of the witnesses' expertise and to prove to the court that the practitioner has sufficient expertise to give opinion evidence in the matter. In certain situations where the admissibility of an expert's opinion is vigorously challenged, the opposing party may request that the challenge be considered by the judge in the absence of the jury, a proceeding, known as a 'voir dire'; here the medical witness remains in the witness box and answers the questions raised by both parties and the judge, who seeks to determine if the issue is one capable of reasonable expert opinion and also whether the witness is sufficiently qualified to give expert opinion on the matter. If the decision of the judge is that the witness may give such evidence, the jury is recalled and the case proceeds as if the interruption had not occurred.

Occasionally during examination-in-chief the judge may ask the forensic practitioner particular questions that are directed at elucidating or clarifying some point of their evidence. The witness should note these questions by the judge most carefully. In most circumstances, the judge is attempting to ensure that the jury can understand the evidence that the witness has given. If a witness finds that the judge is asking a number of questions on matters relating to evidence that they have already given, the judge probably considers the witness's previous answers confusing or too technical in nature. The witness should use the opportunity offered by the judge's questions to clarify the evidence and to deliver parts of it again in a manner such that lay people would find easier to understand. When the party calling the witness considers that they have obtained from the witness all the evidence that they need for their case, examination-in-chief comes to an end. As the court process is adversarial, the opposing party now has their opportunity to question the witness.

Cross-examination by the opposing party often involves the witness being asked questions that may attempt to minimise or neutralise the effect of the witness's previous evidence. Occasionally an expert may be asked no questions or the cross-examination used to reinforce an aspect of the witness's answer in examination-in-chief. However, in most cases the questions in cross-examination are designed to show up discrepancies in the witness's prior evidence, to obtain further evidence from the witness, to obtain concessions from the witness regarding unexplored details of the examination-in-chief, or to attack the witness's credibility or truthfulness.

This cross-examination may take various forms, depending on the nature of the defence that is being raised. The opposing counsel will have had access to the witness's statements made prior to the court case, and in addition will have taken detailed notes of the evidence given during the examination-in-chief. These notes may well include a record of specific words and phrases used by the witness in their previous answers. The extent and nature of cross-examination are extremely variable, and much depends on the nature of the defence that is being raised by the accused person. Several approaches and techniques are used in cross-examination, and a medical witness may experience one or more of these in any particular case. The questions may be open or leading, tending to suggest a particular answer. It is not uncommon for counsel to put forward a hypothetical situation in which a particular set of events is alleged by them to have occurred and to ask the witness whether such a scenario might explain the facts observed. Questions based on hypothetical situations must be treated very carefully by the forensic witness. Given the hypothetical nature of the situation advanced by the cross-examiner, many of the answers that the witness give will apparently be at odds with the answer to the same question in relation to the case alleged by the party that called them. In answering such questions, the witness should include wherever possible the elements of the hypothesis that distinguish the answer from the answer that would have been given had the question been framed around the circumstances alleged by the party that originally called the witness. For example, a medical witness in examination-in-chief may have described a knife wound in the skin as coming to a point at each end of the wound and then gone on to express an opinion that the knife that had caused the wound probably had a double-edged blade. In cross-examination the hypothetical question might be phrased, that if we assume that the blade in question was in fact single-edged, how might it have been moved to cause a wound that came to a sharp point at each end. In answering this question, the medical witness should refer to the hypothetical situation specifically in their answer, so that it is clear to the court that the witness in expressing an opinion is predicating their opinion upon the hypothetical situation that has been presented in cross-examination. It may well be that in the above example the witness is unable to conceive of a way in which a single-edged blade could cause such an injury. However, it may be that some particularly complex manipulation of a weapon could result in such an appearance, in which case the witness should explain the necessary complicated act required for the hypothetical situation to be possible.

In many cases a cross-examiner may not address issues head-on, but may merely suggest to the witness that it is impossible to be absolutely certain about particular inferences and opinions. Sometimes in this situation the cross-examiner is merely setting the scene for the evidence of those experts who may intend to present a contrary view. They often do not present that contrary view during cross-examination in case the witness has an effective counter-argument. Instead they rely on the fact that an expert medical witness is often unable to be absolutely certain of all their opinions, and then reinforce the possibility of error by producing another witness with an alternative view. In such a situation, it is up to the original party who called the medical witness to cross-examine this defence expert appropriately in relation to the new opinion.

There are a number of other techniques that barristers employ during cross-examination to suit particular situations. Some questions to a medical witness in cross-examination may in fact be disguised statements to a jury. Such questions are difficult to deal with because they are not questions and therefore not capable of being answered. Courts generally take a dim view of such questions and they may indeed be formally objected to. It is important, however, that when a witness is asked a particular question in cross-examination that they answer that question only and do not go on to answer any related matters that they were not asked about. Extending the scope of an answer is an extremely dangerous practice for a witness, and can cause considerable confusion in court as the witness may get themselves into areas about which evidence has not been permitted.

Considerable latitude is available to the cross-examiner as to the manner in which questions are put and the range of material that can be covered. A forensic healthcare witness should expect cross-examination to be intellectually challenging, particularly when performed by an experienced barrister who has been specifically advised by other medical experts regarding potential points at issue. However, a competent professional forensic witness is almost invariably treated with respect and courtesy in cross-examination and is unlikely to be subjected to rude or abusive questioning.

After cross-examination, the party who originally called the witness may re-examine. Re-examination allows the witness to explain their evidence and to redress any damage done to their original evidence as a result of the cross-examination. If a witness has given competent evidence during the examination-in-chief and has withstood the challenges of cross-examination well, it is unlikely that re-examination will be required. Indeed, the fact that re-examination is not undertaken implies that the barrister who originally called the witness is satisfied with the witness's evidence. Even when the witness has been successfully challenged in cross-examination, the lack of re-examination implies to the court that the matters raised in cross-examination were not relevant or worthy of redressing. During the re-examination, matters that have been previously raised, including those raised in cross-examination, can be further explored, but usually no new evidence is permitted at this stage.

Further cross-examination and further re-examination of a witness can occur but this is unusual. Witnesses who have completed their evidence are excused from further attendance at the court, although occasionally they are required to remain to assist the court at a later stage.

In addition to questions from the barristers and the judge, questions may be asked by the jury, through the jury foreman, with permission of the judge.

These procedures in a criminal matter continue until each of the witnesses called by the prosecution have been heard and cross-examined. After this, the defence calls witnesses and at the completion of all the evidence, the prosecution and then the defence present a final speech to the jury. While the medical witness is giving evidence, they are there to assist the court in its determinations. At times, the nature of questioning of a medical witness may appear to be intensely personal. But while the aim of the barrister may be to attack and lower the standing of the medical witness, the legal scrutiny is not primarily directed at the witness but rather at the whole of the evidence that pertains to the case in question. As a result, it is essential that the witness retain a calm and even demeanour throughout all forms of legal questioning. Whether the witness's expertise is being magnified or belittled by a barrister, they should treat the questions equally and remain calm and level-headed. The true effectiveness of a witness lies in the way in which what they say is believed by the jury. A witness, who is angry and defensive, or boastful and conceited, becomes less believable in the eyes of the jury. Such a situation is to be avoided at all costs. A calm and moderate response in the face of powerful and potentially damaging questioning is one of the greatest protective responses an experienced forensic medical witness can develop.

There are a number of modifications to this standard procedure that can occur in certain situations. Recently there has been increasing use of procedures involving what is termed concurrent evidence or 'hot tubbing'. Here the expert witnesses are called together and form a small panel in the court with questions put to them as a group. This approach has been increasingly used in coroners' courts and even in some civil and administrative proceedings. However, it is rarely used in criminal hearings where tactical matters associated with expounding on critical issues often predominate.

Communication is a critical skill for both barristers and expert witnesses. In the case of criminal trials in the higher courts, communication to the public is a major concern of any forensic practitioner. The language of medical notes and medico-legal reports finds its way into the language used in giving evidence. For a jury to comprehend and draw the appropriate inferences from a medical witness's evidence, the language must be accessible. Lawyers are always concerned to ensure that the judge and jury understand the language used by medical witnesses. However, it must be remembered that a lawyer who has been working on a particular case for some time is likely to have come to understand much of the specialist language of the medical evidence. It is difficult for such lawyers to put themselves in the position of a lay jury member and as a result both the lawyer and the expert witness may overestimate the knowledge that jury members might have.

Jury members vary in the extent of their specialist knowledge. The educational attainment of a jury spans a wide range. A jury might be composed of individuals with no secondary or tertiary education, or of individuals with tertiary qualifications in medically related disciplines such as anatomy or biochemistry. During the course of a trial, it is important for both the medical witness and the lawyers to gain an impression of the success or failure of the communication of issues to a jury. For the medical witness, this is not as difficult as it may appear. Witnesses can use various techniques to increase their communication to a lay jury. These techniques are those used in an ordinary medical consultation with patients, during which the practitioner explains to the patient the nature of the disease or illness and the issues associated with it. If medical witnesses keep in mind that a jury is no different from many of their patients and indeed can span the intellectual knowledge range of their patients, they should have little difficulty in getting their message across. If, however, the medical witness engages in a technical discussion or argument with particular lawyers, there is a risk that the jury, ignorant of such matters, will feel left out and as a result will ignore the technical material being discussed.

Despite this it is important not to underestimate a lay jury. The range and depth of coverage of scientific and medical forensic matters by the media has educated members of the community in a variety of technical issues at varying levels. Indeed, many matters of forensic science and forensic medical importance are presented both in documentaries and in fictional portrayals. Knowledge of lawyers and medical practitioners of the existence of such information in the general media can be of great value in assisting in the process of communication to lay people in court and particularly to juries.

Communication in the courtroom usually takes the form of words delivered as evidence by the witnesses. But this is not the only way to achieve good communication. The use of charts, videos, diagrams, photographs and physical models should always be considered. Where evidence relating to the human body is concerned, the medical witness often has the best physical model available: their own body. In order to ensure that the anatomical locations of injuries are understood by a jury, it is useful for the witness to indicate the position of the injuries by reference to their own body.

A well-informed jury that has had the medical or scientific issues clearly explained to them in an accessible and intelligible way by a witness is in the best possible position to evaluate the evidence and come to a valid conclusion. Healthcare practitioners should always remember that it is coroners, lay juries or judges who assess their evidence: the opinion of their medical or scientific peers or the parties' lawyers does not determine the forensic outcome of the medical work that they have done.

To communicate successfully takes careful planning and preparation. In many ways preparing to give evidence in court is similar to preparing a lecture.

The information must be presented to the audience in such a way as to retain their interest in what is said and to permit them to comprehend and analyse what they see and hear. The development of analogies that can be used to explain complex medical and scientific notions in lay terms is useful. Such explanatory analogies are a feature of the oratory of good communicators, and part of the armoury of experienced forensic healthcare practitioners.

The presentation of evidence in court is generally the endpoint of forensic healthcare practice and, regardless of the quality of the scientific work performed, how the results are communicated may be just as important in ensuring that the evidence is taken into account. As a result effort put into preparing to give evidence may reap particular benefit for justice outcomes.

Long-term preparation

Long-term preparation merges with the original forensic work performed in a particular case. It includes ensuring that the work has been appropriately carried out and that the original documentation and notes are complete in all relevant particulars. Mistakes and omissions made at this time cannot usually be rectified without considerable embarrassment to the witness, and the need for such amendments may seriously damage the witness's credibility in the eyes of the court. It is important, even at this early stage, to canvass the possible need for court attendance as a witness and the likely civil issues or criminal charges involved. Notes, potential exhibits and relevant materials should be stored in a secure place for retrieval during the later stages of pre-trial preparation. At this time the potential witness should ensure that their contact details are known by legal representatives and investigators so that they can be given the earliest possible notice of any meetings, conferences and court attendances.

Medium-term preparation

At the completion of the substantive casework together with the compilation of medical notes and records, the main preparatory work commences. Initially this should include presentation of the case material to peers so as to gather feedback on the quality of the casework performed, obtain advice on relevant recent advances in the area, and experience informal cross-examination on the opinions you have expressed and the conclusions you have reached. The medical literature should be reviewed at this time and articles dealing with the subject matter of the case obtained and analysed. If special illustrations or models are considered to be useful in communicating the evidence in court, they should be prepared and their use canvassed with the lawyers.

At the completion of these processes, the medical witness collates the notes and materials. Well-prepared witnesses can give evidence confident that:
- they have all they need to communicate their findings;
- they understand what the legal system requires of them;
- the legal representatives understand the nature of the evidence they can give.

Short-term preparation

If the earlier preparation has been adequate, short-term preparation should be limited to reviewing the materials, organising the illustrative materials, assembling any equipment, and ensuring that the court attendance has been included in the diary work schedule. A few days before appearing at court to give evidence, the witness should read their original statement carefully and cross-reference the material in it with their notes, the relevant photographs, charts, radiographs and information obtained from literature searches. At the completion of this review process, the witness should be able to find any relevant item of information quickly in their notes. The models, charts and other illustrations should be packaged appropriately for transport to court and for subsequent storage by the court as exhibits. If the witness has given evidence in the matter before, perhaps at a preliminary hearing, it is advisable to obtain a transcript of the evidence given on that occasion. This transcript should be studied carefully prior to giving any further evidence.

Logistics of appearing as a witness

The process of giving evidence as an expert witness can be stressful, so the practitioner should be fully prepared for all eventualities. Then, as each issue arises, they are in a position to respond immediately and appropriately to the matters raised.

Punctuality is mandatory. The practitioner should make sure of the time and date when they are required to attend court. In order to do this, the doctor may need to contact the party calling them and to make arrangements for an appropriate time to give evidence. The doctor should also make sure that they are aware of the location of the court and the particular courtroom where they will be giving their evidence. This logistic planning should cover matters such as transport to the court, court sitting times, and the telephone numbers and addresses of the parties calling the doctor as a witness.

Before attending court, the medical witness should collect all notes, reference materials and audio-visual aids, and assemble them in such a way that the material can be easily accessed and referred to during their evidence. It may be convenient to use a ring file or similar binder to hold the relevant documents and materials for a case. This allows the material to be organised in advance, so that the witness is completely familiar with it. It is important to take all photographs, x-rays, charts and other print-outs that form part of the material upon which the witness is to give evidence, even if these are copies. The originals will probably be already present in court and it may not be clear in the pre-trial phase whether the witness will be able to refer to the copies in their own case file. However, even if the doctor is not permitted to refer to this material during evidence, it is important to have the material available for review prior to giving evidence and to be able to respond to any associated issues that might arise during evidence.

One of the main organisational matters a medical witness must attend to relates to their notes and records. Whilst a barrister has the bar table upon which to arrange documents and materials, the witness has often just a small lectern on which to arrange their notes. For most witnesses this small space is all that is required as they are asked to give nearly all their evidence from personal recollection without reference to written materials. In contrast the forensic expert witness may have to juggle a medical report, a set of personal notes, hospital records, photographs and radiographs on a tiny area. To cope well in this situation requires a high degree of organisation of the witness's materials. The witness should be so familiar with their materials that finding information in them, while being examined, is a swift and efficient process that causes minimum disruption to the flow of evidence.

While the giving of evidence in court does not ordinarily require the witness to perform analyses or physical examinations, occasionally an expert witness is asked to look at an exhibit such as a radiograph or a physical object such as a dental impression and to demonstrate a feature of it to the court. Normally the court will have the required equipment, such as examination gloves, available for the witness, but this is not always the case. The forensic practitioner should take to court such items of equipment. Not only is it useful to the court if the medical witness is prepared in this way, but it demonstrates the witness's professionalism with regard to their court work. Useful items might include: examination gloves, a pocket calculator, a magnifying glass, a ruler, a pointer, and pens and pencils.

Before entering the witness box it is essential that mobile telephones are switched off. There is nothing that irritates a court more than to hear a mobile telephone ring. Such an event is likely to earn a rebuke from the judge, and to some people indicates a lack of respect for court proceedings on the part of the witness.

Refreshing memory

Few of us have a photographic memory, but it is astonishing how much detail can be remembered accurately for a few days after an intensive reading of our notes and the medico-legal report. Refreshing one's memory is more than simply reading through the material: the reading must be performed intelligently and interactively with other associated material such as photographs. This re-reading provides an opportunity to re-evaluate the basis upon which initial opinions were made. It allows the expert witness to think through the ways in which a finding or observation could best be described to the court. Choice of euphemisms, analogies and appropriate examples of like situations should be thought out at this stage, so that they can be easily and fluently delivered from the witness box. As well as becoming re-acquainted with the written material in the notes and reports previously made, this is the time to cross-reference the features in photographs with the statements made in the report and the entries in the notes. It is important that in doing this, that the original notes are not tampered with by making additions, deletions or modifications. It is crucial that the notes are maintained exactly as they were when originally made: any later interference may render them inadmissible and therefore inaccessible to the witness during their oral evidence.

Revision of medical knowledge

All healthcare professionals are required to maintain and develop their medical and scientific knowledge. Many of the basic aspects of medical science can be forgotten or become unfamiliar as our range and depth of specialist knowledge grows. It is a great mistake to allow knowledge of basic medical science to fade. While a witness may be a leading specialist in a particular esoteric field of medicine or dentistry, demonstration of their lack of knowledge of a fundamental area of anatomy, physiology or biochemistry will stand out in the minds of the jurors and may raise doubt as to their competence. Clearly it is not possible to retain all matters that are covered in the early years of medical or dental training, but part of a witness's pre-trial preparation should include a revision of those areas so that they are in the best position to explain the basis for their opinion and the nature of the scientific principles that underlie it.

Beside the principles of medical science, specialist areas also need to be considered. Research and development in medicine and medical science continue to progress from year to year. A considerable time may elapse between the preparation of a medico-legal report and the presentation of those matters before a court. In that time, developments may have occurred in that field of medicine, and new scientific papers may have been published. It is essential that witnesses be aware of the changes in knowledge in their speciality and of new developments in that and related fields.

In some cases, issues that lie outside the witness's own speciality are involved. For example, in a case involving surgery, a surgeon giving evidence may be completely up-to-date in the specialist principles of diagnosis and treatment surrounding the case in question. However, if the case potentially involves issues about anaesthetics or intensive care, the surgeon might need to revise aspects of these specialist areas and learn about recent developments. In doing this the medical witness is not changing their speciality or field of expertise, they are instead merely ensuring that the associated relevant areas of basic medical science and specialist medical practice are within their immediate knowledge. If they are well prepared and permitted by the court they will be able to deal appropriately with any general issues on these topics that arise during their evidence.

It is important to remember that the whole of an expert's evidence may be tested and challenged by a barrister who has in turn been advised by a leading expert in the witness's field of expertise. As a result the barrister may have access to a specialist medical report, medical textbooks and journal articles that pertain to a particular area of the witness's evidence. In order to meet such challenges, the medical witness must be aware of the current medical literature and be familiar with the standard texts and opinions. This is not to say that they must necessarily embrace the current medical opinion on a topic, but they should be sufficiently informed to be able to contribute intelligently to the debate in court and to apply their view appropriately to the particular facts in the case. Medical witnesses can prepare themselves by refreshing their knowledge on matters that may arise in a case by means of relevant background research and reading. While it is not always possible to predict which matters will be contentious in a case, a clear understanding of the relevant law relating to the issue before the court, coupled with peer review and consultation with colleagues, provides the best method of ensuring that the witness has considered most of the relevant issues.

Medico-legal analysis

It is not sufficient for a forensic practitioner who has been called to give evidence to consider only matters pertinent to their discipline. In addition the forensic expert witness must be aware of the courts' requirements and the particular legal and associated issues that are relevant to the particular case. The expert does not have to become a lawyer in order to do this, but they should be aware of the legal principles at issue. In a criminal matter where the expert witness is appearing on behalf of the prosecution, they should be aware of the charge the defendant faces and the elements that make up the alleged offence. In addition, the witness needs to be aware of the potential general or specific defences that might be appropriate to such a charge and how such defences might be introduced during the court proceedings. With these matters in mind, the witness in preparing to give evidence should identify in their own evidence points of possible or probable contention with regard to fact or opinion and consider these areas in advance. Having given them due consideration in advance they will be in the best position to deal with the issues as they arise, rather than having to consider possibilities in the heat of the moment. It is, of course, dangerous to assume that an expert witness reviewing material in pre-trial preparation will consider all of the potential legal issues that might arise in relation to their evidence. All that is required in practice is for the doctor to turn their mind to the essential forensic issues that may hinge upon their evidence.

Pre-trial conference

Barristers and experienced forensic medical witnesses agree that some form of pre-trial conference with expert witnesses can be of great value. Unfortunately, there is considerable variation in the frequency of such pre-trial conferences; however, they can be advantageous to witnesses and legal counsel alike. Some of the issues that can be clarified in pre-trial conferences include: the witness's qualifications and fields of expertise and the content and implications of their evidence

Because of the importance of expert opinion evidence, the lawyers need to convince the court that the witness is indeed an expert in these areas. Assessment and evaluation of a witness's expertise is one of the major purposes of a pre-trial conference. The conference allows the barrister to meet the witness and to find out not only their formal qualifications but also the extent and depth of their knowledge in a particular area. At the same time, the barrister is able to determine at what point the witness's expertise is likely to be exceeded and to discover any hidden areas of expertise the witness has which have not otherwise been disclosed. The barrister is in the best position to explain to the medical witness what level of proof will be required to show that a witness is indeed an expert in a particular area. The medical witness who is aware of this is in the best position to explain the extent of their knowledge and experience to the court.

Entering the court

An expert witness may often be required to attend court at a time when it is in sitting hearing other evidence. Unless they have been specifically authorised in advance, the witness should not enter the courtroom but wait outside with the other witnesses until called, or until the party who has called them to court comes out of the courtroom to talk with them. In many cases, especially in criminal cases, there may be an order for the exclusion of witnesses in force, which means that only the witness who is actually giving evidence is permitted to remain in the courtroom. This is done to prevent witnesses hearing each other's evidence and being influenced by it. These rules may be relaxed in the case of expert witnesses, whose task may be specifically to evaluate the evidence of others and to give their medical opinion based on it. However, the medical witness should not assume that this is the case, and should not enter the court unless specifically invited to do so by the parties or by the court itself.

Conversations outside the court

The principle regarding witnesses hearing each other's evidence extends to witnesses discussing their evidence outside the courtroom before, during or after they have given evidence. The court wishes to hear from each witness as to their own information unmodified by conversations with other witnesses. A medical witness waiting outside the court, therefore, should refrain from talking to other witnesses about the case. General conversations regarding the weather or the nearest restaurant are acceptable. However even such innocent conversations may be misconstrued as collusion and may be raised in court to discredit the witness's evidence. Even if the witness can convince the court that all they were discussing was the weather, the allegation is an unnecessary interruption to court proceedings and one that may damage the witness's reputation.

This matter is even more important where a witness is in the midst of giving evidence when the court adjourns. During the break the medical witness should not communicate with other witnesses, the media or other persons regarding the evidence they have given, the questions they were asked, or the evidence they are to give at a later stage. If the lunch break or end-of-day adjournment occurs during cross-examination of a witness, they may have been made aware of a number of the defence issues in the case. These issues must not be communicated to the other witnesses who have not yet been called.

On completion of a medical witness's evidence, the party calling them usually requests that the court excuses them from further attendance. If this is done, they may leave the court precinct. Again they must not communicate regarding the evidence they gave or the questions they were asked with other witnesses, especially with other expert witnesses. Such conversations may place the other witness in a difficult position regarding their own evidence.

With regard to the issue of communication, it should be remembered that there is no formal property in a witness. If the party calling you, or the opposing party, wishes to talk to you in advance about matters in relation to the evidence that you will be giving, you are not prevented from doing so. However, there is no obligation upon a witness to discuss their evidence with any party. The only obligation is to answer the questions put to them in the witness box. In practical terms, however, most expert witnesses are there to assist the general process of the court and there is little point in obstructing either party. As a matter of legal courtesy, if an opposing party wishes to discuss the evidence a witness will give in advance, they should inform the party calling that witness of their intention to do so.

Appearance and behaviour

The manner in which evidence is elicited in court and subsequently received and analysed by a jury is influenced by a variety of factors. Clearly, the qualifications and expertise of a witness has a bearing on to what degree a jury accepts what they say. Apart from these obvious professional considerations, there is no doubt that a whole variety of non-professional factors influence the jury's attitude towards a witness. A court is not simply a place where scientific truth is analysed; it is a place where the community, in the form of a lay jury, decides the issues, and the witnesses are evaluated by both professional and social criteria. An expert witness who wants their evidence to have maximum impact needs to be aware of the social as well as the professional factors that influence the way in which their evidence is received. Studies have shown that juries expect expert witnesses to have certain physical characteristics and to behave in certain ways. If a medical witness departs from these accepted cultural standards because of personal idiosyncrasy or deliberate choice, then their evidence may be given less credence by a jury, regardless of its scientific validity.

How the witness looks, behaves and interacts with the people in the court all affect the attitude of a jury toward them. The ideal attributes of medical witnesses are a series of contradictions. They must not be boring, neither must they be flamboyant entertainers; they must not display left-wing politics, they must not display right-wing politics; they must not dress too informally, they must not dress too formally. Finding the middle ground can be difficult. However, there are some general principles that are of considerable use in this area.

Dress

Juries expect the medical witness to fulfil their own views of how a professional should dress. Juries, like patients, may be suspicious of a healthcare professional who wears a T-shirt or jeans, or intimidated by one who wears a very formal dark pin-striped suit and a bow tie. Most members of the community believe that professionals should be smartly dressed. Thus a specialist giving rarefied information on complex surgical techniques may dress somewhat formally, whereas a practitioner giving evidence relating to everyday medical or dental practice may dress in a more casual or middle-of-the-road fashion. For men, an ordinary suit or sports jacket and trousers, and for women, a smart skirt and blouse, with or without a jacket, seems to be the most appropriate. Clothing that is controversial for any reason is best avoided. Stories abound regarding what jurors have said about people and their clothing: 'I don't trust a doctor who wears a bow tie', and so on. While the witness should not simply blend into the background their dress should not be distracting to a jury such that it draws attention away from what they are saying. It may go against a witness's personality, but a slightly casual version of formal dress seems to be the most appropriate clothing for the expert witness.

Entering and leaving the court

The first time a jury sees an expert witness is when they are called into court and they walk from the entrance of the courtroom to the witness box. Those first few seconds are all important. Some members of the jury will be making up their minds whether they have faith in this witness on the basis of their dress and manner. As a result, witnesses should think carefully about their deportment in the court. Court officials bow formally whenever they enter or leave the court. Strictly speaking, it is unnecessary for those not associated with the court to do this. However, it has become accepted practice for most people who have dealings before the court, including expert witnesses, to do the same. It certainly does no harm to conform to this simple custom. The expert witness should make sure they are available near the doorway to the court, so that when they are called they can enter the courtroom immediately. When walking to the witness box, they should carry themselves in a business-like manner, concentrating their gaze on the witness box itself and avoiding the temptation to look all around the court to see who is there. It is often useful to visit the courtroom prior to giving evidence to become familiar with the layout and the position of the witness box. It is important not to dawdle or become distracted while walking to the witness box, and at the same time not to give the impression of haste.

When a witness has completed giving their evidence, in most instances they will be formally excused by the judge from further attendance, or otherwise asked to stand down. It is only after this that the witness should close their file, put away their notes and leave the witness box. The witness should then leave the court in the same manner in which they entered it, walking in a calm and dignified fashion regardless of the experience they have had in the witness box. There are occasions when a medical witness has had an uncomfortable time and is longing to leave the courtroom. Simply rushing out in these circumstances gives everyone the impression that things have gone so badly that the witness wants to get away as soon as possible. If, however, the witness's departure is calm and dignified, it may go some way to redressing an uncomfortable time in the witness box. It is important when leaving the court not to engage in any trivial or social conversation with other individuals, including barristers, solicitors, members of the public and the press. Social conversation should take place outside the court. If one of the barristers or solicitors wishes to talk to a witness after their evidence has been given, they will leave the court and meet the witness outside.

As we have seen expert witnesses may have to bring a number of items into court. In some cases, these include bulky charts and presentation aids that are hard to handle in the confined space of the witness box. The usher may be able to assist, and if the medical witness mentions the problem to the usher when they are being called into court, the court staff will assist with the arrangements.

The witness box

When the witness has arrived in the witness box, all eyes in the court are focused on them. The witness is asked to state their name and then to take the oath or affirmation. This is the first time that the medical witness's voice has been heard in the courtroom, and first impressions can be important for the jury. It is also the first time that the expert has heard their own voice speaking in the court-room. When they tell the court their name, they get some feedback as to the acoustics of the room and the volume at which they must speak in order to be heard by all people present in the court.

The taking of the oath is a moment of great formality and importance in the eyes of the court. It is hard to know how a jury views the taking of an oath, but in any event the medical witness should treat it with the utmost seriousness. Even if the medical witness is aware of the wording of the oath, they should always allow themselves to be led through it by the court. Each phrase should be declared loudly and clearly, and in a manner that implies that the witness understands the terms of the oath. It does not require a theatrical performance, but the jury should be left with the impression that the forensic expert's only concern is to tell the truth. As well as the manner of speaking, their stance and attitude need to be appropriate. The oath is spoken to the judge, magistrate or tribunal chairman who should be faced at all times. The witness should not slouch or fidget or look around in a distracted fashion, and the Bible or other religious work should be held up in a formal but not rigid pose.

While a witness is being sworn in, all people present in the court should remain completely silent and not move or create any form of disturbance. Indeed, a court usually waits for silence and the attention of all people before the oath is administered. No person should enter or leave the court whilst the oath is being administered. As a result of these requirements, the eyes of most people in the court and, in particular, the jury are focused on the witness who is taking the oath. Once the oath has been completed and the witness's evidence is being given, a slightly more relaxed atmosphere prevails.

The aim of the barristers for both parties is to seek from the witness evidence that supports their own client's view and to ensure that the evidence is addressed appropriately to the jury. If the witness gives evidence that does not support their client's case, then the significance of that evidence needs to be minimised in the eyes of the jury. An effective technique is for a barrister to request that the witness gives answers that are favourable to their client directly to the jury whilst answers that are unfavourable are directed to the barrister so that the jury loses eye contact with the witness. The witness should of course address all answers to the jury and the judge, as it is they who have to evaluate and decide upon the evidence. In jurisdictions where witnesses are expected to give their evidence standing, a successful technique is for the witness to stand so that their toes point at the judge and jury rather than at the barristers asking the questions. The effect of this stance is that when the barrister asks a question the witness is side-on to the barrister and is looking at the barrister over their shoulder. When the witness replies they tend to turn and give their answer in the direction in which their feet are pointing. In jurisdictions where witnesses give their evidence seated the witness should ensure that their knees are pointed at the jury so that the same effect is achieved.

There are other important physical factors in relation to stance when giving evidence. While the witness should maintain a relaxed attitude rather than taking up a military-style posture, it is important that the witness does not slouch in the witness box either when giving their answers or during any interruptions or minor breaks in the delivery of evidence. Similarly, the witness should not fidget or fiddle with objects whilst giving their evidence. It is all too easy to use a pen as a pointer to illustrate a feature on a chart or photograph and then to continue holding and fiddling with the pen, which may be a source of great distraction for the jury. If a pointer or other aid is used, it should be replaced on the witness box shelf immediately it is no longer required. The maintenance of a professional physical attitude whilst giving evidence should not be underestimated. The development of a few simple habits and effective techniques can vastly improve the quality and effectiveness of evidence given by a witness.

Report writing

The usual way in which investigation findings are recorded is by means of a written medico-legal report. In the case of post-mortem examinations, the work of the forensic pathologist, the forensic odontologist and the forensic anthropologist may be contained in a single document either in the body of the text or as appendices to the main report or in discrete separate reports. These reports may be required to conform to a standard structure or pro-forma although most specialist investigators would be likely to include greater detail in their report than the pro-forma would require.

The transcription of medico-legal reports into a brief of evidence usually requires a report to be provided as text only. In contrast, modern medical, dental and scientific reports often include graphic elements such as photographs, radiographs, tables, charts or diagrams. This restriction to text in reports for court can be limiting with respect to the communication and recording of findings. As a result, investigators often use handwritten notes or body charts as well as photographs to improve the documentation of their findings. It is essential that the existence of such additional materials be recorded so that they can be made available to the courts. Today these expanded forms of documentation are more commonly presented to court and specialist investigators should not feel limited by the old reliance on textual reports alone.

The timely completion of an accurate and informative final autopsy report is an essential aspect of post-autopsy procedures. Such reports have to be clear and understandable to the various people who require autopsy information. Unfortunately the different audiences make it difficult to phrase an expert report in appropriate terms. For example, a family member may need to have information expressed in non-medical language, while the deceased's medical specialist may require more precise medical terminology. In the case of medico-legal reports where people from different backgrounds will be reading the report, real communication problems can arise.

Even though, strictly speaking, a forensic pathologist or dentist is working for the coroner, they must keep in mind that their report may eventually make its way into the criminal or civil justice systems.

Three kinds of reports figure prominently in medical evidence before coroners' courts. The first is the medical report from the treating medical practitioners of the deceased person. Such practitioners will usually have access to the patient's prior medical history, which provides a longitudinal perspective on the health and medical management of the deceased. General medical practitioners, in particular, may be in a position to provide insights to the court about the general health and wellbeing of the deceased prior to death, as well as of any previous or current medical conditions that may have played a role in the death. For instance, the practitioner may have looked after a person with thalassaemia major for many years and been in a position to observe their decline in health to a point where major specialist medical interventions were necessary to keep the person alive. The doctor may be able to give a perspective on the course of the disease, the person's vulnerability to infection, and the need for particular forms of treatment, whether orthodox or experimental.

The second type of medical report received by a coroner as a result of the death investigation relates to the medical investigation of the dead body.

Generally it is an autopsy report dealing with the findings of a pathological examination. It is often a composite report dealing with a variety of medical and scientific investigations carried out on the body of the deceased or the environment in which the deceased was found. In addition to information relating to general pathology findings, the report may contain the results of other specialist medical investigations, such as dental examinations, radiological imaging of the body and/or toxicological or pharmacological analysis of body tissues. In some post-mortem examinations of a body it may be necessary for a pathologist to refer certain body organs for specialist pathological examination. A brain may be retained for neuropathological examination or the heart retained for examination by a specialist cardiac pathologist. The results of these additional specialist pathological investigations are often contained within the general autopsy report or received by the coroner as attachments to the general autopsy report.

The other form of medical report that is provided routinely to the coroner's court is that of an independent assessor or technical expert, whether a specialist physician, pathologist, psychiatrist (in the form of a psychological autopsy), pharmacologist, toxicologist, dentist or other specialist medical or scientific assessor who could help the coroner to understand the quality and appropriateness of medical treatment provided to the deceased prior to death, the mechanism and mode of death or the identity of the deceased person. Such experts also have the potential to assist with insights into the possible medical causes of death as well as unravelling the often complex circumstances in which the death occurred.

In preparing a medico-legal report it is usual for the investigator to append a curriculum vitae to the report. It need not be lengthy but should communicate to the reader the general professional background of the doctor, highlighting any of its aspects that may be particularly pertinent to the inquest. For instance, if the practitioner has experience in a particular form of medicine that is at issue in the inquest, has attended training in a relevant clinical technique, has given papers at professional gatherings on the subject or been supervised by a prominent practitioner in the area, such matters should be referred to therein. Should the practitioner have written published material that is germane to the hearing that too might alert the coroner to the authoritative status of the report writer. Clarity in the curriculum vitae aids the coroner and the legal representatives in understanding the scope and limitations of an expert's expertise.

In setting out their finding, the investigator who is requested to perform a specialist examination must make a careful record of the time and date that they were originally asked to provide this service. Practitioners should also note where they were when they were called and who called them. A record should also be kept of the time and date of their arrival at any relevant location, including the place at which they performed the examination and the address and specific location where they performed each part of the forensic medical examination. The time and date of the forensic examination should also be noted; if more than one individual is examined over a period of time, the exact time of the commencement and completion of each examination should be specifically recorded. If a case involves several linked medical examinations, after the completion of all of the examinations, the time and date of the completion of the examination series and of the compilation of the notes should also be documented. Upon leaving the place of the examination, the examiner should again record the date and time. In some cases, a practitioner is requested to attend several locations, sometimes for the purpose of examining the scene of a crime. The time of attendance at and departure from each scene should also be recorded in the notes.

It is important that there be a record of the date and time when the notes were compiled. The notes should have been made within a reasonably short time of the examination when the findings were still fresh in the examiner's mind, so there is no basis for concluding that the practitioner could have been confused later on as to the examination findings. The court is more likely to accept notes as being contemporaneous if the date and time the notes were completed is included in the notes themselves, assuming that the date and time noted are reasonable given the circumstances in which the examinations occurred.

If an examiner allows another person such as a mortuary technical officer, nurse or technician to assist with any aspect of an examination, that fact should be recorded, together with the nature of the assistance supplied. There may be situations where the courts require that the persons who assisted a forensic practitioner in the course of an examination give evidence about what they saw or did. This situation might occur, for example, when a forensic technical officer assists with the collection and packaging of forensic specimens taken during an autopsy. This legitimate process should not restrict a practitioner from using appropriate assistants during an examination, but the nature of the assistance, and the name, status and details of the person who provided it, should be clearly set out in the notes and the medico-legal report.

In many situations the practitioner often becomes involved with a number of other persons before, during and after the examination, including nursing and paramedical staff. These additional people are sometimes collectively referred to as observers. In many cases these observers will be professional co-workers but in some situations they may be bystanders with an indirect involvement in medical examination. Such persons may include nursing staff who assist in the medical examinations, social workers, family members including parents, counselors, victim support persons, police and other investigators. The practitioner should record in their notes the names of all persons who were present and observed elements of the examination. The role and status of each observer should be noted, and if they took part in the investigation procedures the nature of their role and their actions should be described.

In any investigation it is important for there to be a clear record of the subject's full name, address, age, date of birth and gender. In some cases it may be necessary to record details of next of kin, or, in the case of children, the names of parents or guardians. Telephone numbers and other personal identifying details are not usually required, but they may be useful if medical follow-up seems appropriate. Where details such as telephone numbers are recorded, it is sufficient if they appear in the examiner's own notes rather than in the final report released to the court. While this may seem to be a departure from the principle that the notes and report should contain the same information, the restriction on such personal details of a patient in the report is often desirable. This is because in some cases the medico-legal report makes its way to a wide range of individuals, and the resulting effective publication of a patient's telephone number could cause them embarrassment and lead to possible harassment.

The accurate recording of a medical history or circumstances surrounding a death or injury is fundamental to any examination. Often the medical and circumstantial history may be obtained from a family member or from police investigators. The medical history and circumstances of the event being investigated always constitute the foundation that defines how any subsequent examination or autopsy is to be conducted. This information must be critically evaluated before the examination begins. It is often useful to develop a problem-based approach to an investigation that identifies the issues to be resolved and the information that must be obtained in order to determine the nature and detail of the physical examination required.

While forensic medical examinations concentrate particularly on the examination of the external features of the body for signs of injury, it is important for the examiner to record the clothing, jewellery and other extraneous material that may be present. The recording of these aspects of an examination can be of great value as it may provide investigators with details regarding important features of the circumstances in which the death or injury occurred.

The description of wounds and injuries is critical to any medical examination, whether the subject is deceased or living. Descriptions should be recorded in detail in the medical notes and in the subsequent medico-legal report, using terms that are objective rather than subjective. The use of subjective terms can have value because it allows for quicker communication of the nature and type of injury. However, if an examiner only describes an injury in its interpreted form, further analysis by another forensic medical practitioner may be rendered more difficult. The advantage of a more objective description of a wound is that it does not presuppose the cause thereof. Such an objective description of an injury is of particular use to other medical experts who may be seeking alternative explanations for the cause of the wound.

Descriptions of wounds and injuries should always be given by reference to the patient in the standard anatomical position: the body standing erect and facing forwards, with the arms by the sides and the palms of the hands facing the front. The position of wounds on the body should be located by reference to fixed bony landmarks wherever possible. This is preferable to using soft tissue landmarks such as the umbilicus or the nipples. In the description of a wound, the medical practitioner should take note of its site, its size, its shape, and its surrounds. The colour, contour, course and contents of a wound should also be recorded, as well as its depth and the nature of its borders. Comments about the cause of the wound, based on classification of the wound type, together with an estimate of its probable age, are often appropriate but these may be best situated at the end of the report with the other analyses. This is so that there can be no confusion between the description of facts and opinions by the writer of the report.

The general principle for describing wounds and injuries is that the description in the report made following a complete medical examination should assist in the reconstruction of the events in which the injury occurred. As a result, it is vital that the recording of injuries and other findings should be optimal. Charts, x-rays, photographs and videos should be used where appropriate. Photographs are of great assistance in recording injuries to the body, but they have several major weaknesses. Most surfaces of the human body curve away in three dimensions, and this feature is hard to capture in a two-dimensional photograph. Additionally, the colour of photographs rarely reproduces real skin tones, pigmentation, or the colour of marks and injuries. This feature can have major implications for the recording of bruises: the use of direct flash illumination can 'white out' the centre of a photograph and obscure faint injuries. The use of more specialised techniques of ultraviolet and infrared photography can be of great help in recording faint bruises and other patterned injuries such as bite marks.

During the course of an examination the practitioner may collect various specimens for pathology testing or forensic analysis. They should be placed in appropriate containers, according to their nature and the type of test to be performed. Laboratories vary regarding the type of transport containers they prefer for specimens, and the medical practitioner should take note of this. Some specimens require special preservatives or transport media to preserve them for subsequent laboratory examination.

Regardless of the quality or number of specimens collected during a medical examination, in order for them to have probative value the results of their testing must be admissible as evidence in subsequent court proceedings. Although the rules relating to this are more relaxed in an inquest, the general principle is that for test results to be admitted in evidence, the court must be assured that the specimen was collected, transported and stored appropriately. The coroner must also be certain that the specimen has been correctly identified and labelled and that its integrity has been assured by its being secured at all times. The coroner is usually assured of these matters by identifying a continuous transfer of custody of the specimen from the time it was taken to the time it was examined. This continuous custodial record is referred to as the 'chain of custody'. With information on how a specimen was passed from person to person, the coroner can call all the people who held the specimen to give evidence of their part in its collection, transport and storage, and so prove that the chain of custody remained unbroken. Following the careful labelling and packaging of the specimens, the examiner should record the name of the person who receives them as well as the time and date this transfer occurs.

When it comes to the final preparation of the formal medico-legal statement, a great deal of care and attention must be given to the construction of the paragraphs dealing with the analysis of the findings and the eventual final comments and conclusions. The first few comments at the conclusion of a report can be used to summarise the key examination findings; this can be of great help in setting the scene for the more analytical comments to follow. In the subsequent comments the examination findings can be explained in relation to the alleged causal scenarios that have been described in the history section at the beginning of the report. Significant absences in the examination findings should be commented upon by reference to the circumstantial and medical histories provided. As mentioned above, internal consistency and integrity are critical. If comments are made about a correlation between an injury pattern and circumstantial information, the injury and the information must be described in the report so that it is clear what the evidential basis for the comments is.

Reference

1 Nathan J. (1989) Victorian Reports/Judgements/1989 VR/ *Harmsworth v the State Coroner* – 1989 VR 989 – 9 March 1989.

Recommended reading

1 Bernstein BE, Hartsell TL. (2005) *The Portable Guide to Testifying in Court*. John Wiley & Sons, New Jersey.
2 Brodsky SL. (1991) *Testifying in Court: Guidelines and Maxims for the Expert Witness*. American Psychological Association, Washington, DC.
3 Forbes TR. (1985) *Surgeons At The Bailey: English Forensic Medicine to 1878*. University Press, Yale.
4 Freckelton I. (1987) *The Trial of the Expert*. Oxford University Press, Melbourne.
5 Freckelton I, Selby H. (1993) *Expert Evidence*, 6-volume loose-leaf service, LBC, Sydney.
6 Freckelton I, Selby H. (2013) *Expert Evidence: Law, Practice and Procedure*. 5th edn, Law Book Co, Sydney.
7 Gee DJ, Mason JK. (1990) *The Courts and the Doctor*. Oxford University Press, Oxford.
8 Hand D, Fife-Yeomans J. (2004) *The Coroner: Investigating Sudden Death*. ABC Books, Sydney.
9 Matthews P. (2002) *Jervis on the Office and Duties of Coroners*. 12th edn, Sweet & Maxwell, London.
10 Medical Protection Society. (1992) *Medico-Legal Reports and Appearing in Courts*. Medical Protection Society, London.
11 Ranson DL. (1995) *Anatomical Figuring: Forensic Body Chart Resource*. Victorian Institute of Forensic Medicine, Melbourne.
12 Smith R, Wynne B. (eds) (1989) *Expert Evidence: Interpreting science in the law*. Routledge, London; New York.
13 Tsushima WT, Anderson RM Jr. (1996) *Mastering Expert Testimony: A Courtroom Handbook for Mental Health Professionals*. Lawrence Erlbaum Publishing, Mahwah, New Jersey.

CHAPTER 3

Anatomy and morphology

Mark Leedham[1] and Erin F. Hutchinson[2]

[1] Northern Territory Coroner's Office, Australia
[2] School of Anatomical Sciences, University of the Witwatersrand, South Africa

Dental anatomy and morphology

Identification of the teeth is a basic and essential skill for competence in forensic odontology. Not only must an odontologist be able to recognise normal anatomy, but also abnormal anatomy. Variations in size, shape and number of teeth can all confound accurate identification, but at the same time be unique markers that can aid identification. Some of these variations can be quite rare, and others less so, for example missing third molars. An awareness of dental development in all its aspects, including developmental stages, is crucial.

A proper interpretation of dental anatomy may make the difference between a positive identification and a possible or probable identification, or an inaccurate identification. The normal dental anatomy of teeth is best seen in the various textbooks on teeth. Any of the undergraduate textbooks on dental anatomy should provide a good source of information on the normal appearance of teeth and associated structures. This foundation knowledge is essential before understanding the variations from normal dental morphology. As restorative dentists, we spend considerable time repairing teeth and attempting to restore normal anatomical structure, and yet at the same time the dentition becomes more individualised and distinct for that person. Recognition of normal anatomy is also an essential part of diagnosis in the normal process of a dental examination in the living patient, as dentists chart and record conditions prior to formulating a treatment plan.

Odontologists also need to be able to recognise teeth in abnormal states (e.g. after fire, or chemical attack), and from images (photographs and radiographs), of varying quality. Isolated and altered teeth (from trauma or restoration) can also present particular problems when there is limited context to provide additional information. Odontologists need to be aware of all the possible variations in size, number, shape and position. In addition, odontologists need to appreciate the possible errors of charting, and problems of x-ray interpretation and processing that can inevitably occur and that may affect

Forensic Odontology: Principles and Practice, First Edition. Edited by Jane A. Taylor and Jules A. Kieser.
© 2016 John Wiley & Sons, Ltd. Published 2016 by John Wiley & Sons, Ltd.

their identification. Possible errors in ante-mortem records, from incorrect identification, and from restorative, orthodontic and surgical alterations to teeth need to be taken into account during comparison of ante-mortem and post-mortem records.

Patients with both normal and unusual dentitions will often have sought dental care that results in changes to dental anatomy, tooth shape and number. A common example would be restoration of upper lateral incisors (peg lateral incisors). Many dental anomalies will also result in referral to dental specialists, (oral and maxillo-facial specialists, orthodontists and prosthodontists) for management or removal of teeth. This will be a further and often very useful source of additional information that may aid in identification. In addition, these referrals will be a further source of dental imaging (x-rays and photographs), which can also be particularly useful.

Morphogenetic fields

The most likely teeth to be missing or varied in size are the last teeth in each morphogenetic field (lateral incisor, second premolar and third molar). The concept of a morphogenetic field for teeth was first described by Butler in 1939 [1, 2], and he postulated that there was a 'gradient of variability' in the mammalian dentition, that increased further away from the first (pole) tooth in the field, hence the most distal tooth in each field was the most likely to vary in size, shape and presence. These ideas were subsequently modified [3, 4] to include the idea that a type of cloning was occurring producing further tooth buds (Fig. 3.1). Both the older and more recent theories on morphogenetic fields have recently been reviewed in the light of new knowledge from the fields of genetics and the probable role of environmental factors [5].

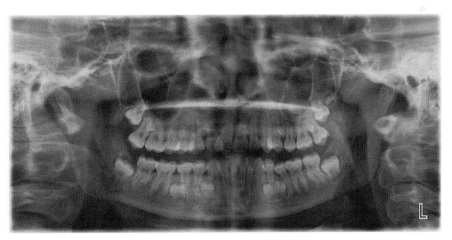

Fig. 3.1 Multiple supernumery teeth (unassociated with a syndrome). There are eight extra teeth. Individual is aged 15 years.

Variations in tooth size, number and shape are determined during the initiation (tooth number) and morphogenetic stages (size and shape) of dental development [6].

Knowledge of various syndromes and conditions that may affect dental development is also essential. While many of these syndromes may be rare, odontologists will come across these anomalies at some time and they can both hinder or aid in identification.

Additional teeth

There does appear to be a hereditary component to tooth number [7], and variation in tooth number is probably due to an interaction between genetic and environmental factors [8]. It has been suggested that no other human tissue shows the variation in developmental stages that is shown in the human diphyodont dentition [9]. It is also believed that over 300 genes may play a role in dental development [10, 11].

Individuals can have extra (supernumery) teeth, or missing teeth. Teeth can be missing for many reasons (e.g. caries and periodontal disease), but also may have never been present. Most commonly a person may have a single extra tooth, but some individuals may have several extra teeth, or very rarely multiple extra teeth.

Additional teeth can be associated with a number of syndromes, but most are extremely rare. Up to 20 syndromes have been reported as associated with missing teeth [12]. The most common syndromes associated with supernumery teeth are cleft lip and palate (Fig. 3.2), cleidocranial dysostosis, (Fig. 3.3) and Garners syndrome [13]. Oligodontia is also very rarely associated with syndromes (Fig. 3.4).

Supernumery teeth can also occur individually in various locations or as multiple supernumery teeth in several locations not associated with syndromes [14].

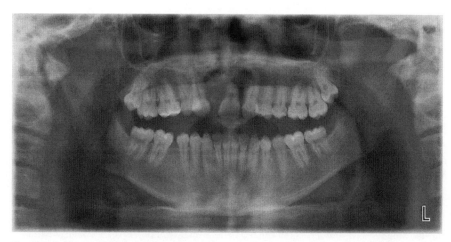

Fig. 3.2 Cleft lip and palate with missing teeth.

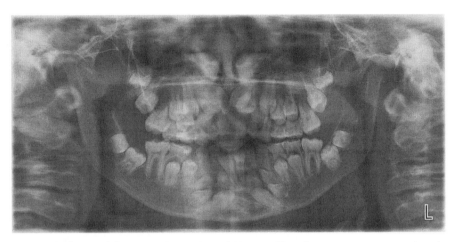

Fig. 3.3 Cleidocranial dysostosis. Patient is aged 12 years. Note the numerous unerupted teeth, including supernumery teeth, and retained deciduous teeth.

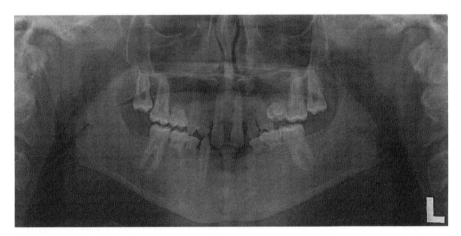

Fig. 3.4 Oligodontia.

The most commonly found supernumery teeth are maxillary midline supernumeries (mesiodens), maxillary fourth molars, maxillary paramolars, mandibular premolars, maxillary lateral incisors (Fig. 3.5), mandibular fourth molars, and maxillary premolars [15].

Supernumery teeth occur more in males than females in a ratio of 2:1 [16], and with an incidence of 0.1–3.2% [14].

Multiple supernumery teeth unassociated with syndromes are rare with few reports in the literature [17]. In cases where supernumerary teeth are observed single supernumeries have an incidence of 76–86%, while two supernumeries occur in 12–23% of cases. In less than 1% of cases where supernumery teeth are present are multiple supernumeries found (Fig. 3.1) [18].

Mesiodens (midline maxillary supernumery teeth) are the most commonly found additional teeth, with a prevalence of 0.15–1.9% (Fig. 3.6). There is

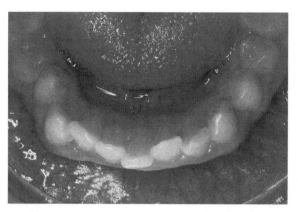

Fig. 3.5 Supernumery lower incisor.

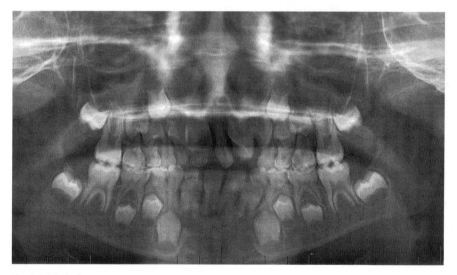

Fig. 3.6 Mesiodens.

also the suggestion that up to 30% of mesiodens may have a familial component [19]. The mesiodens may be found in a variety of positions: vertical,
inverted, transverse, and unerupted (Fig. 3.7) or erupted [20]. Mesiodens
may affect eruption of the incisors (Fig. 3.8a and 3.8b), resulting in their early
detection when the permanent incisors fail to erupt normally, but are often
detected as incidental findings on routine orthopantomogram (OPG) x-rays,
in older age groups. This is particularly so in OPGs taken for assessment of
orthodontic problems (Fig. 3.9) and for assessment of third molars, prior to
possible extraction.

Multiple mesiodens are not uncommon. While most mesiodens occur as individual teeth, occasionally there may be two or more. One study reported that
71.3% occurred as single teeth, and 0.22% of patients had four or more [21].

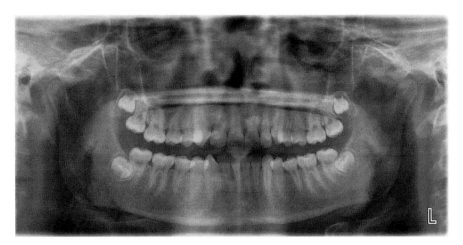

Fig. 3.7 Unerupted, inverted mesiodens.

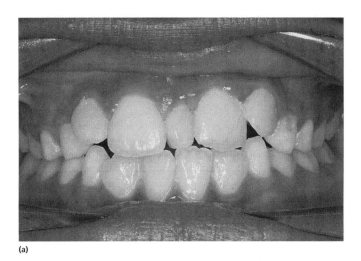

(a)

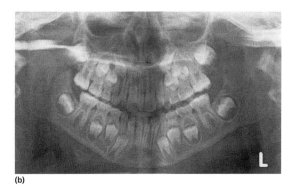

(b)

Fig. 3.8 (a) and (b) Erupted mesiodens (same patient).

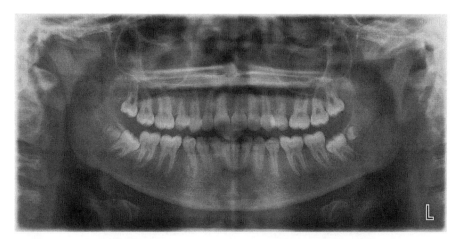

Fig. 3.9 Supernumery lower third molars.

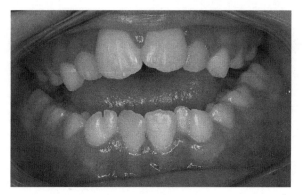

Fig. 3.10 Bilateral fused deciduous lower incisors, with missing lower lateral permanent incisors.

Hypodontia

As noted earlier, the most distal tooth in each morphogenetic field is the most likely tooth to be missing. In addition it is reported that hypodontia is also associated with a reduction in tooth size. Hypodontia is the most common dental developmental anomaly [22]. It has been classified according to severity by Dhanrajani [23], who regarded two to five missing teeth as mild to moderate hypodontia, with six or more teeth missing as severe hypodontia. Oligodontia with large numbers of teeth missing is usually associated with systemic disorders.

Hypodontia within the deciduous dentition is unusual with reported incidences of 0.1–1.5%. Importantly, hypodontia in the deciduous dentition is associated in 75% of cases with agenesis of the following permanent tooth [24]. The most common anomalies in deciduous dentitions are fused or geminated incisors (Fig. 3.10), and these are often associated with missing lateral permanent incisors (Fig. 3.11). In fact, apart from fused and geminated teeth, variation in

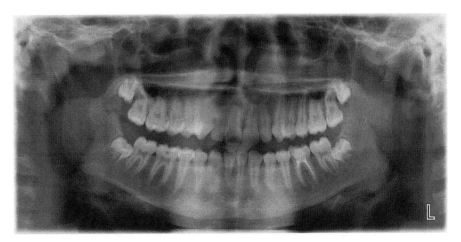

Fig. 3.11 Missing lower incisors.

the deciduous dentition is reported to be lower in prevalence in all aspects compared to the permanent dentition [14].

In the vast majority of cases, agenesis of teeth has a genetic basis. Teeth may of course also be missing as a result of trauma, infection or other dental intervention. There is also the suggestion that, in the last few decades, there has been an increase in the prevalence of missing teeth; however, the evidence is weak [25].

The overall incidence of hypodontia is estimated at 3.5–6.5%, with some variation in different populations. African Negroes and Australian Aborigines are estimated to have an incidence as low as 1%, but it is up to 30% in Japanese people [22]. The most common occurrence is a single missing tooth (80% of cases), a few missing teeth (10%) and multiple missing teeth (less than 1%).

In the permanent dentition, the most common missing teeth are third molars, followed by upper and lower second premolars, upper lateral incisors and lower central incisors [26]. Missing third molars are reported to be between 9–37% in some populations [25].

The most commonly impacted teeth are maxillary canines (Fig. 3.12), third molars and first molars. Impacted teeth are a variation of ectopic teeth, in that they have erupted, or tried to erupt in the wrong place. The incidence of impacted upper canines is very strongly associated with abnormalities of the upper lateral incisor (either agenesis or reduction in size), but also agenesis of the third molars and second premolars [27].

Transposed teeth are teeth within the same quadrant that have changed from their normal position. The most common transpositions are those of the upper canine and first premolar, as well as the lower lateral incisor and lower canine. The incidence is reported at less than 0.4% in one study and spread evenly between the sexes. Transposition in deciduous teeth has never been reported [28].

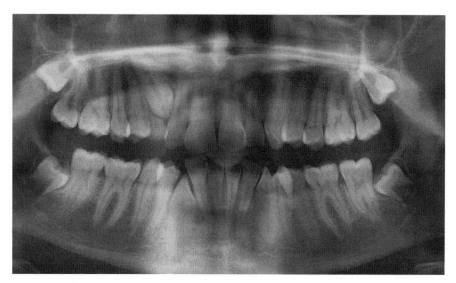

Fig. 3.12 Impacted canine.

Shape anomalies

Taurodontism is an anomaly of tooth shape first described in the early twentieth century. Witkop [29] defined it as 'teeth with large pulp chambers in which the bifurcation or trifurcation is displaced apically and hence that the pulp chamber has greater apico-occlusal height than in normal teeth and lacks the constriction at the level of the cement-enamel junction. The distance from the trifurcation or bifurcation of the root to the CEJ is greater than the occluso- cervical distance'. The mandibular second molar appears to be the most common tooth involved at a rate of 5.6% of individuals examined [30].

Peg lateral incisors

The overall prevalence of peg-shaped maxillary lateral incisors is about 1.8%, approximately 1 in 55 persons [31], with higher rates in Mongoloid (3.1%) than in white (1.3%) populations. Females had a slightly higher prevalence than males, and unilateral and bilateral occurrence was close to the same in both males and females. However, it was noted that among unilateral incidences, some left-sided predisposition existed [31].

Carabelli cusps, as first described by Carabelli in 1842, can vary from a fold on the palatal surface of maxillary molars to a full cusp [32]. They are most commonly seen in people of European extraction.

The most common anomalies seen by dentists are missing and extra teeth, with variations in the position and shape of the teeth adding complexity (Fig. 3.13). The forensic odontologist can use all these variations in dental structure to identify individuals with certainty. We rely on good ante-mortem records, and despite constant recommendations to improve the quality and retention of

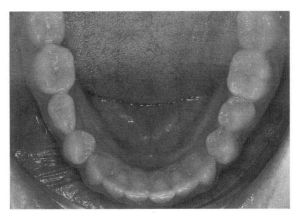

Fig. 3.13 Misshaped lower second premolars.

these records, there are times when the information is inadequate or missing. The skill of the forensic odontologist is not only in interpreting these records, but knowing where else to look for additional information.

Recent research supports the use of dental morphology in identification [33]. Further research may quantify techniques that are more specific and sensitive.

General head and neck anatomy

Temporomandibular joint (TMJ)

Broadly classified as a modified synovial hinge joint, the temporomandibular joint is located between the condyle of the mandible and the mandibular fossa of the temporal bone [34]. The temporomandibular joints collectively contribute as bilateral components of the craniomandibular articulation and are most stable when the teeth are in occlusion [35].

The temporomandibular joint is encapsulated by a synovial capsule, which is described as a thin, slack cuff of collagen fibres. While the capsule does not hinder the movements of the mandible, it is too weak to offer any significant support to the joint [35]. Internally it is attached to the articular disc and lined by a synovial membrane, which secretes synovial fluid for the overall lubrication of the joint [35]. The capsule is strengthened by the lateral temporomandibular ligament, which provides the main form of support to the joint, restricting backward and inferior movements of the mandible and resisting dislocation during functional movements [35]. Additionally, accessory ligaments of the TMJ include the sphenomandibular and stylomandibular ligaments as well as the pterygomandibular raphe. However, the sphenomandibular ligament (a remnant of Meckel's cartilage) is the only accessory ligament thought to provide any support.

In general the TMJ is richly innervated through contributions from auriculotemporal, masseteric and deep temporal nerves of the mandibular division of the trigeminal nerve. The superficial temporal and maxillary arteries, both terminal branches of the external carotid artery, provide blood supply to the joint [34, 35]. The three major sets of movements associated with the temporomandibular joint and facilitated by the muscles of mastication include: elevation and depression (opening/closing), side-to-side (grinding) and protraction/retraction movements [34]. Depression is facilitated by the digastric, mylohyoid and geniohyoid muscles, while the infrahyoid muscles act as stabilisers. Elevation is facilitated by the masseters, medial pterygoids and temporalis muscles. Side-to-side movements are aided by the medial and lateral pterygoid muscles, while protraction is assisted by all four pterygoid muscles.

Infratemporal fossa

Located deep to the ramus of the mandible and antero-medial to the temporo-mandibular joint, the infratemporal fossa communicates with the temporal fossa deep to the zygomatic arch and pterygopalatine fossa through the pterygomaxillary fissure [35]. Major structures associated with this fossa include the lateral and medial pterygoid muscles, branches of the mandibular nerve (including the inferior alveolar, buccal and lingual nerves), the chorda tympani branch of the facial nerve, the otic ganglion, the maxillary artery and the pterygoid venous plexus [34, 35].

Pterygopalatine fossa

Located deep to the pterygomaxillary fissure, the pterygopalatine fossa contains three major structures: the maxillary nerve, the maxillary artery (third part) and the pterygopalatine parasympathetic ganglion [35]. The ganglion transmits branches through to the nose, palate and nasopharynx [34]. The maxillary nerve provides innervation to the posterior, maxillary teeth and passes anteriorly into the orbit. Branches of the maxillary vessels accompany all the nerves [34].

The maxillary nerve first transmits a meningeal branch to the middle cranial fossa before passing through the foramen rotundum into the pterygopalatine fossa. Deviating laterally within the infra-orbital fissure, the nerve passes through the groove and then canal in the floor of the orbit to become the infra-orbital nerve. The zygomatic nerve, a branch of the maxillary nerve, runs above the maxillary nerve to enter the orbit. The posterior superior alveolar nerve also branches off in the fossa. The maxillary nerve is connected to the pterygopalatine ganglion by two branches [34].

The pterygopalatine ganglion is broadly considered to be a relay station between the superior salivatory nucleus, the lacrimal gland and the mucous as well as the serous glands of the palate, nose and paranasal sinuses. The autonomic root to the ganglion is the nerve of the pterygoid canal, formed by contributions from the greater petrosal nerve (branch of the facial nerve) and the deep petrosal nerve (branch of the internal carotid sympathetic plexus) [34]. Postganglionic secretomotor fibres destined for the lacrimal gland join the maxillary nerve, passing in its zygomatic branch en route into the orbit where it joins the lacrimal branch of the ophthalmic nerve [36]. Additional branches of the ganglion include: the medial posterior superior nasal nerves (distributed to the nasal septum), lateral posterior superior nasal nerves, greater palatine nerve (distributed to the anterior 2/3 of bony hard palate, postero-inferior part of lateral wall of nose and medial wall of maxillary sinus), lesser palatine nerve (distributed to the posterior 1/3 of bony hard palate, soft palate), pharyngeal nerve (mucous membrane of the nasopharynx) and some orbital branches [34].

Mandibular nerve

Following its emergence through foramen ovale, the mandibular nerve after a short course divides into a small anterior and a larger posterior branch. Branches from the main trunk of the mandibular nerve include the meningeal branch, which re-enters the middle cranial fossa via either the foramen ovale or spinosum, and the nerve to the medial pterygoid, which gives off a branch passing through the otic ganglion supplying the tensor palatini and tensor tympani muscles [34].

Branches from the anterior trunk of the mandibular nerve, which provide motor innervations, include: two deep temporal branches, the masseteric nerve (gives off a branch innervating the TMJ) and the nerve to lateral pterygoid. The buccal nerve is the only nerve from the anterior trunk that is considered to be sensory in nature [34]. In contrast the branches from the posterior trunk are mainly sensory with the exception of the motor fibres distributed via the mylo-hyoid nerve. These branches include the auriculotemporal nerve, the inferior alveolar nerve and the lingual nerve. Additionally, the chorda tympani branch of the facial nerve joins the lingual nerve, where both nerves provide sensory innervation to the anterior two-thirds of the tongue [34].

Wedged between the tensor palatine muscle and the mandibular nerve just below foramen ovale, the otic ganglion serves as a relay station for parasympathetic secretomotor fibres to the parotid gland. The lesser petrosal branch of the glossopharyngeal nerve brings fibres to the ganglion [34].

Salivary glands

The three major salivary glands associated with the head and neck region include the parotid, submandibular and sublingual glands. The parotid gland is the largest of the three and is located in a region between the ramus of the mandible and the mastoid process [35]. Pyramidal in shape, the gland extends beyond the gonial angle, with the deep surface resting on the ramus of the mandible and masseter muscle and extending beyond the posterior border of the ramus to reach the pharynx [35]. Additionally, emerging from the anterior border is the parotid duct, which in its course pierces the buccinator muscle and opens opposite the second maxillary molar tooth within the oral cavity.

Structures that are found within the substance of the parotid gland include the external carotid artery, retromandibular veins and facial nerve. The lymphatic drainage of the parotid gland is directed to the parotid lymph nodes. The parasympathetic innervation of the gland is from the lesser petrosal branch of the glossopharyngeal nerve.

Located within the submandibular triangle of the neck, the superficial part of the submandibular gland is clearly visible around the inferior border of the mandible. The deeper part of the submandibular gland curls around the posterior border of the mylohyoid muscle. The submandibular duct emerges from the deep part of the gland, wrapping itself around the lingual nerve in its course to terminate on the sublingual papilla in the floor of the mouth [35].

The sublingual gland is the smallest of the three and is located on the hyoglossal muscle in the floor of the mouth. The sublingual gland is divided into anterior and posterior parts with the ducts of the anterior part uniting to form a main duct. The main sublingual duct may either join the submandibular duct or drain directly on to the sublingual papilla. The parasympathetic innervation of both the submandibular and sublingual glands is the chorda tympani branch of the facial nerve [35].

Oral cavity

As the various components of the oral cavity have been covered in some detail in various subsections of this chapter, the tongue will serve as the focus of this section. Comprised of both intrinsic and extrinsic muscles, the tongue serves as the main content of the oral cavity proper.

The intrinsic muscles of the tongue are largely restricted to the substance of the tongue and change its overall shape. These muscles are composed of the transverse (narrower/wider), longitudinal (shorter/thicker) and vertical (thinner/wider) muscle fibre groups. Conversely the extrinsic muscles arise outside the tongue and are largely responsible for the bodily movement of the tongue. They include the genioglossus (protraction and depression), hyoglossus (depression), styloglossus (retraction) and palatoglossus (elevation) muscles.

The overall motor innervation of the tongue is provided by the hypoglossal nerve, which innervates all the extrinsic muscles of the tongue with the exception of the palatoglossus muscle. This muscle is innervated by the cranial part of the accessory nerve through its contribution to the pharyngeal plexus. The sensory innervation is subdivided into general (temperature) and special (taste) sensation. To complicate things further the tongue is subdivided into an anterior two-thirds and a posterior one-third by the sulcus terminalis. The general and special sensation of the posterior third is provided by the glossopharyngeal nerve. The special sensory innervation of the anterior two thirds is provided by the chorda tympani nerve, while the general sensory innervation is provided by the lingual nerve, a branch of the mandibular division of trigeminal. Additionally, the main source of blood supply to the tongue is the lingual artery, a branch of the external carotid artery.

Blood supply and lymphatic drainage of the orodental tissues

Lymphatics of the lower part of the face, as well as the mandibular incisors, is directed to the submandibular lymph nodes via the buccal lymph node groups. The medial portion of the lower lip is directed to the submental groups, while the teeth usually run into the submandibular lymph node groups of the corresponding sides.

Lymphatics from the labial and buccal gingivae of the maxillary and mandibular dentition drain into the submandibular nodes. The lingual and palatal gingivae drain into the jugulodigastric nodes either directly or indirectly via the submandibular nodes. Lymphatics from most areas of the palate as well as the floor of the mouth terminate in the jugulodigastric group of nodes. The soft palate lymphatics drain into the pharyngeal lymph node groups.

The anterior two-thirds of the tongue is somewhat complicated in its overall drainage scheme. The marginal lymph vessels drain the lateral third of the dorsum of the tongue and lateral margin of its ventral surface and these then drain into the submandibular lymph nodes on the corresponding side [35]. The remaining regions drain into the central vessels. The central vessels at the tip of the tongue drain into the submental lymph nodes. Central vessels behind the tip drain into ipsilateral and contralateral submandibular lymph nodes. Lymphatics from the posterior third drain into the deep cervical lymph node groups [35].

General blood supply to the head and neck regions are summarised in Table 3.1 [34, 35].

Osteology of the juvenile and adult craniofacial complex

The general configuration of the craniofacial complex includes the skull, which is subdivided into the cranium and the mandible. The cranium includes the calvaria (neurocranium) and the facial skeleton (viscerocranium). The calvaria comprises the calotte (desmocranium) as the roof and the basicranium as the base [36–38]. The basicranium may also be known as the chondrocranium because of the cartilaginous nature of this region during the earlier stages of cranial growth and development [38].

Neurocranium

The calotte and basicranium, as major contributors to the neurocranial complex, play a significant role in the overall protection and housing of the brain and its associated structures [37]. The anatomy of the calotte is relatively simple, with significant contributions arising anteriorly and laterally from the frontal and parietal bones respectively. The frontal and parietal bones are separated anteriorly by the coronal suture, while the two parietal bones are separated along the sagittal plane by the sagittal suture (Fig. 3.14). The sagittal and coronal sutures

Table 3.1 Summary of the general blood supply to the head and neck regions.

Main artery	Branches	Region supplied
• Common carotid	• Internal carotid • External carotid	• Intracranial supply • Extracranial supply

• External carotid
  (terminal branches)
• Anterior branches
	• Maxillary
	• Superficial temporal
	• Superior thyroid
	• Lingual
	• Facial
		• Superficial and deep
		  structures of the face
		• Superior pole of the
		  thyroid gland
		• Tongue
		• Face

• Posterior branches	• Occipital • Posterior auricular	• Posterior scalp and occipital region • Posterior auricle and ear

• Medial branches
• Maxillary artery first part
  (lateral to lateral pterygoid
  muscle)
	• Ascending pharyngeal
	• Inferior alveolar
	• Middle meningeal
	• Accessory meningeal
	• Deep auricular
	• Anterior tympanic
		• Pharynx

• Second part (Adjacent to
  lateral pterygoid muscle)
	• Artery to pterygoid muscles
	• Master artery
	• Deep temporal artery
	• Buccal artery
		• Supply mainly muscular
		  in nature

• Third part (after the lateral
  pterygoid muscle within
  the pterygomaxillary fossa)
	• Infra-orbital
	• Sphenopalatine
	• Posterior superior alveolar
	• Greater palatine
	• Pharyngeal	

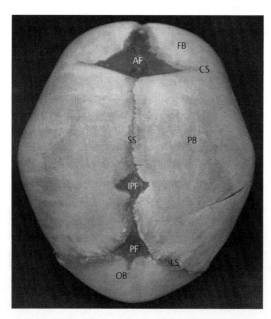

Fig. 3.14 Superior view of the juvenile calotte (FB: frontal bone; PB: parietal bone; OB: occipital bone; CS: coronal suture; SS: sagittal suture; LS: lambdoid suture; AF: anterior fontanelle; IPF: interparietal foramen; PF: posterior fontanelle).

meet at a diamond-shaped antero-medial junction called the anterior fontanelle, which following its closure in juveniles between one and two years of postnatal growth, is known as the bregma (Fig. 3.14).

Additionally the occipital bone, specifically the pars interparietalis, makes a minor posterior contribution to the calotte and is separated from the left and right parietal bones by the coronally oriented lambdoid suture. The lambdoid suture bisects the coronal suture at the triangular-shaped postero-medial junction called the posterior fontanelle which, following its closure just prior to three months of postnatal growth, is then known as the lambda (Fig. 3.14).

Along the infero-lateral border of the calotte on either side of the skull two additional fontanelles are observed. The first fontanelle is the antero-laterally oriented sphenoidal fontanelle, which is located at the junction of the frontal, parietal, temporal and sphenoid bones. Following its closure at six months of postnatal growth, the region associated with this fontanelle is known as pterion (Fig. 3.15). Pterion in the juvenile and adult skull not only marks the junction of these four bones but also the location of the underlying middle meningeal artery. This is clinically significant in cases of depression fractures of this region as the pterion is a weak point in the overall architecture of the skull. The second fontanelle to mark the division between the calotte and basicranium is the postero-lateral mastoid fontanelle and usually closes between 6 and 18 months of postnatal growth (Fig. 3.15).

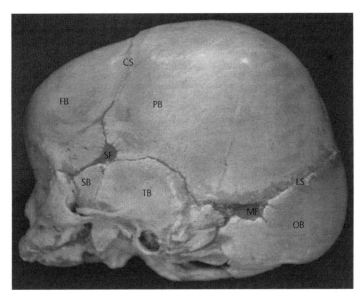

Fig. 3.15 Lateral view of a juvenile cranium indicating the neurocranium components (FB: frontal bone; CS: coronal suture; PB: parietal bone; LS: lambdoid suture; OB: occipital bone; MF: mastoid foramen/postero-lateral fontanelle; TB: temporal bone; SB: sphenoid bone; SF: sphenoid fontanelle/antero-lateral fontanelle).

In contrast to the relatively simple configuration of the calotte, the anatomy of the basicranium is far more complex. The complexity of this area may be attributed to the admixture of intramembranous and endochondral ossification. The general configuration of the basicranium includes contributions along the midline from the occipital bone (juvenile pars basilaris and pars squama) posteriorly and sphenoid bone (juvenile pre-sphenoid and post-sphenoid) anteriorly. Lateral and additional posterior contributions to the basicranium include the temporal bone (juvenile pars tympani, pars petrosa and pars squama), sphenoid bone (greater and lesser wings) and the occipal bone (juvenile pars lateralis) respectively.

Frontal bone

The frontal bone is a major component of the anterior cranial fossa. The overall shape of this bone is described as irregular with a general bowl-shape configuration [39]. This may be attributed to the frontal bone consisting of a squamous portion, which is largely associated with and cradles the frontal lobe of the developing brain, and an orbital plate that contributes to the roof of the bony orbit.

The primary ossification centre of each half of the frontal bone first appears at the junction between the squamous portion of the bone and the anterior portion of the orbital plate, alternatively known as the supercilliary arch. Ossification then spreads as a network of radiating trabeculae, with the squamous portion of the frontal bone progressing faster than the orbital plate region. This initial progression in the ossification of the frontal bone, which is usually completed during week 13 of gestation, only accounts for the part of the supercilliary arch located medial to the future supra-orbital notch [39]. The lateral two-thirds of the arch as well as the infero-lateral zygomatic process commence their development later during the period between 10 and 12 gestational weeks. Additionally the lateral part of the superciliary arch will separate the bony orbital cavity from the temporal fossa and will complete the lateral border of the bony orbit initially. The process of formation of the lateral component of the supercilliary arch also leads to the formation of the linea temporalis and a fissure for the attachment of the membrane of the sphenoidal fontanelle.

In general, the frontal bone is recognisable by 13 gestational weeks of growth. The basic appearance of the frontal bone at this stage of development closely resembles a fragile, dome-shaped bone with the overall antero-posterior length exceeding the medial-lateral width. The anterior edge of the frontal bone is somewhat thickened at the junction between the orbital plate and squamous portion, thus marking the position of the supra-orbital notch or foramen [39]. At this stage of the frontal bone's development, the orbital plate is exceptionally thin in nature. At the conclusion of week 20 of gestation the development of the antero-posterior length of the frontal bone exceeds its lateral width and as such the frontal bone is somewhat slender in its general appearance.

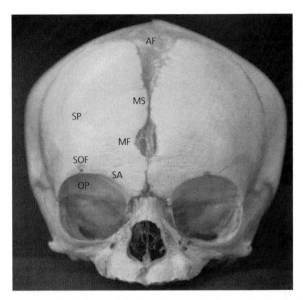

Fig. 3.16 Anterior view of the left and right frontal bones (AF: anterior fontanelle;
MS: metopic suture; MF: metopic foramen; SA: supercilliary arch; SOF: supra-orbital foramen;
OP: orbital plate; SP: squamous portion).

During the last two months of prenatal life, the frontal bone is more substantial in its general appearance. The infero-medial angle of the bone, ultimately forming the adult glabella region, is transversely striated and from this point the medial border is smooth in appearance for a short distance. Additionally, at a location approximately halfway between the frontal eminence (pointed region on the anterior surface) and the medial border of the frontal bone, there may be the occurrence of the metopic foramen. The metopic foramen is continuous with the medial border of the frontal bone by means of a groove or slit in the bone. When both halves of the frontal bone are viewed in situ, this area marks the site of the metopic fontanelle [39] (Fig. 3.16). Continuing with the medial border in a postero-superior direction, the medial edge of the frontal bone adopts a finely serrated appearance and it slopes away laterally to form the anterior margin of the anterior fontanelle (Fig. 3.16).

The coronal margin of the frontal bone, which is essentially a continuation of the medial border, is also observed to have a serrated appearance. This serrated appearance persists along the entire border as far as the lateral edge of the supra-orbital ridge. At this particular junction of the frontal bone, the bone is somewhat thickened for articulation with the zygomatic bone. It presents as an elongated triangular region easily distinguished by the appearance of a groove, whose apex points in a posterior direction (Fig. 3.17). The lateral edge of the supra-orbital margin is sharp, while the medial third of the ridge is smooth, which is also observed in the adult bone [39].

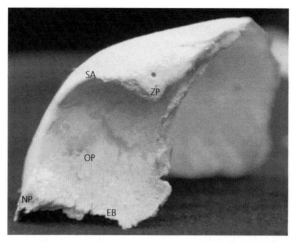

Fig. 3.17 Inferior view of the left frontal bone orbital plate indicating the groove associated with the zygomatic process (ZP: zygomatic process; SA: supercilliary arch; OP: orbital plate; EB: ethmoid border; NP: nasal process).

Postnatally, both the thickened articulations for the maxilla and the nasal bones as well as undulations in the orbital plate become obvious. At birth the frontal bone is composed of two symmetrical halves that are separated by the metopic suture (Fig. 3.16). The metopic suture is broadly considered a constant feature in fetuses and newborns [40]. It is located along the median line of the face and extends from the nasion (anteriorly) to the anterior angle of the anterior fontanelle or alternatively the bregma (postero-superiorly). Closure of the suture usually commences towards the end of the first year of life. In most instances complete closure of the suture is observed at the end of the fourth year of life [40]. However the metopic suture may persist well into adulthood (sutura metopica persistens) as metopism. The frequency of metopism in adults varies between 0–13% and is thought to be influenced by geographical proximity [40]. While the persistence of the metopic suture poses no clinical significance [37], there is evidence to suggest that hypoplasia of the frontal sinuses occurs in more than 50% of individuals presenting with metopism [40].

The frontal sinuses commence development during foetal life either as a mucosal invagination at the anterior end of the middle nasal meatus or from the anterior ethmoidal cells [39]. However pneumatisation of the sinus only commences during the postnatal period of growth, with expansion of the sinuses commencing at approximately 3.5 years of age [39] and while adult dimensions are reached by puberty, growth may persist until approximately 24 years of age [40]. In the adult frontal bone, the sinuses are described as a pneumatic cavity located within the squamous part of the frontal bone and open into the lateral wall of the nasal cavity by means of the ethmoidal infundibulum.

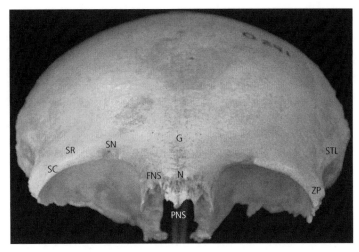

Fig. 3.18 Anterior view of the adult frontal bone (SC: supra-orbital crest; SR: supra-orbital ridge; SN: supra-orbital notch/foramen; FNS: frontonasal suture; PNS: posterior nasal spine; N: nasion; G: glabella; ZP: zygomatic process; STL: superior temporal line).

Following the complete closure of the metopic suture, the frontal bone presents as a single bone dominating the anterior view of the adult skull. Located along the median plane of the frontal bone, essentially the meeting point of the left and right supra-orbital ridges, is the glabella. The glabella is described as the most anterior projecting point in the midline of the forehead at the level of the supra-orbital ridges just superior to the frontonasal suture [41] (Fig. 3.18). The frontonasal suture marks the junction between the frontal bone and the nasal bones. This suture also contributes to the bridge of the nose and, together with the two nasal bones protruding inferiorly from it, is particularly vulnerable to blunt force trauma often resulting in fractures of this region [37]. Located just inferior to the glabella at the junction of the frontonasal suture and the midsagittal plane is the nasion. In addition to its location the nasion is the most superior landmark for the measure of facial height [41] (Fig. 3.18).

Additionally, located along the medial aspect of the inferior border of the supra-orbital ridge is the supra-orbital notch (or foramen if complete). The supra-orbital notch gives passage to the supra-orbital nerve (a branch of the ophthalmic nerve) and at times may be completed by the ossification of a ligament crossing the inferior border of the notch [37]. The supra-orbital region of the frontal bone also serves in the estimation of an individual's sex, owing to its prominence and distinction in males, while the supra-orbital margin/crest is sharp in females and blunt in males [41]. Furthermore, located at the most medial point on the incurve of the superior temporal ridge, just above the zygomaticofrontal suture (junction between the zygomatic and frontal bones) is the frontotemporale point [41] (Fig. 3.18).

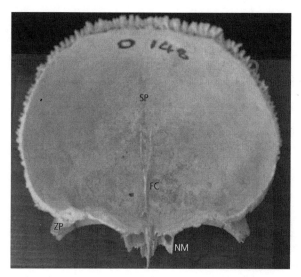

Fig. 3.19 Posterior view of the adult frontal bone (SP: squamous part; FC: frontal crest; NM: nasal margin; ZP: zygomatic process).

The internal surface of the adult frontal bone has an unremarkable morphology. Located along the median plane of the internal surface, the frontal crest arises and anchors the falx cerebri (layer of the dura mater associated with the left and right cerebral hemispheres) (Fig. 3.19). Situated just inferior to the frontal crest is the foramen caecum [37], which transmits the emissary veins of the superior sagittal sinus.

Parietal bone

The parietal bones serve as a dominant feature of the calotte, wedged between the anterior frontal bone and posterior occipital bone. The parietal bones articulate laterally with the squamous part of the respective temporal bones and are separated along the midline of the calotte by the sagittal suture. The highest point of the skull, the vertex, may be located within this region [37, 41]. The external surface of each parietal bone is convex in shape while the concave internal surface cradles the parietal lobe of each cerebral hemisphere [37].

The parietal bones develop by means of intramembranous ossification from two centres originating near the parietal tuberosities [38]. These centres are observed to rapidly unite and ossification gradually progresses in a radial manner towards the outer margins of each bone [38]. During week 20 of gestation, the development of the parietal eminence on the most lateral aspect of the bone commences at the location where the two ossification centres have met [42]. At the conclusion of this week, the parietal bone appears as a delicate, ellipsoidal membranous disc with a thickened central eminence and a radiating fine network of trabeculae emerging from the central eminence [39].

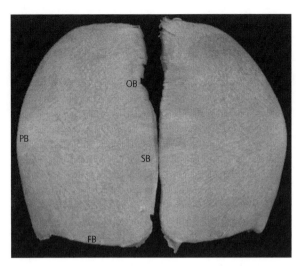

Fig. 3.20 Superior view of the juvenile parietal bones (OB: obelion; SB: sagittal border; FB: frontal border; PE: parietal eminence).

During week 24 of gestation, the individual borders and margins of the parietal bone begin to straighten and the angles assume their characteristic shapes [39]. The frontal border is slightly concave with finely serrated edging and reaches its conclusion at the sphenoidal angle, which is directed acutely anteriorly [39]. The sagittal border of the parietal bone runs directly posterior from the rounded frontal angle for approximately two-thirds of its length where it reaches the obelion (Fig. 3.20). The obelion marks the point along the sagittal border of the parietal bone where a parietal notch may occur. Proceeding posteriorly from this point, the serrations in the sagittal border assume a fringe-like appearance as the border slopes away towards the rounded occipital angle at the posterior fontanelle [39]. The occipital border is also finely serrated and one or two slits in the border do commonly occur. The inferior border of the parietal bone is the squamosal border, which is divided into two sections. These include a posterior blunt portion and an anterior curved portion, accommodating the mastoid and squamous portions of the temporal bone respectively [39].

During the period of 24 gestational weeks to birth, the parietal bone increases in size. At the site of the parietal notch, in the region of the obelion, the occurrence of either a fissure (incisura), small parietal fontanelle or parietal foramina of varying sizes has been documented. Additionally notches on either side of the sagittal suture, usually in the area of the obelion, may enlarge to form a sagittal fontanelle (third fontanelle or fontanelle oblique) [39]. The incidence of the sagittal fontanelle is between 50 and 80% in skulls at birth and has been shown to have a higher incidence in Down's syndrome cases and other abnormalities [39]. In general the sagittal fontanelle and associated fissures disappear shortly before or at birth, but in rare cases may persist until as late as nine months of life [39].

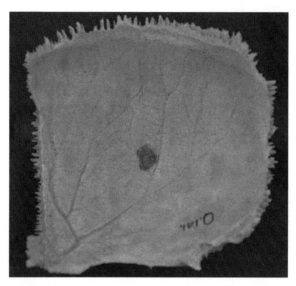

Fig. 3.21 Internal surface of an adult parietal bone indicating the impressions created by the middle meningeal artery.

The adult parietal bone is roughly quadrangular in shape with a protruding lateral surface and a concave internal surface. There are also small perforations along the surface of the bone, particularly in the region of the sagittal suture [37], which transmit emissary veins from the superior sagittal sinus to the scalp. On the external surface there are two parallel curved ridges, namely the superior and inferior temporal lines, which serve as attachment sites for the superior border of the temporalis muscle and its associated fascia [37]. Additionally, impressions for the branches of the middle meningeal artery may be observed along the internal surface of the bone (Fig. 3.21). In the overall estimation of sex, the female skull is more gracile, smaller and smoother when compared to males [41]. Furthermore, it has a tendency to retain the childhood characteristics of frontal and parietal bossing, which is not retained in males [41].

Occipital bone

The occipital bone contributes to the posterior and the middle cranial fossa. During the prenatal development of the occipital bone, four main components may be distinguished namely, the pars squama, left and right pars lateralis and the pars basilaris (Fig. 3.22).

The prenatal pars squama is subdivided into two components, the pars interparietalis superiorly and the pars supra-occipitalis inferiorly (Fig. 3.22) [43, 44]. The pars inter-parietalis develops by means of intramembranous ossification, while the pars supra-occipitalis develops by means of endochondral ossification [39, 44]. However, there is some debate as to the method of ossification in the

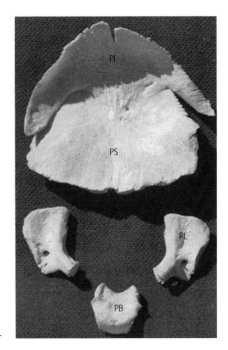

Fig. 3.22 Sub-components of the occipital bone complex. Pars squama (PI: pars interparietalis; PS: pars supra-occipitalis) (above), PL: pars lateralis (middle) and PB: pars basilaris (below).

area located between the highest nuchal line and the superior nuchal line, termed the torus occipitalis transversus [45, 46].

The overall morphological arrangement of the supra-occipitalis consists of a central component flanked by left and right segments [47]. The central segment is separated from the left and right segments by vertical sutures, which extend from the inter-parietal-supra-occipital suture (separating the membranous inter-parietal and cartilaginous supra-occipital components) to the posterior margin of the foramen magnum [47]. The central component forms more than half of the posterior margin of the foramen magnum [47]. Additionally, in the membranous space extending from the centre of the squamous portion to the posterior margin of the foramen magnum, a spicule of bone, that is the process of Kerckring, has been identified [39, 47]. One hypothesis surrounding the origin of this process is that it arises as an overgrowth of periosteal bone from the pars inter-parietalis [39].

The left and right segments of the supra-occipitalis are incompletely divided into upper and lower divisions by a superior horizontal suture located at the level of the inferior nuchal line [47]. The lateral segments of the supra-occipitalis articulate with the inferior angle of the parietal bone and the mastoid part of the temporal bone laterally, the central segment medially, the inter-parietal bone superiorly and the pars lateralis of the occipital bone inferiorly at the inferior horizontal suture [47].

At the commencement of the fifth month of development, all the membranous ossification centres associated with the pars inter-parietalis appear to have fused

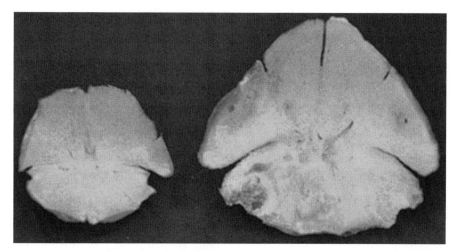

Fig. 3.23 Pars squama of the occipital bone indicating the degree of curling in the borders of the bone and fusion of the pars interparietalis and pars supra-occipitalis.

and a trabecular meshwork is in place covering the external surface of the pars squama [48]. A fan-shaped bone results from the ossification of the secondary centres as well as the appearance of a distinct border along the internal surface of the primary inter-parietal bone [48]. Additionally, in the midline, the root of the inter-parietal bone has grown to reach and fuse with the bony trabeculae that cover the internal surface of the supra-occipital bone [48]. At the conclusion of the sixth month of development the inter-parietal part of the pars squama consists of many radiating trabeculae, and the border between the primary and secondary parts is still visible on the internal surface [48] (Fig. 3.23). Additionally, the supra-occipital part of the pars squama appears as a solid bony plate with roughened surfaces, resulting from the migration of the inter-parietal trabecular meshwork along the internal and external surfaces of the pars squama [39, 43]. At this stage of foetal development, the structural integrity of the pars inter-parietalis, and to a lesser degree the supra-occipitalis, is exceptionally fragile (Fig. 3.23). This is particularly evident within a forensic setting where the edges of the bone are observed to 'curl or fold inwardly', following the maceration of cadaveric tissues and further preparation of the associated skeletal elements. The curling of the squamous edges is indicative of a lower degree of ossification, with the degree of curling serving as an indication of the advancement of ossification. Additionally it is found to be less prominent in the area of the supra-occipitalis and in skeletal elements in more advanced stages of ossification.

As the general pattern of ossification of the pars inter-parietalis is postulated to be highly variable, the incidence of variations is inevitable [39]. The most common variant is the occurrence of the os inca otherwise commonly referred to as the os inter-parietale or os wormian [48]. It is thought that the inca bone arises as a result of the multiple ossification centres of the inter-parietal

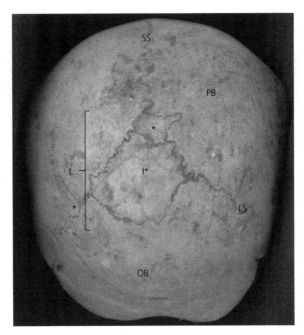

Fig. 3.24 Occurrence of inca bones in the occipital region of the calotte (SS: sagittal suture; PB: parietal bone; LS: lambdoid suture; OB: occipital bone; L: lambda; I*: inca bones along the lambdoid suture).

bone failing to fuse, ultimately resulting in one of several varieties of the inca bone [48]. These varieties range from a single separate inca bone to multiple bones located within the lambdoid region and usually closely associated with the lambdoid suture [46, 49]. The inca bone usually presents as a triangular bone separated from the remainder of the pars inter-parietalis by a transverse suture or the mendosal suture (incomplete suture separating the pars interparietalis and pars squama) (Fig. 3.24) [48, 50, 51]. Some studies describe the morphology of the inca bone commonly presenting as elongated with the rare occurrence of a rounded shape [50]. There have also been suggestions of an increased incidence of inca bones in individuals presenting with craniosynostosis and other cranial developmental abnormalities [51].

The general spread of ossification associated with the pars lateralis leads to the formation of flattened quadrilateral plates [39], which may be oriented by placing the long axes in an antero-posterior configuration (Fig. 3.25). Due to the orientation of the quadrilateral plates the wedge-shaped posterior border of the plate will lie adjacent to the pars supra-occipitalis, the thickened medial border will form the lateral border of the foramen magnum and the lateral border of the plate will form the inferior border of the mastoid fontanelle (Fig. 3.25). Additionally, the general appearance of the quadrilateral plates in foetuses between 20 and 30 gestational weeks may be confused with the blade of the scapula.

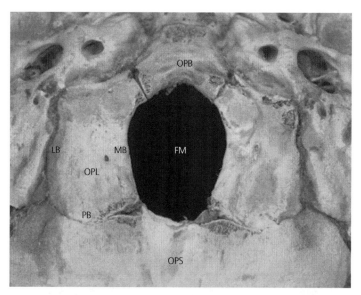

Fig. 3.25 Pars lateralis of the occipital bone in situ (OPB: pars basilaris; FM: foramen magnum; OPS: pars squama; MB: medial border; PB: posterior border; LB: lateral border; OPL: pars lateralis).

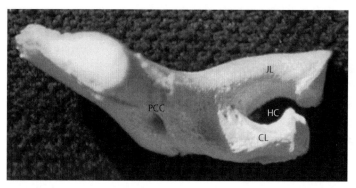

Fig. 3.26 Medial surface view of the pars lateralis indicating the incomplete hypoglossal canal and associated condylar and jugular limbs (JL: jugular limb; HC: hypoglossal canal; CL: condylar limb; PCC: posterior condylar canal).

In neonates the lateral border of the quadrilateral plate extends antero-laterally to form the occipital border of the jugular foramen. During the first postnatal year, the bone located immediately posterior to the jugular foramen may extend laterally to form the quadrangular-shaped jugular process [39]. Furthermore a second bony extension, the condylar limb, is observed as the anterior extension of the medial border. Both the jugular and condylar limbs contribute significantly to the formation of the hypoglossal canal (Fig. 3.26) [39]. The condylar limb through its inferior orientation houses the occipital condyle, and contributes to the posterior two-thirds of the adult occipital condyle. Located

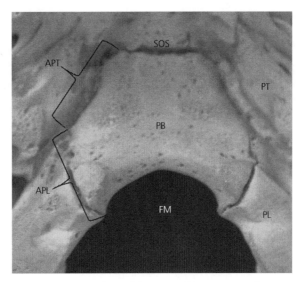

Fig. 3.27 Inferior view of the pars basilaris of the occipital bone (SOS: spheno-occipital synchondrosis; PT: petrous part of temporal bone; PL: pars lateralis; FM: foramen magnum; PB: pars basilaris; APT: articulation for petrous temporal bone; APL: articulation for pars lateralis).

just posterior to the occipital condyle on the condylar limb, the posterior condylar canal may be observed during early foetal development (Fig. 3.26). Additionally, the condylar limb of the pars lateralis develops a hook-like extension during the first three years of postnatal growth. This hook-like protuberance extends superiorly to meet with the jugular limb, thus completing the hypoglossal canal [39]. During the prenatal stages of the hypoglossal canal's development, both the condylar limb and the jugular limb are closely associated with the pars basilaris through articulation on reciprocal surfaces located along the posterior border of the pars basilaris.

The fourth and most anterior component of the occipital bone is the pars basilaris or basiocciput. Originating from the exoccipital cartilages of the cranial base, the basiocciput commences its ossification during the twelfth week of development [39, 52]. The basiocciput is recognisable from the third prenatal month as a spindle-shaped bone, but by the fourth month is more triangular in shape [39]. The base of the basiocciput forms the majority of the anterior border of the foramen magnum (Fig. 3.27). In the earlier stages of the basiocciput's development the base is 'v'-shaped. Over a two-week period this shape will soften and assume a u-shaped appearance [39]. As the base changes shape the articulation points for the jugular and condylar limbs of the pars lateralis become more pronounced, particularly along the inferior surface of the bone (Fig. 3.27) [39]. During a two-week period, the sides of the basiocciput assume a parallel orientation and in turn the bone adopts a more quadrangular shape. At seven months of development, as the lateral margins expand and in turn become more angulated at the midpoint of the bone, the pars basilaris will assume a trapezoidal shape [39]. One of the more common philosophies used in ageing the pars basilaris based on its shape, and states that if the width is less than the sagittal length, then the individual is less than 28 weeks of development and vice versa [53].

In contrast to the prenatal pars basilaris, the postnatal equivalent is far more robust. The inferior surface is flattened, while the intracranial surface assumes a slightly more concave appearance extending along the longitudinal axis of the bone. The intracranial surface presents with numerous nutrient foramina giving this surface a more pitted appearance [39]. Additionally, the inferior surface of the pars basilaris has an anteriorly located pharyngeal tubercle for the attachment of the posterior pharyngeal raphe [39]. This tubercle is usually only identified from about the second year of life [39]. Located immediately anterior to the pharyngeal tubercle is the fossa pharyngea [39]. This fossa may also be referred to as the fovea bursa and is thought to close during the third prenatal month [39]. Additionally, located along the inferior surface of the clivus or body, a median occipital condyle may be present [54, 55]. The incidence of this process is relatively rare with a 14% occurrence rate.

The anterior border of the pars basilaris forms the posterior surface of the spheno-occipital synchrondrosis. This surface of the pars basilaris is identified in the early postnatal stages of development by its 'D'-shape appearance, with the straight edge being associated with the intracranial surface of the pars basilaris. Furthermore a transverse supplementary fissure associated with the anterior border is sometimes present and may present as either complete or incomplete [56]. In cases where the transverse supplementary fissure is complete there is usually the presence of an independent ossicle named the basioticum (or anterior centrum) of the basi-occipital [56]. Other anomalies associated with this area of the occipital bone in particular may include hypoplasia of the basiocciput or persistence of the spheno-occipital synchondroses [56].

In contrast, the base or posterior border of the pars basilaris is thickened and forms a semi-lunar curve, with each of the horns contributing the final third to each of the occipital condyles located inferiorly [39]. The posterior border will reach adult size at about two years of age. The lateral border of the pars basilaris at this stage of foetal development is subdivided into two parts, roughly identified at the point where the horns of the base extend laterally midway along the body/clivus. The anterior component articulates with the petrous part of the temporal bone (Fig. 3.27) [39]. The posterior component is identified by two distinct facets for the articulation of the jugular and condylar limbs of the pars lateralis (Fig. 3.28) [39].

The adult occipital bone is morphologically distinct and associated with both the occipital lobes of the cerebral hemispheres as well as the cerebellum. The internal surface of the squamous part of the occipital bone is concave in appearance with a centrally located protuberance: the internal occipital protuberance (Fig. 3.29). The internal occipital protuberance is considered to be a significant

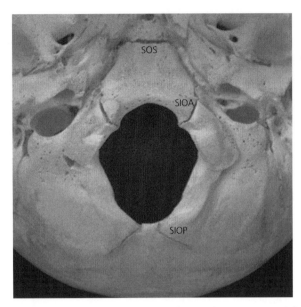

Fig. 3.28 Fusion points of the pars lateralis, pars basilaris and pars squama of the occipital bone (SOS: spheno-occipital synchondrosis; SIOA: sutura intra-occipitalis anterior; SIOP: suture intra-occipitalis posterior).

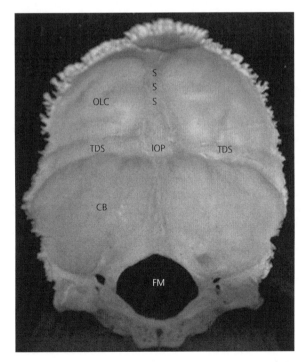

Fig. 3.29 Internal surface of the adult occipital bone (SSS: superior sagittal sinus impression; TDS: transverse dural venous sinus impression; IOP: internal occipital protuberance; FM: foramen magnum; CB: cerebellum impression; OLC: occipital lobe cerebrum impression).

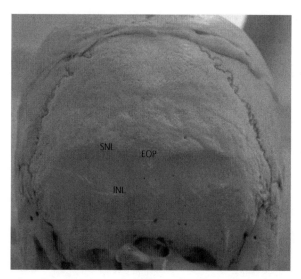

Fig. 3.30 External surface of the adult occipital bone (EOP: external occipital protuberance; SNL: superior nuchal line; INL: inferior nuchal line).

junction not only as it demarcates the meeting point of the superior sagittal, straight and transverse dural venous sinuses at the confluence of sinuses, but it also serves as an attachment site for the tentorium cerebelli (Fig. 3.29). This layer of dura mater marks the division between the occipital lobes of the cerebrum and the cerebellar hemispheres.

The external occipital protuberance, which corresponds with the positioning of the internal occipital protuberance, may be described as a bony point marking the attachment site of the nuchal ligament of the head and neck region (Fig. 3.30) [37]. Incidentally, it also marks the point of the inion, described as a point at the base of the external occipital protuberance [41]. The external occipital protuberance also marks the level of the superior nuchal line, which along with the inferior nuchal line serve as attachment points for muscles of the head, neck and back regions (Fig. 3.30) [37]. The opisthocranion, which is the most posterior point on the skull and is often confused with the external occipital protuberance, is a floating point used in the overall assessment of the maximum cranial length in conjunction with the glabella [41].

Furthermore, the foramen magnum which is found at the epicentre of the squamous, lateral and basal parts of the occipital bone, serves as the site for a number of anthropological landmarks. These include the opisthion, basion and endobasion. The opisthion is a landmark located at the midpoint of the posterior margin of the foramen magnum, while the basion is a landmark located at the midpoint of the anterior margin of the foramen magnum [41]. Additionally, the basion is the most distant point from the bregma and is used in the measure of the height of the skull. The endobasion is the most posterior point of the anterior border of foramen magnum and is placed internal to the basion [41].

Temporal bone

The temporal bone significantly contributes to the middle cranial fossa as well as the lateral walls and base of the skull [37]. The temporal bone may be subdivided into four, namely the petromastoid, squamous, tympanic and styloid components (Fig. 3.31).

The petromastoid component of the temporal bone may be further subdivided into the petrous and the mastoid parts. The petrous part occupies the lateral aspect of the cranial base between the greater wing and body of the sphenoid bone and the basiocciput [39]. Additionally, it is the primary location for the inner and middle ear cavities and their associated structures. The mastoid portion is located posterior to the external auditory meatus, articulating with both the squamous part of the occipital bone and the parietal bone [39].

During week 20 of gestation, the petrous part of the temporal bone is first recognised, and within a forensic context is the most durable and easily retained component. It's described as irregular in shape with the retention of the rounded anterior cochlear end and a more expanded canalicular end, both first identified in the otic capsule [39]. As the petrous part is largely associated with structures of the auditory apparatus, the internal acoustic meatus may be identified along its medial surface (Fig. 3.32). Located just posterior to the internal acoustic meatus is the subarcuate fossa, which is large and wide [39]. Superior to the subarcuate fossa, the exposed curves of the anterior and posterior semi-circular canals lie at right angles to each other (Fig. 3.32).

The superior surface of the petrous part is smooth in appearance and serves as the location for the facial foramen (passage of the facial nerve into the tympanic cavity) [39]. Located just inferior to this, the lateral surface of the petrous part forms the irregular medial wall of the future middle ear cavity. The oval

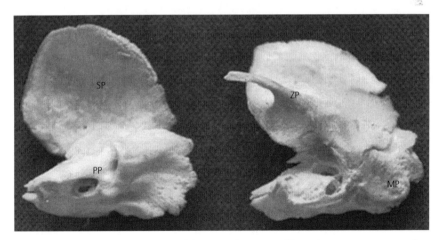

Fig. 3.31 Internal and external views of the juvenile temporal bone (SP: squamous part of temporal bone; PP: petrous part; MP: mastoid part; ZP: zygomatic process).

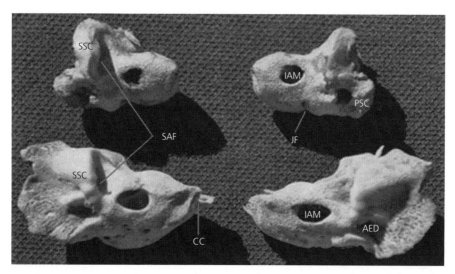

Fig. 3.32 Internal and external views of the petrous part of the temporal bone (SSC: superior semi-circular canal; SAF: sub-arcuate fossa; CC: carotid canal; IAM: internal auditory meatus; PSC: posterior semi-circular canal; JF: jugular fossa; AED: Aperture for endolymphatic duct).

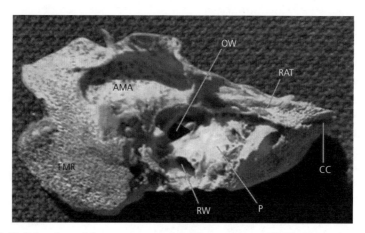

Fig. 3.33 Medial surface of the petrous part of the temporal bone (AMA: aditus to mastoid antrum; EMR: expanded mastoid region; OW: oval window; RW: round window; P: promontory; RAT: roof of auditory tube; CC: carotid canal).

window of the inner ear cavity is located in the middle of the lateral surface (Fig. 3.33). Just superior to the oval window is a minute aperture leading to a groove, the partially formed facial canal, which bends postero-inferiorly over the oval window. The fossula of the fenestra cochlea is located just postero-inferior to the oval window and is best identified by the presence of the posterior facing round window of the inner ear cavity (Fig. 3.33) [39].

The inferior surface of the petrous part of the temporal bone is slightly grooved anteriorly for the passage of the internal carotid artery. However, during the early stages of growth, the carotid canal is not yet formed. Posterior to the groove for the internal carotid artery is the smooth jugular part of the bone. The last regions of the canalicular part of the petrous part to ossify are the posterior and lateral canals and the lateral aspect of the superior canal. This is because they continue to grow for some time after the rest of the internal ear has reached maximum size [39]. This whole area of the canalicular part of the petrous temporal bone will spread in a posterior direction towards the future mastoid part of the bone.

During the period of 20 gestational weeks to birth, the ossification of most of the extra-capsular areas of the petrous bone takes place by extension from the outer periosteal layer of the capsule. The facial foramen during this time will be enclosed by a plate of bone which is continued laterally as the tegmen tympani (thin plate of bone covering the middle ear). The tegmen tympani is thought to ossify during week 23 of gestation and contributes largely to the roof of the middle ear, antrum and part of the wall of the auditory tube [39].

The canal for the facial nerve arises by extension from the otic capsule. Initially the facial nerve appears to lie in a groove on the lateral wall of the canalicular part of the capsule. During week 26 of gestation, the facial nerve in conjunction with the stapedius muscle and associated vasculature are partially enclosed in a bony sulcus [39]. The facial canal under normal circumstances is observed to close during the first year of life. However, in cases where the membranous bone fails to close completely, this leads to dehiscence (splitting/incomplete closure) of the facial nerve canal in approximately 25% of cases, which persists throughout life [57].

Additionally, between the oval and round windows of the lateral surface of the petrous part of the temporal bone, the promontory (bony protuberance), related to the basal turn of the cochlea, forms a bulge in the lateral wall. The inferior edge of the lateral surface also forms a semilunar ledge, which in time will serve to support the inferior parts of the tympanic ring [39]. During the period between 24 and 29 gestational weeks, a further petrosal ledge known as the jugular plate extends laterally and contributes significantly to the floor of the middle ear cavity.

During the period of 30 gestational weeks to birth, the subarcuate fossa and internal auditory meatus are observed to be equal in size, with the aperture for the endolymphatic duct located just inferior to them [39]. Furthermore, the extracapsular parts of the petrous temporal bone expand further and a tongue-like extension of bone is observed to curve inferiorly from the anterior part of the semilunar ledge to form the entrance of the carotid canal. The developing jugular fossa and the expanding mastoid process are located just posterior to this. The mastoid process will only develop fully after birth [37] and with the assumption of an upright sitting position. During this period the development of the main tympanic cavity is complete. The epitympanum, which is defined as the superior space leading posteriorly to the mastoid antrum and anteriorly to

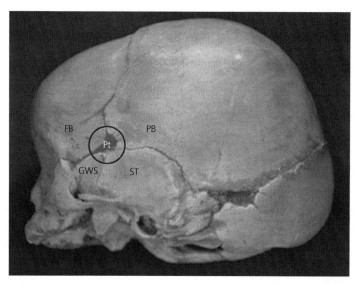

Fig. 3.34 Lateral view of the juvenile skull indicating the location of the pterion (Pt), a shared junction between the frontal bone (FB), parietal bone (PB), squamous part of the temporal bone (ST) and the greater wing of the sphenoid bone (GWS).

the double canal for the auditory tube and tensor tympani muscle, has completed its development [39]. The pneumatisation of the extracapsular parts of the petrous temporal bone begin. This process is effectively accelerated only after birth when the amniotic fluid of the middle ear cavity is replaced by air and may continue throughout infancy and early childhood. Effectively there are three principal groups of air cells associated with the petrous temporal bone, which are formed during prenatal development and continue to grow postnatally until puberty. The air cells include those opening into the mastoid antrum, the main auditory cavity and those associated with the auditory tube [39].

The squamous component of the temporal bone (pars squama) forms part of the lateral wall of both the cranial cavity and the middle ear and is closely associated with the pterion (Fig. 3.34) [39, 52]. The pars squama is described as a thin, narrow, plate-like bone located just lateral to the upper parts of the malleus and incus. It is shortened along its vertical axis (supero-inferiorly) and serrated both posteriorly and anteriorly. Within a forensic setting this component of the temporal bone is subject to a high degree of damage.

During week 20 of gestation, the pars squama is usually recognisable with the assumption of more adult proportions and is described as a delicate, almost flat semi-circular plate with finely serrated edges. One of the more identifiable features of the bone is the zygomatic process (Fig. 3.35). This process projects anteriorly from a thickened root below which is a small curved plate that will become the mandibular fossa (Fig. 3.35). The zygomatic process is far more durable within a forensic context. Located just postero-inferior to the root of the zygomatic

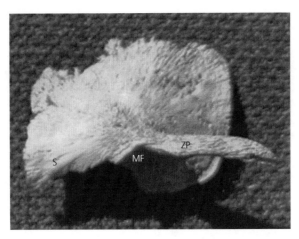

Fig. 3.35 Lateral surface of the juvenile squamous part of the temporal bone (S: scutum; MF: mandibular fossa; ZP: zygomatic process).

process is the scutum (a protective covering or shield), a triangular extension with a sharp inferior angle that later becomes pneumatised (Fig. 3.35). On the medial surface, the scutum is delineated superiorly by a ledge of bone that fuses with the tegmen tympani of the petrous temporal bone postnatally [39].

The tympanic part of the temporal bone, located immediately inferior to the squamous component and anterior to the mastoid part of the temporal bones, may be described as a quadrilateral plate [39]. The external acoustic meatus that accommodates the tympanic membrane is formed by the posterior part of the temporal bone's tympanic division. Projecting antero-inferiorly from the tympanic plate is the styloid process of the temporal bone.

The primary ossification centre of the tympanic ring is observed near the malleus with a series of secondary ossification centres following [57]. The appearance of the secondary ossification centres effectively establish the c-shape of the ring, with the anterior limb of the developing annulus more developed than the posterior limb (Fig. 3.36). Furthermore as the tympanic cavity is expanding during this time medial to the ring, there is an excavation of the ectodermal plate to establish the external auditory canal. Effectively the tympanic ring will continue to grow until week 35 of gestation when its adult diameter is reached. As the tympanic ring is never closed along its superior axis, this opening gives rise to the incisura tympanica where the pars flaccida of the tympanic membrane is thought to attach in adults [57]. During this advanced stage of prenatal growth, the tympanic bone commences its attachment to the adjacent squamous plate in the postero-lateral segment of the tympanic bone [57].

At the 20th gestational week, the tympanic ring is recognisable in isolation. It is deficient at the superiorly oriented tympanic incisure, which is effectively framed by the anterior and posterior horns of the ring. The anterior horn of the ring is considered to be more morphologically distinct than its posterior

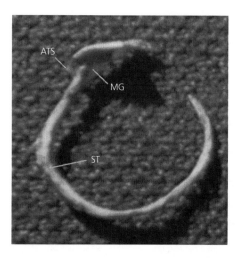

Fig. 3.36 Perinatal tympanic ring indicating the anterior tympanic spine (ATS), mallear gutter (MG) and sulcus tympanicus (ST).

counterpart. Medially just inferior to the larger anterior horn is a transverse groove, the mallear gutter, which ultimately accommodates the anterior process of the malleus [39]. Located just superior to the mallear gutter is the crista spinarum, a sharp ridge delineating the mallear gutter and whose respective ends form the anterior and posterior tympanic spines. The inferior, inner end of the mallear gutter protrudes as the anterior tympanic tubercle (Fig. 3.36). The posterior tympanic tubercle may be located approximately halfway along the posterior limb of the tympanic ring.

The inner surface of the tympanic ring is grooved by the sulcus tympanicus, a structure delineating the attachment of the tympanic membrane (Fig. 3.36). At the commencement of the 35th gestational week, the tympanic ring has attained almost full adult dimensions. There is a localised fusion of the posterior segment of the ring to the squamous part of the bone. At term, the ring is slightly more robust and usually fusion with the squamous part of the tympanic bone has taken place at the open end of the ring. The anterior horn attaches postero-inferiorly to the root of the zygomatic process, while the posterior horn fuses with the pointed end of the scutum [39]. The fusion of the tympanic ring to the squamous part of the temporal bone effectively forms the lateral wall of the tympanic cavity [57]. There is a small protuberance observed in the anterior ring which forms the superior boundary of the inter chordae anterius (where the tympanic ring attaches to the squamous temporal bone). This landmark may be observed throughout life [57]. During the period of 35 gestational weeks to birth, it is possible to look through the ring into the tympanic cavity of a dry skull and observe the auditory ossicles and associated round and oval windows (Fig. 3.37).

The ossification centre for the base of the styloid process appears in the perinatal period of growth. Appearance of subsequent ossification centres for the main part of the styloid process occurs during the third and fourth years of life [57].

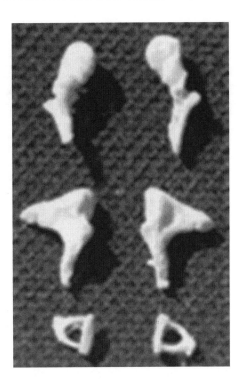

Fig. 3.37 Bony ear ossicles of the middle ear cavity, which include the malleus (above), incus (middle) and stapes (below).

The postnatal growth of the temporal bone essentially encompasses the fusion of the squamotympanic and petromastoid parts of the temporal bone along various segments. First, the bony ledge on the medial surface of the pars squama fuses with the reciprocal ledge of the tegmen tympani at the internal petrosquamous suture. Through this fusion the scutum will effectively become the lateral wall of the epitympanic recess of the middle ear. Subsequently during this time the scutum also becomes increasingly pneumatised.

The second event in the fusion sequence occurs when the external petrosquamous (squamomastoid) suture is formed by the fusion of the posterior border of the squamous part fusing with the mastoid section of the temporal bone [39]. This particular suture may persist well into adulthood. Gradually the squamous part of the temporal bone extends inferiorly and, in so doing, covers the anterior part of the petromastoid and contributes to the rapidly growing mastoid process [39]. The mastoid process will, during this time, gain momentum in its growth through the assumption of an upright sitting position placing strain on the sternocleidomastoid attachment site [37]. Additionally the lower part of the tympanic ring fuses with the semilunar ledge at the lower border of the tympanic cavity.

The first year of life encompasses the anterior and posterior tympanic tubercles enlarging and growing towards each other across the ring. The eventual fusion of the two tubercles creates a second opening, the foramen of Huschke, located immediately below the main auditory meatus (Fig. 3.38) [39].

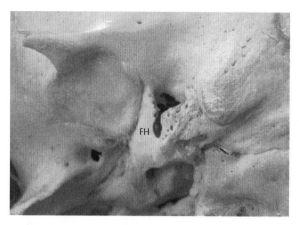

Fig. 3.38 Infero-lateral view of the foramen of Huschke.

During the same period, the tympanic plate grows laterally, thus gradually converting the ring into the bony external auditory meatus. Subsequently fingers of bone are observed to grow inward from the edges of the foramen of Huschke, resulting in its closure by roughly five years of age [39].

Additionally, as the bony meatus grows laterally, further displacing the tympanic ring from the external osseous opening, it will result in considerable change in the overall orientation of the tympanic membrane. At birth the tympanic membrane adopts a horizontal orientation with the growth of the external auditory meatus; the membrane adopts a more vertical disposition by approximately the fourth or fifth years of life [39]. The growth of the tympanic plate also extends posteriorly and inferiorly to enclose the base of the styloid process in its vaginal sheath. It also extends a tongue of bone to enclose the anterior border of the carotid canal, which will eventually fuse with the petrous base, but may still be viewed as late as puberty. On the inferior surface of the petrous temporal bone an edge of the tegmen tympani protrudes between the growing tympanic plate and the glenoid fossa, dividing the squamotympanic fissure into a petrotympanic part posteriorly and a petrosquamous part anteriorly.

The foetal components of the temporal bone persist into adulthood. Two notable features of the squamous part include the zygomatic process and the supramastoid crest [37]. The supramastoid crest is fairly obvious in males but insipid in females. Located just posterior to the zygomatic process are two prominences separated by the mandibular fossa. The anterior prominence is the tubercle of the root of the zygoma, which provides attachment for the lateral ligament of the temporomandibular joint and the posterior prominence provides a buttress against which the head of the mandible rests [37].

Located immediately posterior to the mandibular fossa is the tympanic plate [37]. Additionally the porion, a landmark used in anthropometric assessments, is located on the uppermost lateral point in the margin of the external auditory meatus [41]. Originating immediately posterior to the tympanic plate is the slender styloid process, which extends in an anterior and inferior direction and is of variable length. In the adult temporal bone, the styloid process provides attachment to two ligaments (stylohyoid and stylomandibular ligaments) and three muscles (styloglossus, stylopharyngeus and stylohyoid) [37].

The mastoid part of the temporal bone, characterised by a stout inferior projection, is separated from the tympanic annulus (ring surrounding the external auditory meatus) by the tympanomastoid fissure. The tympanomastoid fissure carries the sensory auricular branch of the vagus nerve which innervates the pinna and skin of the external auditory canal [37]. The mastoid process in adults contains air cells that are connected to the middle ear. As the mastoid process is underdeveloped in the infant, the facial nerve is at risk of injury, considering the nerve emerges from the skull through the stylomastoid foramen. Additionally, the anthropological point, the mastoidale, may be located as the lowest point on the mastoid process [41].

The petrous part of the temporal bone is mainly associated with the medial aspect of the cranial base and on its superior surface has a sharp ridge extending the length of the bone [37]. The tentorium cerebelli, a horizontally oriented layer of dura mater separating the cerebral from the cerebellar hemispheres, is attached to the ridge forming the cover for the posterior cranial fossa. Anterior to the ridge the irregular bony surface of the petrous temporal bone has one prominent protuberance, the arcuate eminence beneath which is the epitympanic recess of the middle ear [37].

Sphenoid bone

The sphenoid bone rests on the precipice between the neurocranium and the viscerocranium articulating with skeletal elements belonging to both areas. In general the sphenoid bone offers contributions to both the anterior and middle cranial fossae.

In general the body of the sphenoid bone ossifies by means of endochondral ossification. Two sets of centres are associated with the body, namely the anterior pre-sphenoid and the posterior post-sphenoid groups (Fig. 3.39) [52]. Fusion between the two sets of centres at the synchondrosis intrasphenoidalis takes

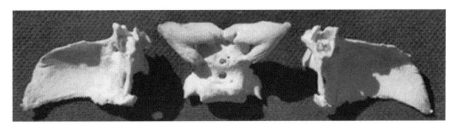

Fig. 3.39 Fused pre-sphenoid and post-sphenoid components of the central body alongside the left and right greater wing complexes of the sphenoid bone.

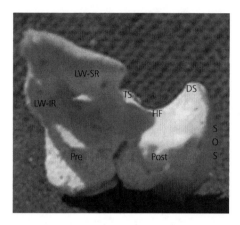

Fig. 3.40 Lateral view of the pre-sphenoid and post-sphenoid components of the central body of the sphenoid bone (LW-SR: lesser wing superior root; LW-IR: lesser wing inferior root; Pre: pre-sphenoid; Post: post-sphenoid; TS: tuberculum sellae; HF: hypophyseal fossa; DS: dorsum sellae; SOS: articular surface for the spheno-occipital synchondrosis).

place at the tuberculum sellae, which is the junction of the prechordal and chordal regions of the skull base (Fig. 3.40) [39].

The post-sphenoid part of the body is recognisable usually by 20 gestational weeks as a roughly quadrilateral shaped bone [39]. At this stage of development, the overall width of the post-sphenoid is twice the length, with two lateral alar projections extending in a postero-inferior direction. The centre of the superior surface appears concave along the antero-posterior axis forming a shallow hypo-physeal fossa from which the blunt alar processes extend in a lateral direction (Fig. 3.40) [39]. The anterior and posterior surfaces of the body may be divided by deep central fissures, indicating the dual origin of the associated ossification centres (Fig. 3.40). During the later stages of development, the alar processes become separated inferiorly from the main part of the body by the laterally oriented carotid sulcus. The alar processes develop anteriorly directed sharp projections, which articulate with the pre-sphenoid part of the body, and the posterior processes will ultimately form the lingulae [39].

During the 24th gestational week, the main pre-sphenoid centres have fused together to form the medial wall of the optic foramen. Formation of the interoptic region, which will become the jugum sphenoidale, is variable and may be formed either by extension of the pre-sphenoid centres or by formation of the median unpaired rostral centre [39]. This lower part of the body of the sphenoid will eventually form the crest, rostrum and ethmoid spine [39]. The anterior wall of the sella turcica presents at this stage of development as a cartilaginous structure and gradually ossifies in the last trimester by the posterior and medial growth of the pre-sphenoid centres. These extend from the superior to the inferior surface of the body, but may only be fully ossified by the end of the first year of life [39].

The pre-sphenoid part of the body may be described as an inverted 'y-shaped' bone with the main single stem facing anteriorly and the two limbs assuming a posterior orientation. The superior surface is relatively smooth while the infe-rior surface bears a blunt finger-like projection pointing antero-inferiorly (Fig. 3.41) [39]. The posterior limb has three main surfaces that include the

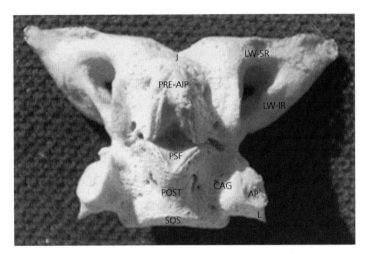

Fig. 3.41 Antero-inferior view of the sphenoid body and fused lesser wings (LW-SR: lesser wing superior root; LW-IR: lesser wing inferior root; J: jugum; PRE-AIP: pre-sphenoid antero-inferior projection; PSF: post-sphenoid fissure; POST: post-sphenoid; CAG: carotid artery groove; AP: alar projection; L: lingual; SOS: surface for the spheno-occipital synchondrosis).

supero-anterior and the supero-posterior surfaces, which are set at right angles and articulate with the lesser wings (Fig. 3.41). The third surface associated with each posterior limb is the infero-posterior surface, which is situated at a right angle and forms the upper boundaries of the cruciform space between the pre- and post-sphenoid parts of the body.

At the commencement of the 16th gestational week, the optic foramen is almost entirely surrounded by bone. There is a small linear process, described as the antero-inferior segment of the optic strut (posterior root/crus posterior), which extends from the lesser wing and fuses with the post-sphenoid centre of the body (Fig. 3.41). This fusion ultimately leads to the formation of the infero-lateral border of the optic foramen. At this stage of development the optic foramen assumes a keyhole shape, with the ophthalmic artery assuming occupancy of the narrow portion and the larger optic nerve being more superiorly oriented in the wider part of the keyhole. At 20 gestational weeks, the formation of the optic canal commences by means of the formation of a second or postero-superior strut, which joins the lesser wing to the pre-sphenoid centre of the body [39]. During this period of development, the ophthalmic artery migrates superiorly above the second strut and is incorporated into the dural sheath of the optic nerve. This effectively results in the optic strut, for a short period of time, being composed of two segments enclosing a transitory foramen between them, which on its closure forms the cranial opening of the optic canal [39].

During the 20th gestational week, the lesser wing of the sphenoid bone is recognisable as a small flat piece of bone adopting the shape of an arrow head with the tip of the wing pointing laterally (Fig. 3.42). The superior root/anterior crus is somewhat flatter and wider in presentation when compared to the inferior root/posterior crus of the lesser wing. During the later stages of development, the distinction between the two roots of the lesser wing is more obvious, with the superior root developing a posteromedial projection, which articulates with the pre-sphenoid part of the body (Fig. 3.42) [39].

The greater wings of the sphenoid bone are derived by means of both intramembranous and endochondral ossification [38,39,52]. The foramen rotundum is only considered complete once the laterally located centre for intramembranous ossification and the medially located centres of endochondral ossification associated with the greater wing have united (Fig. 3.43) [39].

The margins of the foramen ovale are largely represented by a medial process and a lateral tongue of bone, which fuse behind the mandibular division of the trigeminal nerve. The fusion of the medial process and lateral tongue of bone may

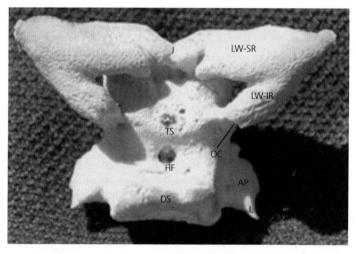

Fig. 3.42 Superior view of the lesser wings and body of the sphenoid bone (J: jugum; LW-SR: lesser wing superior root; LW-IR: lesser wing inferior root; TS: tuberculum sellae; HF: hypophyseal fossa; DS: dorsum sellae; OC: optic canal; AP: alar process; L: lingula).

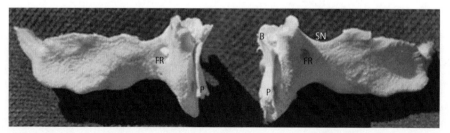

Fig. 3.43 Anterior view of the greater wings of the sphenoid bone (SN: semi-circular notch; FR: foramen rotundum; B: articulation point for the body; P: pterygoid plates).

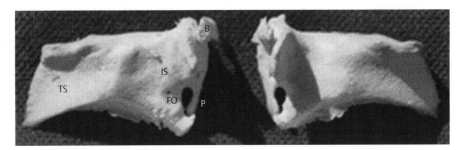

Fig. 3.44 Inferior view of the greater wings of the sphenoid bone indicating the incomplete foramen ovale (FO) and its association with the pterygoid plates (P) and body articulation point (B) (TS: temporal surface; IS: inferior surface).

take place either late in foetal life or may be delayed until the first year of postnatal life. However there are instances where fusion may never take place and the foramen remains open to the petrosphenoid suture [39]. The fusion of the posteriorly located foramen spinosum is usually complete by the second year of life

In general the morphology of the greater wings and pterygoid plates is recognisable during the 20th gestational week. The greater wing may be divided into a posteromedial third and an anterolateral two-thirds by a line running through the foramen rotundum anteriorly and a fissure running for a variable distance into the bone towards it from the posterior surface [39]. The medial surface of the greater wing is complex in nature as it provides for the attachment of the alar processes of the sphenoid body. The incomplete foramen ovale is observed on the posterior surface of the bone, where the foramen spinosum is also incomplete (Fig. 3.44). There are three surfaces associated with the lateral surface of the greater wing. The first surface is the anterior surface and is distinguished from the other surfaces as it takes on a thicker appearance and turns upwards at right angles to form part of the lateral wall of the bony orbit (Fig. 3.44). The superior border of the anterior surface just above the opening of the foramen rotundum forms a very distinct semilunar notch at the medial end of the superior orbital fissure (Fig. 3.44) [39]. This serves as an ideal landmark when the necessity arises to side the greater wing of the sphenoid bone (Fig. 3.44). In addition, the gently concave superior cranial surface, which is the second surface associated with the greater wing, tapers down towards the thin, serrated lateral and posterolateral borders (Fig. 3.45). In contrast to the slightly concave superior surface of the greater wing, the inferior surface adopts a reciprocal convex nature [39]. The lateral and medial pterygoid plates project inferiorly from the medial aspect of the inferior surface and have a tendency to be closer in proximity along the anterior axis of the surface than posteriorly (Fig. 3.45). In addition the lateral pterygoid plate extends slightly further in a posterior direction (Fig. 3.45).

Within a forensic context the components of the sphenoid bone maintain a high degree of structural integrity and are often among those osteological elements recovered in a relatively intact state. While the general appearance of the

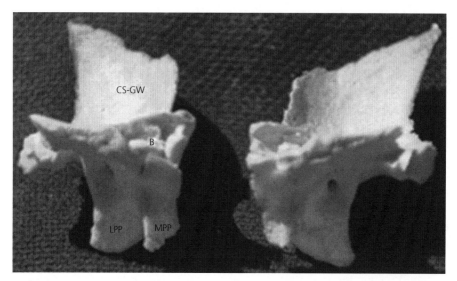

Fig. 3.45 Medial surface view of the left and right greater wings of the sphenoid bone complex (CS-GW: cranial surface or greater wing; B: articulation point for body; LPP: lateral pterygoid plate; MPP: medial pterygoid plate).

various components of the sphenoid bone appears to be relatively consistent and reliable in terms of timing, the general fusion sequence of these components is highly varied. The fusion sequence of the sphenoid bones may be tentatively summarised as follows from birth:

- At birth the sphenoid bone may be represented by three parts, namely the body with the attached lesser wings and two separate greater wings each with their attached pterygoid plates.
- Alternatively, at birth the fusion of the pre-sphenoid and post-sphenoid may be delayed resulting in the sphenoid presenting in five separate components namely, the lesser wing/pre-sphenoid combination, post-sphenoid and two separate greater wings with attached pterygoid plates.
- The third combination that may present at birth is found less commonly. This combination consists of the presphenoid bone fusing to the lesser wings and the post-sphenoid bone fusing with the greater wings, rendering the general appearance of the sphenoid bone as two major parts.

At the conclusion of the first year of life, all components of the sphenoid bone are consistently found to have fused, resulting in a single sphenoid bone complex.

During the perinatal period of growth, the jugum sphenoidale is undeveloped as the lesser wings are separated by a cleft, which will be filled with bone during the first year of life. The general antero-posterior growth of the jugum is found to be variable in nature and is reflected in the reciprocity of the widths of the jugum and sulcus [39]. The posterior margin of the jugum, otherwise known as the limbus sphenoidale, may remain separate from the underlying pre-sphenoid for a variable number of years leaving a cleft between them. Under normal circumstances the two structures, namely the limbus sphenoidale and the pre-sphenoid, have fused by adulthood.

The pneumatisation of the sphenoid sinus is usually observed during the sixth month of life and is found to be an extension of the nasal cavity into the conchal area, which spreads into the pre-sphenoid part of the sphenoid body [39]. The pneumatisation of the sphenoid sinus may spread into the basisphenoid by 4 years of age and with further occurrences in 50% of individuals aged 8 years and 90% of individuals aged 12 years. The dosum sellae and posterior clinoid processes have been found to be pneumatised in approximately 20% of individuals aged between 12 and 20 years. During this progression of pneumatisation, the sphenoidal conchae gradually attach to the ethmoid bone by means of resorption of the intervening cartilage, effectively anchoring the sphenoid complex to the ethmoidal complex. The time of this fusion is characteristic of the sphenoid bone and may vary between 4 years of age and as late as puberty.

The adult anatomy of the sphenoid bone is somewhat simpler. In isolation the adult sphenoid bone closely resembles the shape of a butterfly, with a central body and greater and lesser wings. Intracranially the lesser wings are joined centrally by the jugum which is continuous posteriorly with the tuberculum sellae (Fig. 3.46) [37]. Extending medially along the posterior border of the lesser wings is the anterior clinoid process (Fig. 3.46). Located just antero-inferior to the anterior clinoid processes is the opening for the optic canal that transmits the optic nerve and ophthalmic artery for each bony orbit.

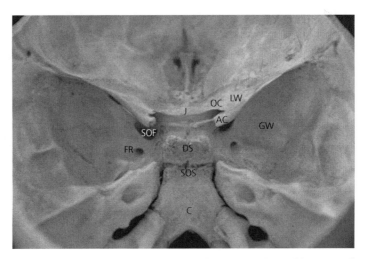

Fig. 3.46 Posterior view of the intracranial surface of the adult sphenoid bone complex (J: jugum; OC: optic canal; LW: lesser wing; GW: greater wing; AC: anterior clinoid process; SOF: supra-orbital fissure; FR: foramen rotundum; DS: dorsum sellae; SOS: spheno-occipital synchondrosis; C: clivus).

The greater wings of the sphenoid bone are clearly visible both intracranially and extracranially. Additionally, the greater wings of the sphenoid bone have a number of foramina associated which include [37]:

- Superior orbital fissure: located between the greater and lesser wings of the sphenoid bone and a dominant feature of the bony orbit. The SOF transmits the oculomotor nerve (CNIII), the trochlear nerve (CNIV), the abducent nerve (CNVI) and the ophthalmic divisions of the trigeminal nerve (CNV$_1$) as well as the superior and inferior ophthalmic veins.
- Foramen rotundum: associated with the greater wing, transmits the maxillary nerve (CNV$_2$).
- Foramen ovale: associated with the greater wing, transmits the mandibular nerve (CNV$_3$).
- Foramen spinosum: associated with the greater wing of the sphenoid bone, transmits the middle meningeal artery and the nervus spinosus.

Furthermore the medial and lateral pterygoid plates are seen as inferior extensions of the greater wings of the sphenoid bone. The pterygoid plates offer attachment to the medial and lateral pterygoid muscles as well as the cartilaginous part of the pharyngotympanic tube [37].

In addition the body of the sphenoid, while presenting as a solid structure, contains the sphenoid air sinuses that open into the spheno-ethmoidal recess of the nasal cavity. The intracranially oriented superior surface of the sphenoid body is hollow in shape as it accommodates the pituitary gland. The gland is covered superiorly by a layer of dura mater that spans the distance between the anterior and posterior clinoid processes. The anterior surface of the body articulates with the ethmoid bone of the nasal cavity as well as the vomer bone, while the posterior surface articulates with the clivus of the occipital bone at the spheno-occipital synchondrosis [37].

Viscerocranium

The second major division of the craniofacial complex is the viscerocranium. Three major apertures associated with this area include the centrally located nasal cavity, two bony orbits and the oral cavity.

Zygomatic bone

Considered a prominent feature of the cheek, the zygomatic bone is wedged between the frontal bone (superiorly), the maxilla (infero-medially) and the greater wing of the sphenoid bone (supero-medially) (Fig. 3.47). Posteriorly, the temporal process of the zygomatic bone articulates with the zygomatic process of the temporal bone. The articulation between these two bony points laterally forms the zygomatic arch and the lateral border of the infratemporal fossa (Fig. 3.47). The zygomatic bone also forms the lateral border of the bony orbit. In general the zygomatic bone is irregular in shape with three surfaces, two processes and five borders.

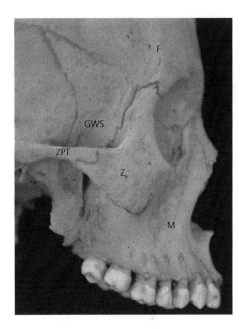

Fig. 3.47 Lateral view of the right zygomatic bone in situ (F: frontal bone; M: maxilla; Z: zygomatic bone; ZPT: zygomatic process of temporal bone; GWS: greater wing of sphenoid).

The bone initially appears as a triangular squama with the temporal process far more advanced in its development when compared to the frontal process. During the ninth gestational week, the zygomatic bone already resembles the adult bone, appearing as an inwardly curved quadrilateral with four angles [39]. The border between the cranial and ventral angles forms the part that will articulate with the maxilla. Additionally the development of the temporal process is more advanced at nine gestational weeks. However, it will not complete the zygomatic arch posteriorly until late into foetal life and in some instances only at birth.

At the beginning of the 20th gestational week, the zygomatic bone closely resembles its adult counterpart although its proportions are somewhat different (Fig. 3.48). In addition, the zygomatic bone is large and robust. Perinatally, the zygomatic bone is described as a gracile, tri-radiate bone with slender frontal, temporal and maxillary processes, projecting from a small curved body (Fig. 3.48) [39].

The three surfaces of the zygomatic bone have the same relationship to each other as observed in the adult bone but the borders vary owing to the small facial height. Along the inferior border of the zygomatic bone, approximately a third of the way from its medial end, there is a prominent notch, which marks the future angle between the antero-inferior and postero-inferior borders (Fig. 3.48) [39]. The postero-medial border just touches the frontal bone and then articulates with the greater wing of the sphenoid bone. There is a significant non-articular area below this point, which marks the area where the inferior orbital fissure is relatively large at this stage and the inferior part of the border articulates with the maxilla obliquely along the middle of the orbital floor (Fig. 3.49) [39].

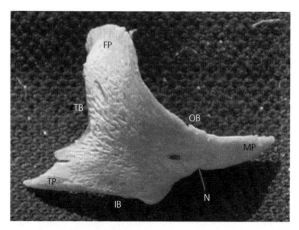

Fig. 3.48 Lateral view of a right zygomatic bone (FP: frontal process; MP: maxillary process; TP: temporal process; OB: orbital border; IB: inferior border; TB: temporal border; N: zygomatic notch).

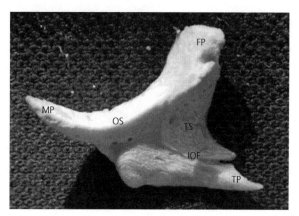

Fig. 3.49 Medial view of the right zygomatic bone (FP: frontal process; TP: temporal process; MP: maxillary process; OS: orbital surface; TS: temporal surface; IOF: inferior orbital fissure).

During infancy and childhood, the zygomatic bone's growth and development is inherently linked with that of the maxilla, with increases in height and width to accommodate the deciduous dentition. This causes a change in the position of the articulation between the maxilla and the angulation at the zygomatic notch on the inferior border. The infra-orbital zygomaticomaxillary suture changes position from the middle to the lateral side of the orbital floor, and the antero-inferior and postero-inferior borders become more defined. At the completion of the eruption of the deciduous dentition, the zygomatic bone has achieved its adult proportions. Both the tuberculum marginale and the eminentia orbitalis become palpable during the second or third years of life, and about the same time the ends of the frontal and temporal processes become serrated [39]. In addition to the previously discussed features of the zygomatic bone, there is also the occurrence of the zygomaticofacial foramen and canal located on the lateral surface of the bone. The zygomaticofacial canal normally contains the zygomaticofacial nerve [37]. The zygomatic bone within a forensic setting has a high recovery rate, which has been attributed to the general robusticity of the bone as early as the juvenile stages of growth.

Furthermore, the adult zygomatic arch extends anteriorly from the region of the temporomandibular joint, which is formed by the articulation of the zygomatic process of the temporal bone and temporal process of the zygomatic bone. As the arch forms the lateral border of the infratemporal fossa, the temporalis muscle contained within the fossa passes medial to the zygomatic arch [37]. The general contour of the arch is normally smooth, but as the arch is a protruding feature of the viscerocranium, it is subject to damage by blunt force trauma to the cheek. Subsequently trauma to the arch may result in fractures of the arch and force fragments of bone medially into the temporalis muscle resulting in trismus [37]. Additionally, trauma in the form of fractures to this region may result in displacement of the bone leading to orbital haematoma as well as diplopia (double vision) [37].

In a forensic context the anthropological landmarks associated with the zygomatic bone, include the zygion and ectoconchion [41]. The zygion is considered to be the most lateral point of the zygomatic arch and is usually determined instrumentally. The ectoconchion is a point where the orbital length line, parallel to the superior border, meets the outer orbital rim. It is also considered to be the point of maximum breadth on the lateral wall of the bony orbit [41].

Lacrimal bone

Located along the antero-medial aspect of the bony orbit, the lacrimal bone is one of the most delicate bones of the craniofacial complex. The lacrimal bone has a highly variable morphology with only two surfaces and four borders (Fig. 3.50) [39].

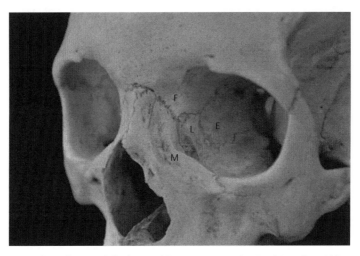

Fig. 3.50 Antero-lateral view of the lacrimal bone in situ (L: lacrimal; E: ethmoid bone; M: maxilla; F: frontal bone).

The main part of the lacrimal bone is the first to form, followed by the crista, then the hamulus and finally the orbital part [39]. The orbital part is very small when compared to the facial part in foetuses between 20 and 32 gestational weeks. However, by birth, the two parts are nearly equal in size [39].

The perinatal bone is long and slim supero-inferiorly with the facial and orbital parts separated by the lacrimal crest, and may only articulate with the orbital plate of the ethmoid bone after birth [39]. At birth the lacrimal bone closely resembles the shape of a leaf. There are two periods of significant growth in the length of the nasolacrimal duct, which in turn has a significant influence on the overall growth of the lacrimal bone. Both these periods of growth coincide with the eruption of the deciduous dentition and the second permanent molars. Additionally, there are reports of failure of ossification of the lacrimal bone resulting in either a rudimentary or completely absent lacrimal bone. In such instances the medial wall of the bony orbit is then occupied by the ethmoid bone or maxilla [39].

When in isolation, the lacrimal bone is commonly mistaken for a bone fragment and owing to the extremely fragile nature of the bone is often severely damaged. This in turn makes the juvenile lacrimal bone exceptionally difficult to study. The adult lacrimal bone is quadrilateral in shape and is sutured to the frontal bone superiorly, the maxilla anteriorly and the ethmoid bone posteriorly [37]. Additionally, at approximately the vertical centre of the lacrimal bone, the posterior lacrimal crest is present. Anterior to the crest is a vertical groove, which houses the lacrimal sac. The lacrimal sac leads to the nasolacrimal canal containing the nasolacrimal duct [37].

Anthropological landmarks include the dacryon, the lacrimale and the maxillofrontale landmark points. The dacryon is described as the point on the medial wall of the orbit at the junction of the lacrimomaxillary suture and the frontal bone [41]. The lacrimale is the point of intersection on the posterior lacrimal crest with the frontolacrimal suture [41]. The maxillofrontale is described as the point of intersection of the anterior lacrimal crest with the frontomaxillary suture [41].

Ethmoid bone

The ethmoid bone is located antero-medially within the anterior cranial fossa, articulating with the ethmoidal notch of the frontal bone medially and the lesser wings and body of the sphenoid bone posteriorly (Fig. 3.51). In general, the ethmoid bone is described as irregular in shape consisting of a horizontally oriented cribiform plate, a midline perpendicular plate and two lateral labyrinths (Fig. 3.51) [39].

During the period of five to six months of prenatal development the ethmoid and frontal paranasal sinus systems begin their development as air cells budding out from the superior and middle nasal meati of the nasal cavity to invaginate the ectethmoid part of the nasal capsule [39]. Ossification in general spreads into the superior nasal concha and then slowly into the intercellular septa as far as

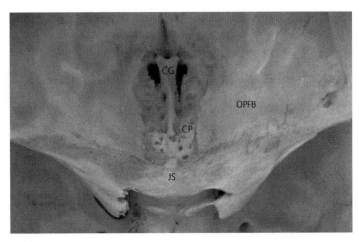

Fig. 3.51 Intracranial view of the ethmoid bone within the anterior cranial fossa (CG: crista galli; CP: cribiform plate; JS: jugum sphenoidale; OPFB: orbital plate of frontal bone).

the orbital laminae, which will form as the external surfaces of ethmoidal cells. At the conclusion of six months each labyrinth is almost completely ossified [39]. However ossification may be delayed until birth [38].

At birth the ethmoid bone consists of the two bony labyrinths held together by the cartilaginous cribiform and perpendicular plates (Fig. 3.52) [39]. In the perinatal period, an individual labyrinth may be identified by its characteristic adult morphology. However, owing to the fragile state of the bone at this stage of development, it is rarely recovered within a forensic setting. The labyrinth is a slim rectangular-shaped structure, with a wrinkled medial side forming the superior and middle concha (Fig. 3.52). The lateral side of the labyrinth is the smooth orbital plate, which forms a somewhat continuous covering precluding the anterior end where open air cells are usually visible [39].

During the first year of life, the perpendicular plate ossifies from the median centre and by the second year of life fuses with the ethmoidal labyrinth [38]. The cribiform plate ossifies from both the perpendicular plate and the ethmoid labyrinth [38]. From four to eight months post-partum, the internal parts of the cribiform plate originating from the median centre and the external part arising from the bony labyrinth unite, commencing in the posterior third [39]. The crista galli ossifies during the second year of life [38], either by extension from the internal part of the cribiform plate or from a separate centre of ossification [39]. In general the growth in the length and width of the cribiform plate ceases by between 2 and 3 years of age, when the cribiform plate fuses with the labyrinths [38]. Following this the width of the labyrinths can only increase by surface deposition during further pneumatisation on the orbital side of the labyrinth [39]. The most anterior group of air cells sometimes gives rise to the frontal air sinuses, which start to pneumatise the frontal bone during early childhood. Pneumatisation

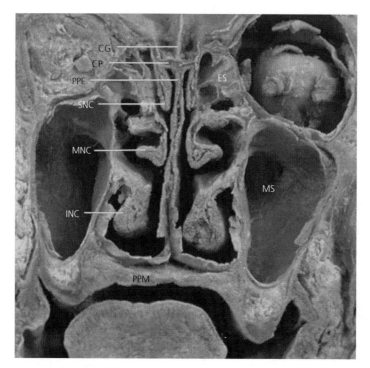

Fig. 3.52 Coronal section through the adult cadaver nasal cavity (CG: crista galli; CP: cribiform plate; PPE: perpendicular plate of ethmoid bone; SNC: superior nasal concha; MNC: middle nasal concha; INC: inferior nasal concha; ES: ethmoidal sinus; MS: maxillary sinus; PPM: palatine process of the maxillary bone and floor of nasal cavity/roof of oral cavity).

may spread further into the uncinated process and ethmoidal air cells may also invade the sphenoid, maxilla and lacrimal bones [39].

In general, the complexity of the ethmoidal bone precludes studying it in its entirety since it is hidden within the superior aspect of the nasal cavity. However certain parts of the bone may be identified in situ. These include the cribiform plate which transmits olfactory nerve fibres to the superior olfactory region of the nasal cavity and the superiorly directed crista galli which anchors the dural falx cerebri anteriorly [37]. While the perpendicular plate in its contribution to the nasal septum subdivides the nasal cavity into a left and right chamber, the superior and middle nasal conchae serve as dominant features of the lateral wall (Fig. 3.52). Within forensic circumstances the recovery of the ethmoid bone is difficult owing to the irregular shape and fragile nature of the bone, especially in the prenatal and juvenile stages of growth.

Inferior nasal concha

Located just inferior to the middle nasal concha of the ethmoid bone on the lateral wall of the nasal cavity, the inferior nasal concha may be described as a detached part of the ethmoid bone (Fig. 3.52). The inferior nasal concha is generally described as being boat shaped, presenting with two ends and two surfaces with associated borders [39]. The general shape of the bone may also be attributed to the confined space occupied by the bone within the nasal cavity in general.

Alternatively referred to as the inferior nasal turbinate, the inferior nasal concha is derived from a single ossification centre associated with the lateral nasal capsule [38]. While endochondral ossification commences from as early as the 16th gestational week [39], it generally only begins during the 20th gestational week [38] and rapidly progresses inferiorly. The inferior nasal concha loses continuity with the nasal capsule during ossification and as such develops as an independent bone [38]. Subsequently, during the seventh month of development, there is the appearance of a second plate of bone, which appears at the inferior border of the first ossification centre. As development progresses, the bony plate develops and spreads superiorly as a corrugated mass of bone and covers the medial surface of the upper plate of the developing inferior nasal concha [39]. In addition to the overall morphological development of the inferior nasal concha during the seventh month of development, there is also the appearance of three processes associated with the bone, namely the maxillary, the ethmoid and the lacrimal processes of the inferior nasal concha [39]. The maxillary process is the first to appear during the seventh month of development, followed by the ethmoid and lacrimal processes during the eighth month [39].

At birth, the inferior nasal concha bears all the characteristics of the adult bone, although more wrinkled in nature and with the processes of the superior border being less obvious. During adolescence, the inferior nasal concha frequently fuses with the maxilla. However, it may also fuse with the uncinated process of the ethmoid bone (Fig. 3.52) [39].

In adults, the inferior nasal concha is a hollow bone with its convex surface protruding into the inferior part of the nasal cavity. It is sutured along the lateral wall of the nasal cavity to an inferior extension of the lacrimal bone anteriorly, the maxilla in the middle and a superior extension of the palatine bone posteriorly [37]. In general the inferior nasal concha, owing to its morphology, is often mistaken within a forensic setting for a fragment of bone and especially within a juvenile context, is rarely recovered intact.

Vomer bone

Dominating the inferior aspect of the nasal septum and continuous with the floor of the nasal cavity, the vomer is described as being trapezoidal in shape with two surfaces and four borders [39].

Ossification of the vomer bone commences during the eighth gestational week with the appearance of an ossification centre on each side of the midline. This results in two slender strips of bone that are widest in the middle and taper off towards their respective ends (Fig. 3.53) [39]. At the conclusion of the 12th gestational week, the ossification centres of each bony strip have united below the septal cartilage and formed a groove for the nasal septal cartilage [38].

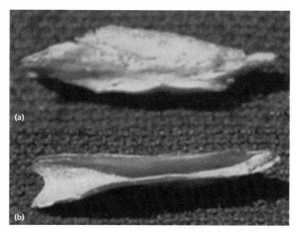

Fig. 3.53 Lateral (a) and superior (b) views of the vomer bone.

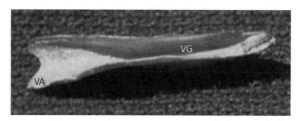

Fig. 3.54 Superior view of the vomer bone (VA: vomerine ala; VG: vomerine groove).

The overall shape of the vomer bone, at this stage of its development, may be described as V- or U-shaped, and with the progression of growth will adopt an overall Y-shape between 19 and 23 gestational weeks (Fig. 3.53) [39].

The vomerine groove, which extends from the sphenoid posteriorly to the premaxilla region anteriorly, supports the inferior border of the septal cartilage, of which the posterior part will ossify later as the perpendicular plate of the ethmoid bone [39]. It is the support of and subsequent alteration in the morphology of the nasal septum that ultimately influences the change in the shape of the vomer bone with development.

At the beginning of the 24th gestational week, the vomer assumes a boat-shaped appearance and consists of two leaves of bone joined inferiorly into a single lamina with a flattened base (Fig. 3.53) [39]. Each leaf has a feathery free edge, which is pointed and directed almost vertically in an anterior direction. Posteriorly the two leaves fan outwards, opening up the posterior aspect of the vomer and creating a scoop-shaped posterior end that concludes in the vomerine alae (Fig. 3.54) [39].

The postnatal growth of the vomer is inherently connected to the growth of the nasal septum and the facial skeleton [38,39]. The downward spread of the ossification of the perpendicular plate reaches the vomer during the early stages of childhood and contact between the two structures induces further ossification at the open edges of the vomerine groove [39]. At 10 years of age, the posterior edge of the nasal septum has reached adult proportions in approximately 80% of individuals. During puberty the superior edges of the left and right vomerine leaves fuse, converting the vomerine groove into a canal [39]. In early adulthood there is a fusion of the vomer with the perpendicular plate of the ethmoid bone, with later compaction, thinning and increases in height observed [39].

Incomplete ossification may lead to perforations in the vomerine bone or possible narrowing of the cavity between the two sides. Most variations in the overall shape of the vomer bone have an influence on the occurrence of the clinical condition of deviated septum.

In the adult skull the vomer forms an anchorage for the posterior bony part of the nasal septum and is identified by the V-shaped aperture at its posterior extremity [37]. The flange or ala occurring on either side of the posterior aspect of the vomer bone makes contact with the medial extensions or vaginal processes of the medial pterygoid plates [37]. The alae meet in the midline to form a central plate, which is in contact superiorly with three structures, namely the sphenoid bone posteriorly, the ethmoid bone in the middle and the septal cartilage anteriorly. Inferiorly the vomerine plate makes contact with the perpendicular plates of the palatine and maxillary bones [37].

Nasal bone

Fundamentally forming the bridge of the nose, the frontal bones are also seldom recovered intact and in most instances may be mistaken for a bony fragment arising from an alternative source. During the 12th gestational week, the nasal bone may be identified from its adult morphology although it does differ somewhat in size and overall proportions. An obvious articular surface on the medial border of the nasal bone for the opposite nasal bone does not develop until late in foetal life [39].

At birth the nasal bone is surprisingly robust, the borders are smooth and a vascular foramen is visible in the lower half of the bone. The overall length of the bone is double that of the breadth across the lower part of the nasal bone, with the overall shape being highly variable in nature (Fig. 3.55) [39]. During the first year, the bone lengthens in its inferior part so that by puberty it is three times as long as it is wide. Both the serrated superior border and the nasal spine develop after the age of 3 years. The nasal bone grows by means of a combination of apposition and resorption along the outer and inner surfaces respectively, resulting in a high degree of morphological variation throughout its growth period [39].

Maxilla

The maxilla is considered to be a dominant feature of the viscerocranium, contributing significantly to all three associated apertures (Fig. 3.56). As a result of its positioning within the viscerocranial complex, the general osteology of the maxilla consists of a body from which four distinct processes extend [39].

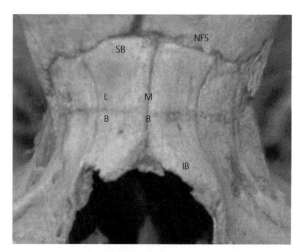

Fig. 3.55 Anterior view of the nasal bones (NFS: nasofrontal suture; MB: medial border, IB: inferior border; LB: lateral border; SB: superior border).

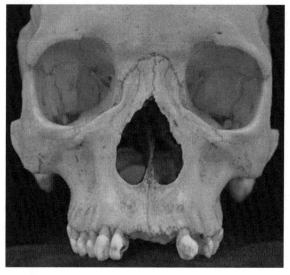

Fig. 3.56 Anterior view of the adult maxillary bone indicating its common association with the bony orbits, nasal cavity and oral cavity.

During gestational weeks 11 and 12, there is the appearance of the incisive fissure separating the premaxilla from the maxilla and the maxillopalatine suture separating the maxilla from the posterior palatine bones (Fig. 3.57). The incisive fissure assists in accommodating the increased volume of tissue during the development of the dentition. This is while the maxillopalatine suture functions in the antero-posterior growth of the bony palate [39].

The prenatal maxilla towards the end of the prenatal period of development consists of a small main body, the nasal notch, the infra-orbital margin

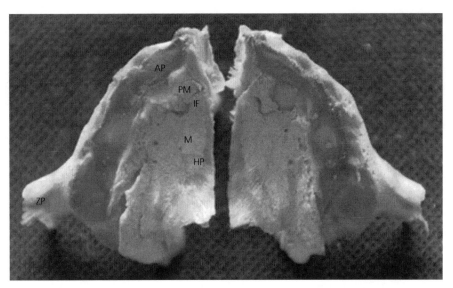

Fig. 3.57 Inferior view of the palatine, alveolar and zygomatic processes of the maxilla (AP: alveolar process; ZP: zygomatic process; HP: palatine process; PM: premaxilla; IF: incisive suture; M: maxilla).

and all four processes that are recognisable [39]. The frontal process is triangular in shape and lies on the side wall of the ectethmoid part of the nasal capsule in front of the epiphanial foramen, with the lacrimal bone above and the paraseptal cartilage below. The derivation of the frontal process from the premaxilla and maxilla sometimes shows a cleft [39]. The zygomatic process points dorsolaterally but at this stage of development, there is a wide interval between it and the zygomatic bone (Fig. 3.57). The alveolar process is an irregular, cresentic groove with rough edges filled with developing tooth germs (Fig. 3.57) [39]. The palatine process, at this stage of development, is represented by a shelf of bone extending from the inner alveolar area towards the midline. It is divided into maxillary and premaxillary parts, but none of these parts makes contact with the opposing bone or the palatine bone posteriorly (Fig. 3.57). The infra-orbital nerve, a branch of the maxillary division of the trigeminal nerve, lies in a groove in the bone of the orbital floor (Fig. 3.58). During the later stages of growth, the infra-orbital groove is closed over in the anterior part of the orbital floor and the nerve then emerges through the infra-orbital foramen [39]. The maxillary sinus commences development between weeks 10 and 12 of gestation while the initial position of the maxillary sinus is located above the floor of the nasal cavity and supero-medial to the infra-orbital foramen. The position of the sinus changes as pneumatisation proceeds into the ossifying maxilla.

The palatal process comprises a thin plate of bone until the later stages of prenatal development. After this, the medial surface anterior to the incisive

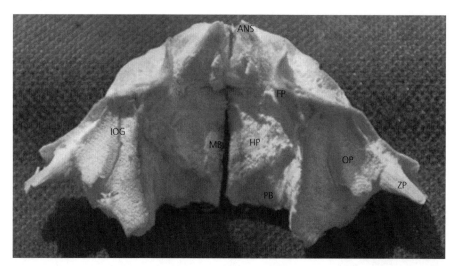

Fig. 3.58 Superior view of the left and right unfused maxillary bones (ANS: anterior nasal spine; FP: frontal process; MB: medial border; HP: palatine process; PB: posterior border; OP: orbital plate;ZP: zygomatic process; IOG: infra-orbital groove).

canal increases its height as it assumes the role of the interdental septum between the central incisor tooth germs [39]. The growth of the whole alveolar process is complex and develops in close relationship to the developing deciduous and permanent tooth germs. The alveolar tooth crypts develop in an antero-posterior direction with the lingual lamina in advance of the buccal lamina [39]. The interalveolar septa are the last parts to complete each crypt. Proceeding in an antero-posterior direction, at 11 gestational weeks the crypts of the deciduous incisors start formation and septa form between the tooth germs at approximately 13 gestational weeks [39]. At approximately 17 to 18 gestational weeks, the dental crypts of all the teeth from the central incisors anteriorly to the first molars postero-laterally are complete.

The perinatal maxilla has a very small body in order to accommodate the tooth germs as it is close to the orbital floor. Although at this stage of development the air sinus is very small, its bony outline is evident as a spindle-shaped depression in the lateral wall of the nasal cavity immediately lateral to the inferior concha [39]. During prenatal development, the sinuses are filled with amniotic fluid and do not become aerated until approximately ten days after birth. In addition within the prenatal maxilla, a prominent infra-orbital foramen is visible on the anterior surface of the maxilla and may still be open superiorly and continuous with the groove in the floor of the orbit [39]. The perinatal frontal process bears a resemblance to a lance, with the anterior lacrimal crest prominent on the external surface (Fig. 3.59). The zygomatic process is slender and extends postero-laterally from above the infra-orbital foramen and consists almost entirely of a triangular articular surface for the zygomatic bone (Fig. 3.59) [39].

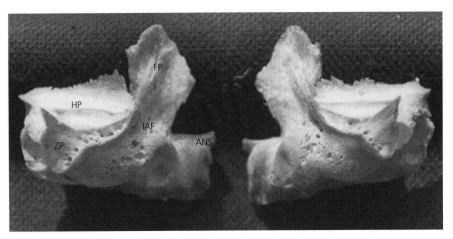

Fig. 3.59 Lateral view of the juvenile maxilla (FP: frontal process; ANS: anterior nasal spine; IAF: infra-orbital foramen; HP: palatine process; ZP: zygomatic process).

The palatal process is thin except at the medial border. Located between the central incisors there is a smooth interdental septum behind which the incisive canal runs almost vertically. Posteriorly, the bone becomes thinner as it forms the main component of the intermaxillary suture [39]. The incisive fissure on the palatal surface extends from the incisive fossa medially to a varied position laterally, and may be continuous with a fissure on the nasal aspect of the frontal process or end in the alveolar bone. Additionally, the calcified crowns of the deciduous dentition cause prominent bulges on the antero-lateral surface of the alveolar process and the inferior view of the process is dominated by the curve formed by the alveolar crypts, which envelop the palate [39].

In terms of overall shape definition, the first three dental crypts are triangular and arranged in a cuneiform pattern. The first molar crypt is rectangular in shape while the deciduous molar crypt is still somewhat incomplete and continuous posteriorly with the infratemporal fossa [39]. The infratemporal surface of the body is only distinguishable late in foetal life as it lies postero-inferior to the orbital floor and superior to the alveolar process. Both these structures are late in their ossification posteriorly.

The maxillary tuberosity does not exist during childhood as its place is occupied by posterior extensions of the alveolar processes. Following the eruption of the second and third molars the tuberosity is more defined and becomes closely related to the pyramidal process of the palatine bone [39].

The postnatal growth of the maxilla is rapid and intrinsically linked to different functional areas of the anterior part of the skull. Thus increases in the size of the eyeballs and nose both influence the development of the main part of the body [36, 39]. The growth of the nasal septum carries the maxilla antero-inferiorly, more anteriorly during the first decade and more vertically in the second. The major mechanism of maxillary growth is apposition and this occurs mainly at the alveolar region, the facial surface and the posterior border [39]. The contained air sinus enlarges by resorption and deposition of bone surfaces and by 4 years of age, pneumatisation has expanded laterally to the infra-orbital foramen and inferiorly to the attachment of the inferior nasal concha [39]. At approximately 8 years of age, the maxillary air sinus has reached beyond the infra-orbital foramen and at 12 years of age is found at the same level as the floor of the nasal cavity inferiorly, and has expanded laterally to the molar teeth. During puberty the maxillary air sinus has expanded below the floor of the nasal cavity. Incidentally, during this period of growth, the general size and shape of the sinus is somewhat variable in nature.

Furthermore, with the influence of the dentition on the overall growth of the maxilla, the time of closure of the incisive suture is very variable. The facial aspect of the suture is observed to close during infancy. However, the internal aspect in the region of the incisive canal between the two maxillae is slow to fuse and approximately 30% of the suture in this location may remain unfused in adolescence [39]. The posterior palatal aspect of the suture may close laterally as early as the perinatal period during which the palatal processes fuse with the alveolar bone. The medial part of the suture may remain open into adulthood with the earliest age of eradication of the suture occurring at 25 years [39].

The maxilla, as a result of its location within the craniofacial complex, is often compromised as a result of either trauma or pathology. The most commonly associated fracture patterns associated with the maxilla are the three main types of Le Fort fractures [58]. These extensive mid-facial fractures are rarely present in a classic form and often present in a comminution/fragmentation pattern [58]. Furthermore the general proximity of the maxillary paranasal sinuses to the dentition may also present with complications following the occurrence of impacted third molars towards the posterior bony hard palate.

Within a forensic context, the juvenile and adult maxillary bone is exceptionally well preserved despite its propensity for damage in cases of trauma. As a result, the maxilla is the site for a variety of anthropological landmarks of the facial skeleton, which may include [41]:

- Incision: at the incisal level of the maxillary central incisors.
- Alveolare: the upper alveolar point at the apex of the septum between the maxillary central incisors. Incidentally it is also used as the most inferior landmark in the measurement of facial height.
- Prosthion: often confused with the alveolare, it is described as the most anterior point in the midline of the superior alveolar process.

Anthropological landmarks involving the bony hard palate include [41]:

- Alveolon: a point on the bony hard palate where a line drawn through the termination of the alveolar ridges crosses the median line.
- Staphylion: the point in the midline of the posterior bony hard palate (interpalatal suture) where it is crossed by a line drawn tangent to the curves of the posterior margin of the palate.

- Orale: the point on the bony hard palate where the line drawn tangent to the curves in the alveolar margin at the back of the two medial incisor teeth crosses the midsagittal plane. Incidentally, it is on the opposite side of the bone from the alveolare.

In the overall assessment of the palate, the prosthion and alveolon are used in the assessment of the external palatal length, while the orale and staphylion are used in the assessment of the internal palatal length [41]. Paired craniometric points involving the maxilla include:

- Alare: the instrumentally determined most lateral point on the nasal aperture taken perpendicular to the nasal height.
- Orbitale: the most inferior point in the margin of the orbit and one of the points used in determining facial height.
- Ectomolare: the most lateral point on the outer surface of the alveolar margins, usually opposite the middle of the maxillary second molar tooth and commonly used in the overall assessment of maxillary breadth.
- Endomolare: the most medial point on the inner surface of the alveolar ridge opposite the middle of the second maxillary molar tooth and used in the assessment of palatal breadths.

Palatine

Located immediately posterior to the maxilla, each palatine bone consists of two plates: namely the horizontal and perpendicular plates, which are set at right angles to each other [39]. The orbital and sphenoidal processes of the palatine bone are attached to the superior border of the perpendicular plate, with a pyramidal process extending posterolaterally from the junction of the two plates [39].

The left and right palatine bones fuse in the midline of the palate and subsequently articulate with the maxillae, inferior nasal conchae, ethmoid and sphenoid bones respectively. The palatine bones in conjunction with the vomer also contribute to the skeleton of the posterior choanae, which act as a passage between the nasal cavity and nasopharynx [39].

During the 20th gestational week, the palatine bone may be distinguished in isolation as it assumes the morphological features of its adult counterpart. In the prenatal period of growth, the thin horizontal plate of the palatine bone, the future posterior third of the bony hard palate, is almost square in shape. The medial border is slightly thickened for the sagittal suture and the palatine crest may be seen running transversely across the oral surface [39]. The perpendicular plate is approximately the same height as the width of the horizontal plate and is also observed to be very thin at this stage of growth. On the nasal surface of the palatine bone, the conchal crest is present for articulation with the posterior end of the inferior nasal concha and is located just above the perpendicular and horizontal plates. The groove leading down to the greater palatine foramen, which transmits the greater palatine neurovascular bundle, is obvious on the maxillary surface [39]. Additionally, there is a notch that separates the sphenoid and orbital processes, with the sphenoid process being the larger of the two and directed laterally and the orbital process inclined medially. The postero-laterally extending pyramidal process is somewhat larger in adults, but even at this stage of development already bears the same recognisable morphology [39].

Up to approximately 3 years of age, the horizontal and perpendicular plates of the palatine bone are equal in size. However, following this the growth rate of the perpendicular plate increases to keep pace with the rapid increases in facial and nasal cavity growth during childhood. At the commencement of puberty the height is approximately twice the width of the horizontal plate [39].

In addition to the general growth of the individual palatine bone, the bone also contributes to the posterior third of the bony hard palate. Postnatally the growth of the palate at the midpalatal suture slows and effectively ceases between two and four years of age [39]. Appositional growth of the palate at the alveolar margins continues to widen the palate posteriorly until approximately 7 years of age. Increases in the general height of the palate appear to cease after 9 years of age with increases in length continuing into adult life [39]. In some instances growth at the maxillopalatine suture have been observed to continue until the age of 13 to 15 years. Following this, sutural growth ceases while appositional growth is observed to continue [39]. The growth in the width of the palate at the midpalatine (sagittal) suture may continue until approximately 16 years of age in girls and 18 years in boys.

While the palatine bone contributes significantly to the growth and general structure of the bony hard palate, within a forensic context it is seldom recovered. The palatine bone in its overall contribution to the anthropological dimensions of the bony hard palate is discussed in conjunction with the maxilla.

Mandible

Aside from the ossicles of the middle ear, the mandible is the only other bone of the craniofacial complex to enjoy independent movement. As a structure of the viscerocranium, the mandible is a dominant feature of the oral cavity, contributing significantly to the antero-lateral border. Additionally the mandible plays a pivotal role in the general mastication functioning of the oral cavity. It provides attachment to the muscles of mastication and tongue, as well as serving as the bony scaffold for the deciduous and permanent dentition sets.

The mandible is considered a composite structure derived from a combination of intramembranous and endochondral ossification. As the mandible during its prenatal development consists of two separate hemi-mandibles a centre for each half of the bone appears between weeks 6 and 7 of gestation lateral to Meckel's cartilage in the ventral part of the first pharyngeal arch [39, 59, 60]. The mandibular division of the trigeminal nerve is thought to be the catalyst in this process and as such is essential in the overall induction of ossification [39, 60–62].

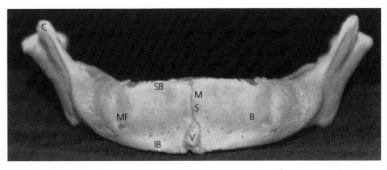

Fig. 3.60 Anterior view of a juvenile mandible (SB: superior border/surface; MF: mental foramen; IB: inferior border/surface; MS: symphyseal surface; V: ventral cartilage island; B: body of mandible; C: coronoid process).

The coronoid process of the mandible differentiates within the temporal muscle mass during the seventh gestational week and is observed to start uniting with the ramus of the mandible during the eighth gestational week [39, 61]. At approximately 10 gestational weeks, the ventral end of the Meckel's cartilage, spanning the mental foramen and the mandibular symphysis, starts to ossify, forming islands of cartilage that will eventually form part of the symphyseal region of the mandible (Fig. 3.60) [39, 60, 63]. Posterior to the mental foramen and extending to the lingula of the mandible, Meckel's cartilage starts to disappear, ultimately forming the malleus and incus bony ossicles and the sphenomandibular and anterior malleolar ligaments [62, 63].

During the period of 12 to 14 gestational weeks, a set of secondary cartilages develop in the region of the condylar and coronoid processes and the small cartilage nodules of the ventral end of Meckle's cartilage are observed at the symphysis (Fig. 3.60) [60, 63]. At approximately 16 gestational weeks the temporomandibular joint is clearly defined and the hyaline cartilage is associated with the posterior end [62].

In the initial stages of development, the cone-shaped condylar cartilage extends anteriorly well into the ramus of the mandible. However, by 16 gestational weeks the cartilage has started its conversion to bone [29, 61]. At 20 gestational weeks, the condylar cartilage assumes the shape of a narrow strip of cartilage immediately beneath the condyle of the mandible. The coronoid cartilage is rapidly converted to bone and all traces of cartilage associated with the coronoid process have disappeared by 24 gestational weeks [39].

In the symphyseal region of the mandible, ossification commences at approximately 28 gestational weeks and is usually fused with the anterior part of the opposing hemi-mandible during the first year of life (Fig. 3.60) [39, 60, 61, 63]. However the condylar cartilage maintains its role as a main growth centre well into the third decade of life, essentially directing the overall growth of the mandible in response to a variety of factors (Fig. 3.61) [39, 59, 63].

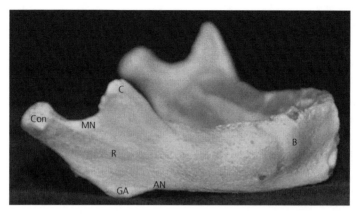

Fig. 3.61 Lateral view of the juvenile mandible (Con: condylar process; MN: mandibular notch; C: coronoid process; R: ramus; GA: gonial/mandibular angle; AN: antegonial notch; B: body).

In general, the perinatal mandible is represented by a body and ramus just under half the length of the body and extending in a posterior direction (Figs. 3.60 and 3.61). The ramus is nearly horizontally aligned, with the head of the mandibular condyle almost perfectly aligned with the superior surface of the body [39, 59, 63, 64]. The external surface of the body of the mandible is flattened anteriorly at the level of the canine and first molar crypts, the body assumes a rounded shape just above the base of the crypt. The mental foramen is two-thirds of the way above the inferior border of the mandible and is roughly aligned with the deciduous canine and first molar crypts (Fig. 3.60) [59]. Additionally the opening of the mental foramen is anteriorly directed, but does assume a more lateral disposition with the growth of the mandible into adulthood [65, 66]. The mental spines and the mylohyoid line are clearly visible on the internal surface of the mandible and offer attachment to the genioglossus, geniohyoid and mylohyoid muscles respectively [59].

The overall angle between the ramus and the body of the mandible at this stage of growth is obtuse and ranges between 135° and 145° (Fig. 3.61) [39, 64]. The articular surface of the mandibular condyle is directed posteriorly, with a shallow mandibular notch separating it from the anterior coronoid process of the mandible (Fig. 3.61). A prominent mandibular foramen and its associated bony flap, the lingula, are observed on the internal surface of the ramus [39, 63]. The inferior edge of the symphyseal surface curves laterally, creating a gap between the two symphyseal surfaces of the respective hemimandibles [63].

Postnatally the mandible undergoes considerable change in both shape and overall dimensions as a result of the development and subsequent replacement of dentition sets as well as a change in masticatory demand [59]. During the first year of life there is the fusion of the symphyseal surfaces of the two respective hemi-mandibles. The fusion commences along the antero-inferior surfaces of the hemi-mandible and proceeds postero-superiorly, with overall completion usually being observed during the first six months of life [39]. However fusion may be prolonged until as late as the end of the first year [63]. Along the posterior aspect of the mandible the condyle plays a significant role in the overall growth of the mandible postnatally [59, 61, 63]. The condyle directs the antero-inferior growth of the mandible from the cranial base (Fig. 3.61).

The inferior junction between the body and ramus of the mandible, that is the gonial angle, is observed to change orientation postnatally, becoming more acute with the overall growth of the mandible (Fig. 3.61). Alveolar bone is deposited on the superior surface of the body as the deciduous dentition develops, but following the establishment of the occlusal plane stabilises and maintains a constant relationship with the lower border of the mandible [39]. The resultant decrease in the gonial angle, and the rapid increase in the height of the ramus, result in the ramus assuming a more upright position with growth (Fig. 3.61) [63]. In addition to changes in the position of the ramus relative to the body, the body of the mandible is also observed to significantly widen (Fig. 3.62).

At birth the mental foramen first aligns with the deciduous canine and first molar dental crypts; as the body of the mandible lengthens with general growth, the position of the foramen changes, ultimately aligning the foramen with the first and second molars [39]. The mental foramen also alters its vertical position with the changes in the depth of the alveolar processes. At birth the mental foramen points antero-inferiorly, but during childhood changes to a more posterior orientation. Incidentally, the chin also alters its general morphology during childhood, with its depth increasing considerably after the eruption of

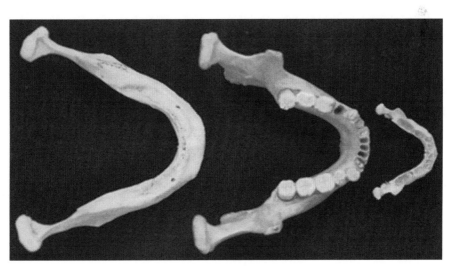

Fig. 3.62 Superior view of changes in the mandibular arch width with age (Left: edentulous mandible; Middle: adult mandible; Right: perinatal mandible).

the incisor teeth. In general the concavity of the chin region changes somewhat from very shallow at about 4 years of age to the distinctly concave shape observed at 14 years of age.

While the growth of the juvenile mandible centres around the development and eruption of the dentition sets and changes in mastication, changes in the adult mandible morphology are largely centred on the loss of the dentition. Thus the most significant change in the morphology of the adult mandible is the resorption of the alveolar ridge when the dentition is lost.

The mandible within a forensic context is highly resilient and as such is often retained following mass disasters and other traumatic events. As such the following anthropological landmarks are associated with the mandible [41]:

- Gnathion: the lowest median point on the lower border of the mandible.
- Pogonion: the most anterior point in the midline on the chin.
- Infradentale: the apex of the septum between the lower central incisors.
- Condylion laterale: the most lateral point on the condyle of the mandible.
- Gonion: the midpoint of the angle of the mandible between the body and the ramus.

Additionally, the mandible is also used in the estimation of sex in unidentified individuals. The chin is square in males and rounded with a midline in females [41].

References

1 Butler PM. (1939) Studies of the mammalian dentition. Differentiation of the post-canine dentition. *Proceedings of the Zoological Society of London* **B109**, 1–36.

2 Kieser JA. (1986) Odontogenic polarity and Butler's field theory. *Medical Hypotheses* **20**, 103–107.

3 Dahlberg AA. (1945) The changing dentition of man. *Journal of the American Dental Association* **32**, 676–690.

4 Osborn JW. (1978) Morphogenetic gradients: fields versus clones. In: Butler PM, Joysey KA (eds) *Development, Function and Evolution of Teeth*. Academic Press, London, pp. 171–201.

5 Townsend G, Harris EF, Lesot H et al. (2009) Morphogenetic fields within the human dentition: a new, clinically relevant synthesis of an old concept. *Archives of Oral Biology* **54**, 34–44.

6 Brook AH, Jernvall J, Smith RN et al. (2014) The dentition: the outcomes of morphogenesis leading to variations of tooth number, size, and shape. *Australian Dental Journal* **59**, (suppl s1) 131–142.

7 Fleming PS, Xavier GM, DiBiase AT et al. (2010) Revisiting the supernumery: the epidemiological and molecular basis of extra teeth. *British Dental Journal* **208**, 25–30.

8 Brook AH. (2009) Multilevel complex interactions between genetic, epigenetic and environment factors in the aetiology of anomalies of dental development. *Archives of Oral Biology* **54**, S3–S17.

9 Brook AH, Hughes T, Townsend GC et al. (2013) The development of the dentition as a complex adaptive system. *American Journal of Physical Anthropology* **150**, (suppl 56) 89–89.

10 Jernvall J, Thesleff I. (2012) Tooth shape formation and tooth renewal evolving with the same signals. *Development* **139**, 3487–3497.

11 Thesleff I. (2014) Current understanding of the process of tooth formation: transfer from the laboratory to the clinic. *Australian Dental Journal* **59**, (suppl s1) 48–54.

12 Rajab LD, Hamdan MA. (2002) Supernumery teeth: review of the literature and a survey of 152 cases. *International Journal of Paediatric Dentistry* **12**, 244–254.

13 Hattab FN, Yasin OM, Rawashdeh MA. (1994) Supernumerary teeth: Report of three cases and review of the literature. *ASDC Journal of Dentistry for Children* **61**, 382–393.

14 Brook AH. (1974) Dental anomalies of number, form and size: their prevalence in British schoolchildren. *Journal of the International Association for Dentistry in Children* **5**, 37–53.

15 Luten JR. (1967) The prevalence of supernumery teeth in primary and mixed dentition. *ASDC Journal of Dentistry for Children* **34**, 346–353.

16 Gallas MM, Garcia A. (2000) Retention of permanent incisor by mesiodens. *British Dental Journal* **188**, 63–64.

17 Orhan AI, Ozer L, Orhan K. (2006) Familial occurrence of nonsyndromal multiple supernumerary teeth. A rare condition. *Angle Orthodontics* **76**, 891–897.

18 Scheiner MA, Sampson WJ. (1997) Supernumery teeth: a review of the literature and four case reports. *Australian Dental Journal* **42**, 160–165.

19 Stellzig A, Basdra EK, Komposch G. (1997) Mesiodentes: incidence, morphology, aetiology. *Journal of Orofacial Orthopedics* **58**, 144–153.

20 Parolia A, Kundabala M, Dahal M et al. (2011) Management of supernumery teeth. *Journal of Conservative Dentistry* **14**, 221–224.

21 Hyun HK, Lee SJ, Lee SH et al. (2009) Clinical characteristics and complications associated with mesiodentes. *Journal of Oral and Maxillofacial Surgery* **67**, 2639–2643.

22 Kırzıoğlu Z, Köseler Şentut T, Özay Ertürk MS et al. (2005) Clinical features of hypodontia and associated dental anomalies: a retrospective study. *Oral Diseases* **11**, 399–404.

23 Dhanrajani PJ. (2002) Hypodontia: etiology, clinical features, and management. *Quintessence International* **33**, 294–302.

24 Kirkham J, Kaur R, Stillman EC et al. (2005) The patterning of hypodontia in a group of young adults in Sheffield, UK. *Archives of Oral Biology* **50**, 287–291.

25 De Coster PJ, Marks LA, Martens LC et al. (2009) Dental agenesis: genetic and clinical perspectives. *Journal of Oral Pathology and Medicine* **38**, 1–17.

26 Galluccio G, Castellano M, La Monaca C. (2012) Genetic basis of non–syndromic anomalies of human tooth number. *Archives of Oral Biology* **57**, 918–930.

27 Peck S, Peck L, Kataja M. (1996) Prevalence of tooth agenesis and peg–shaped maxillary lateral incisor associated with palatally displaced canine (PDC) anomaly. *American Journal of Orthodontics and Dentofacial Orthopedics* **110**, 441–443.

28 Nambiar S, Mogra S, Shetty S. (2014) Transposition of teeth: a forensic perspective. *Journal of Forensic Dental Sciences* **6**, 151–153.

29 Witkop CJ. (1976) Clinical aspects of dental anomalies. *International Dental Journal* **26**, 378–390.

30 Shifman A, Chanannel I. (1978) Prevalence of taurodontism found in radiographic dental examination of 1,200 young adult Israeli patients. *Community Dentistry and Oral Epidemiology* **6**, 200–203.

31 Hua F, He H, Ngan P et al. (2013) Prevalence of peg-shaped maxillary permanent lateral incisors: A meta-analysis. *American Journal of Orthodontics and Dentofacial Orthopedics* **144**, 97–109.

32 Moormann S, Guatelli-Steinberg D, Hunter J. (2013) Metamerism, morphogenesis, and the expression of Carabelli and other dental traits in humans. *American Journal of Physical Anthropology* **150**, 400–408.

33 Ashar A, Hughes T, Kaidonis J, James H et al. (2014) The individuality of the human dentition: implications for forensic odontology. *Australian Dental Journal* **59**, S6.

34 Sinnatamby CS. (2011) *Last's Anatomy: Regional and Applied.* 12th edn, Churchill Livingstone, London.

35 Berkovitz BKB, Holland GR, Moxham BJ. (2009) *Oral Anatomy, Histology and Embryology.* 4th edn, Mosby Elsevier, Edinburgh.

36 Martinez-Maza C, Rosas A, Nieto-Diaz M. (2013) Postnatal changes in the growth dynamics of the human face revealed from bone modelling patterns. *Journal of Anatomy* **223**, 228–241.

37 Kramer B, Allan JC. (2005) *Fundamentals of Human Osteology*. 1st edn, LexisNexis Butterworths, Durban.

38 Som PM, Naidich TP. (2013) Development of the skull base and calvarium: an overview of the progression from mesenchyme to chondrification to ossification. *Neurographics*. **3**, 169–184.

39 Scheuer L, Black S. (2004) *The Juvenile Skeleton*. 1st edn, Elsevier Academic Press, London.

40 Guerram A, Le Minor J, Renger S et al. (2014) Brief communication: the size of the human frontal sinuses in adults presenting complete persistence of the metopic suture. *American Journal of Physical Anthropology* **154**, 621–627. doi: 10.1002/ajpa.22532.

41 Bass WM. (2005) *Human Osteology: A Laboratory and Field Manual*. 5th edn, Missouri Archaeological Society, Springfield.

42 Shapiro R. (1972) Anomalous parietal sutures and the bipartite parietal bone. *American Journal of Roentgenology* **115**, 569–577.

43 Matsumura G, England MA, Uchiumi T et al. (1994) The fusion of ossification centres in the cartilaginous and membranous parts of the occipital squama in human fetuses. *Journal of Anatomy* **185**, 295–300.

44 Matsumura G, Uchiumi T, Kida K et al. (1993) Developmental studies on the interparietal part of the human occipital squama. *Journal of Anatomy* **182**, 197–204.

45 Srivastava HC. (1992) Ossification of the membranous portion of the squamous part of the occipital bone in man. *Journal of Anatomy* **180**, 219–224.

46 Khan AA, Ullah M, Asari MA et al. (2013) Interparietal bone variations in accordance with their ossification centres in human skulls. *Internation Journal of Morphology* **31**, 546–552.

47 Srivastava HC. (1977) Development of ossification centres in the squamous portion of the occipital bone in man. *Journal of Anatomy* **124**, 643–649.

48 Shapiro R, Robinson F. (1976) The os incae. *American Journal of Roentgenology* **127**, 469–471.

49 Pal GP, Tamankar BP, Routal VR et al. (1984) The ossification of the membranous part of the squamous occipital bone in man. *Journal of Anatomy* **138**, 259–266.

50 Da Mata JR, Da Mata FR, Aversi-Ferreira TA. (2010) Analysis of bone variations of the occipital bone in man. *International Journal of Morphology* **28**, 243–428.

51 Wu JK, Goodrich JT, Amadi CC et al. (2010) Interparietal bone (Os Incae) in craniosynostosis. *American Journal of Medical Genetics Part A* **155**, 287–294.

52 Allan JC, Kramer B. (2010) *The Fundamentals of Human Embryology*. 2nd edn, Wits University Press, Johannesburg.

53 Scheuer L, Maclaughlin-Black S. (1994) Age estimation from the pars basilaris of the fetal and juvenile occipital bone. *International Journal of Osteoarchaeology* **4**, 377–380.

54 Prasada Rao PVV. (2002) Median (third) occipital condyle. *Clinical Anatomy* **15**, 148–151.

55 Figueiredo N, Moraes LB, Serra A et al. (2008) Median (third) occipital condyle causing atlantoaxial instablility and myelopathy. *Arq Neuropsiquitr* **66**, 90–92.

56 Wackenheim A. (1985) Hypoplasia of the basi–occipital bone and persistence of the spheno-occipital synchondrosis in a patient with transitory supplementary fissure of the basi-occipital. *Neuroradiology* **27**, 226–231.

57 Eby TL. (1996) Development of the facial recess: implications for cochlear implantation. *Laryngoscope* **106**, 1–7.

58 Pedlar J, Frame JW. (2007) *Oral and Maxillofacial Surgery: An Objective Based Textbook*. 2nd edn, Churchill Livingstone, London.

59 Hutchinson EF, Kieser JA, Kramer B. (2014) Morphometric growth relationships of the immature human mandible and tongue. *European Journal of Oral Sciences* **122**, 181–189.

60 Radlanski RJ, Renz H, Klarkowski MC. (2003) Prenatal development of the human mandible: 3D reconstructions, morphometry and bone remodelling pattern, sizes 12–117mm CRL. *Anatomy and Embryology* **207**, 221–232.

61 Lee SK, Kim YS, Oh HS et al. (2001) Prenatal development of the human mandible. *Anatomical Record* **263**, 314–325.

62 Sperber GH, Sperber SM, Guttmann GD. (2010) *Craniofacial Embryogenetics and Development.* 2nd edn, People's Medical Publishing House, Conneticut.

63 Hutchinson EF. (2010) An assessment of growth and sex from mandibles of cadaver foetuses and newborns (MSc Thesis). University of Pretoria Academic Press, Johannesburg.

64 Hutchinson EF, L'Abbe EN, Oettle' AC. (2012) An assessment of early mandibular growth. *Forensic Science International* **217**, 233e1–233e6.

65 Kieser JA, Kuzmanovic D, Payne A et al. (2002) Patterns of emergence of the human mental nerve. *Archives of Oral Biology.* **47**, 743–747.

66 Kuzmanovic DV, Payne AGT, Kieser JA et al. (2003) Anterior loop of the mental nerve: a morphological and radiological study. *Clinical Oral Implants Research* **14**, 464–471.

.

CHAPTER 4

Forensic pathology

David L. Ranson[1] and Norman Firth[2]

[1] Victorian Institute of Forensic Medicine; and Monash University, Australia

[2] Faculty of Dentistry, University of Otago, New Zealand

The role of the forensic pathologist

The individual discipline of forensic pathology is not a professional field that is found universally throughout the world. Forensic pathology practice in Australia and New Zealand, together with the range of countries that inherited their legal system from the United Kingdom, is generally similar, with services being provided by specialist pathologists who have gone on to sub-specialise in forensic pathology practice. Forensic pathology practice in these jurisdictions is associated with coroners' jurisdictions where the coroner is a legal official statutorily empowered to investigate deaths.

In contrast, many countries outside the traditional English legal system, such as many of the jurisdictions in Europe, have a broader medico-legal system whose medical specialists may not have pathology as their major medical discipline. The specialists in legal medicine in these jurisdictions are often engaged in casework that may include injury assessment for the purposes of civil and criminal compensation as well as a variety of medical administrative matters and assessments for government and the insurance industry. While some European medico-legal specialists may regularly perform medico-legal autopsies, these practitioners are likely to have had further training in forensic pathology than their general medico-legal colleagues. In reality therefore, in both English and continental jurisdictions, most doctors practising as forensic pathology specialists have a wide range of experience in the areas of clinical pathology, and in particular anatomical or histopathology.

Forensic pathologists are sub-specialist pathologists who usually have commenced their training in the field of anatomical pathology or histopathology. The principles of pathology applied in the work of the forensic pathologist are the same as those applied by their clinical pathology colleagues; however, the nature of the work performed by forensic pathologists is different in that they focus on death investigation and the autopsy rather than clinical diagnosis in the living. In addition, there is considerable difference in the mental and analytical

---

Forensic Odontology: Principles and Practice, First Edition. Edited by Jane A. Taylor and Jules A. Kieser.
© 2016 John Wiley & Sons, Ltd. Published 2016 by John Wiley & Sons, Ltd.

processes applied to forensic casework. While the clinical pathologist is contributing directly or indirectly to the medical care given to patients, the forensic pathologist's focus is the end-point of forensic investigations that are part of the judicial process. As a result the information produced by forensic pathologists is usually presented to a criminal or coroner's court rather than to medical staff on a hospital ward round.

In practical terms the forensic pathologist as a death investigator takes on a number of roles that are focused on gathering information regarding the circumstances in which death occurred, performing particular investigations or analysis in relation to the deceased's body and formulating opinions based on the information discovered. On completion of this investigative process the forensic pathologist sets out their findings in a medico-legal report that includes their conclusions regarding the cause of death, the identity of the deceased and the mechanism and circumstances of the death. The report is therefore a combination of medical facts and opinions leading to particular conclusions, and it is necessary that the evidence base for the conclusions must be stated clearly within the report so that the analysis and the deductions reached can be independently verified.

The medico-legal autopsy

Not all autopsies are undertaken for medico-legal purposes. Today in Australia and New Zealand the majority of autopsies would be undertaken at the request of a coroner; however, clinical autopsies undertaken with the consent of the family are still performed at a number of major hospitals. Such clinical autopsies are performed not to determine the cause of death (if the cause of death is unknown the death needs to be referred to the coroner), but instead to identify the extent of the known disease and perhaps the effects of treatments provided.

Other types of autopsy are recognised, such as virtual autopsies where no dissection of the body takes place but instead a variety of imaging techniques including CT scanning, MRI scanning and surface laser scanning are undertaken. Other approaches to death investigation include the psychological autopsy, where a detailed evaluation of an individual's behaviour and social interactions prior to death is used to determine the circumstances of a suspected suicide. In some public health situations, particularly in Third World countries, deaths may be investigated days or weeks after they have occurred and the person's body disposed of. Here a public health investigation of the environment in which the person died as well as an exploration of their terminal illness and medical records is used to try to come to a conclusion regarding the nature of their final illness and its causation.

For practical purposes, autopsies involving dissection include those performed for clinical medical purposes and those performed for medico-legal purposes. The general pathological procedures of both these autopsy types are the same;

however, the emphasis placed on particular components of the autopsy differs. The issue of human identification is a good example of this difference. Identification of a deceased person is rarely an issue in autopsies performed for clinical medical purposes, whereas it is an essential element of medico-legal autopsies with important ramifications for coronial, criminal and civil justice systems.

In addition to the information gathering aspects of an autopsy, consideration needs to be given to occupational health and safety issues that may pose risks to the operators and the community. Taking part in autopsy procedures necessarily involves some personal risk. This is particularly true when the identity and background of the deceased are unknown. Both physical injury and communication of infectious agents are potential hazards. Individuals infected with one of the types of infectious viral hepatitis, HIV or tuberculosis pose special risks; however, it should not be forgotten that commensal organisms can pose a threat to the operators if these organisms are inoculated into their body tissues via a cutaneous injury. In deaths that have occurred as a result of major trauma, foreign materials present on or in the body may puncture protective clothing including surgical gloves, and represent a significant hazard to the examiners. Any object, whether a part of the body or foreign material, that can cause a cutaneous injury needs to be identified in advance and counter-measures instituted. Working with bodies that are very cold or frozen poses a particular risk, as the operator's sense of touch and fine movement may become impaired. Control of the production of fluid splashes and aerosols during the autopsy should be given similar attention, as these can also transmit infectious agents.

As well as physical injury being associated with the risk of transmitting infectious agents to the operator, other physical hazards can occur. The very act of moving heavy bodies and body parts can cause back and limb injuries and these should be avoided by the use of appropriate equipment and assistance. Chemical injuries to an operator can also occur if the body is contaminated, and this can occur in a number of major disaster incidents and industrial deaths. Hydraulic fluids, caustic and corrosive chemicals as well as gas and radiation hazards must be anticipated and counter-measures instituted at the appropriate time during the investigation. Deaths occurring in a setting of military action or terrorist activity may also involve complex, highly toxic chemical contamination as well as explosive hazards from retained weapon projectiles and other explosive devices.

While the goals and aims of autopsies have differed over the centuries, today there is considerable uniformity of purpose with most pathologists agreeing on the value of the procedure for medical and legal purposes. Despite this, public perception of the role of the autopsy is clouded by misleading presentations in the media and by a degree of ignorance and indifference to the procedure communicated to them by some clinical medical practitioners. It is sometimes thought that today's advanced techniques in clinical investigation in the living have rendered the autopsy irrelevant; however, it is not uncommon for medico-legal autopsies to identify a range of pathology that was not identified by clinicians during life.

Key aims of autopsies can include:
- confirmation or determination of the identity of the deceased;
- identification of injuries and natural disease;
- determination of the extent of injuries and their causation;
- determination of the effect of medical treatments;
- evaluation of the mode or mechanism of death;
- determination of the cause of death;
- provision of an educational resource for the medical profession;
- provision of tissues for use in medical research and therapeutic procedures;
- retrieval of trace evidence and other samples for use as evidence in court;
- reconciliation of the findings on/in the body with the features of the death scene;
- reconstruction of the circumstances surrounding the death.

The performance of an autopsy involves a series of medical investigation tasks nearly all of which are similar to those performed in some aspects of clinical medical practice. Indeed the basic elements comprising all medical examinations are similar. An autopsy is a structured investigation where the focus is on solving a range of problems some of which are generally applicable to all examinations while others are specific to the particular death circumstances. This means that the first element of an autopsy is the identification of the goals or purpose of the examination. These goals may differ from case to case and depend upon the basis of the autopsy request. A coroner may have a different purpose in mind to that of the police, the family or a treating clinician. Each may be separately seeking answers to their own questions. It is up to the pathologist performing the autopsy to assure themselves of the questions at issue so that they can orientate their examination appropriately.

Where identification of the body is concerned, the pathologist must plan the autopsy in collaboration with the other investigators including the forensic odontologists, the forensic anthropologists/osteologists and the police. This will ensure that the technical procedures carried out are complementary and do not interfere adversely with each other. For example, in the case of procedures used in facial identification it would be possible for some aspects of facial dissection to interfere with forensic radiology and photographic requirements. If the jaws are resected before skull or dental radiographs are obtained, the relationship of the dental and facial structures cannot be used as a point of comparison with radiographs that may have been taken in life. The sequence of examination procedures is therefore of considerable importance and should never be left to chance.

Whether the autopsy is being performed for forensic or medical reasons, some universal basic goals exist. These include the discovery of significant disease processes and the determination of the pathological states and injuries that have led directly or indirectly to the death. In the case of hospital autopsies, most of the disease processes and the cause of death will be known in advance. The main goal of the hospital autopsy is focused on determining the extent of the disease process and the effects of treatments provided in life. At the same time as investigating the death, the physical autopsy provides an opportunity for the collection of education material for medical teaching and research. These autopsies require that consent for the procedure is given by those having legal control of the body and who in turn must ensure – in some jurisdictions – that relatives do not object. In practice these requirements are met by obtaining the consent of the next of kin. In contrast to this, a medico-legal autopsy can be performed on the instructions of the coroner and without consent being obtained from the next of kin. This situation applies in the case of autopsies that are conducted principally to identify the deceased. There are instances where the next of kin or other relatives can object to a coroner ordering an autopsy, but these are rarely applicable where the identity of the deceased is unknown.

Prior to the examination of a body at a mortuary, the pathologist may have already carried out a superficial examination of the body in the place in which it was found. This is most likely to occur where the identity of the body is unknown and where the death appears to be suspicious. The scope of examination of a body at the scene of death depends on the circumstances, but in most cases some initial information can be gathered from the position of the body, the presence or absence of rigor mortis or post-mortem hypostatic lividity (discolouration of the skin) and the temperature of the body. A body that is fully clothed or otherwise wrapped and partly concealed may be difficult to examine adequately at the scene, and no definitive conclusions regarding identity of the deceased or the nature of the death should be made until the body has been examined fully at autopsy and the necessary follow-up tests have been completed.

The next process involved in an autopsy is the retrieval and evaluation of information relating to the deceased, including the past medical and dental history of individuals who are missing and may be the deceased. The collection of ante-mortem records is a specific phase in the processes involved in disaster victim identification (DVI), and most coroner and medical examiner jurisdictions will have protocols for this procedure. Mass disaster involving loss of life can be conveniently divided into two types: open disasters and closed disasters. Open disasters refer to the situation where there is no record of the names of the individuals who may have been killed: an example of such a situation might be a major train crash. Anyone in the community might be on a particular train and it is not until friends and relatives report them missing that the investigators have an idea of who the deceased might be. In a closed disaster there is a record of all people who might be involved. An example of a closed disaster might be a plane crash where a list of passengers is immediately available from the airline. Clearly the task of identifying individuals involved in a closed disaster is much simpler as the ante-mortem investigation team know where to go to get their information. This ante-mortem information may include family and personal details, such as information regarding their last known activities as well as background information on, for example, their work history, clothing and personal effects and family background. Medical details such as previous radiological examinations, drug history and previous surgical or dental procedures are also important. While in many cases police investigators provide this information, it is often important for the pathologist and odontologist to be able to request particular information from or speak to any dental or medical practitioners who have been involved with these suspected individuals prior to death. The ante-mortem information collected should include actual medical and dental practitioners' files as well as photographs and radiographs of the suspected individuals taken in life.

Before the deceased's body is physically examined for identification purposes, it is necessary to carry out a number of preliminary investigations. This may involve the taking of specialist radiographs, blood tests for infectious diseases and or photographs. Where the body is not too severely damaged the deceased may have their fingerprints recorded or an attempt may be made to have them visually identified by a friend or a member of their family. These preliminary matters may take some time to complete before the physical autopsy can be commenced, and coordination of the whole process is essential at this time.

Post-mortem changes in the deceased

Post-mortem changes are inevitable and vary depending on a number of intrinsic and extrinsic factors. It is therefore not possible to accurately estimate the time of death, but rather use the concept of a 'window of death'. Initially this will be the time between the last known time the person was alive and the time the person was declared dead. Post-mortem changes can be divided into early post-mortem changes, decomposition and skeletalisation.

Early post-mortem changes (algor mortis, livor mortis and rigor mortis) are generally considered to be those occurring in the first 24 hours following death.
- *Algor mortis* is the cooling of a body following death. Usually this involves cooling to the temperature of the immediate environment, but can result in warming in situations where the ambient temperature is greater than that of the deceased. Environmental factors affecting the rate of cooling include fluctuations in the ambient temperature, circulating air, dampness or water immersion. An elevated or reduced body temperature at the time of death will also have an influence. This is influenced by medical factors, for example the presence of infection, thyroid disease, overall health and medications, and also by physical exertion (exercise or struggle during violent confrontation) at the time of death.
- *Livor mortis* is the settling of blood due to gravity following cessation of the circulation at the time of death. It is visible on the external skin as pink or purple discolouration, but will not occur in regions where external pressure initially results in blanching and blood is pushed away from the region. Initial visible changes can occur within about 20 minutes and after 8 to 12 hours the colour becomes a deeper purple and fixed, that is no longer blanches if pressure is applied. Temperature will influence the rate at which livor mortis becomes

fixed. Other influences are the natural skin colour and medical conditions, such as anaemia. The evaluation of livor mortis includes assessment of its location in relation to the position of the body, colour and colour intensity, and whether it is blanching or is fixed.

- *Rigor mortis* is the stiffening of the body after death due to the chemical reaction in skeletal muscle fibres. The fibres do not contract during this process, which commences and may be noticeable 30 minutes after death and reaches a maximum approximately 12 hours later. After 24 hours the skeletal muscle fibres break down and the rigidity is lost, although the process may take several days.

Decomposition

The two main components of decomposition are autolysis and putrefaction. The former is tissue and cellular breakdown as a result of the body's own enzymatic action. The latter involves breakdown by microorganisms. The skin acts as a barrier to putrefaction, so any breach in the skin allows entry of microorganisms into the body and therefore hastens putrefaction. Both autolysis and putrefaction are influenced by temperature. After the early changes described above, decomposition produces visible changes including darkening of the skin, blistering and skin slippage. Gas accumulation is evident by abdominal distension and bloating of the scrotum. Decomposition fluids, reddish in colour, purge from the nose and mouth. Insect activity will hasten the process, which is environmentally dependent. Mummification will occur in a dry environment with low humidity. Darkening and hardening of the skin occurs followed by cracking, flaking and eventually loss of skin and soft tissues leading to skeletonisation.

Radiological examination

Radiographic studies play an important part in the forensic autopsy and are particularly relevant in cases where the identity of the deceased is unknown. Comparison of post-mortem radiographs with clinical radiographs taken in life can result in identity being established with a very high degree of certainty. The shape of the frontal sinuses and dental structures are highly individual features and make post-mortem radiography of the head almost mandatory in autopsies on unknown individuals. It is important to coordinate the radiological examination with the remainder of the autopsy procedures in order to minimise the risk that one process will interfere with another. For example, if the head is first opened with a saw, later radiographs of the frontal sinuses of the skull will be much more difficult to interpret. Similarly, the process of embalming a body may cause artefactual trauma and introduce air and fluids into body cavities, changing the radiological appearance.

While standard radiological views of the head are of value in any exploration of head and neck trauma and identification procedures, today CT scanning has replaced many of the plain film radiographs used in the past. While the resolution of CT is not as high as plain film radiographs, such that fine trabecular bone structure may be lost, they provide a far simpler means of obtaining an image that can be reconfigured electronically to give both surface projections from any angle and transverse planes through any internal structure from any angle. This makes comparison with radiographs taken in life easier as the post-mortem radiographic dataset can be repositioned to represent the view of the radiograph obtained in life.

External examination

The first stage of the physical examination of a body involves a detailed inspection of the outer surface of the body prior to removal of clothing, jewellery and any other wrappings from the body. Each of the items on the body is then carefully removed and further examined for damage, stains and foreign material. The clothing and any possessions are photographed and collected in such a way that they are preserved and protected from further contamination. For forensic and evidential purposes, all items removed from the body must be documented including being described and photographed before being collected in a controlled, safe and secure manner for later possible forensic examination. Among other procedures this involves labelling and logging of specimens in such a way that a continuous chain of custody of the item is maintained from the time of its collection until its appearance in court as an exhibit. Following the removal and collection of surface material the body is inspected and the external surface of each region of the body is systematically examined with photography and descriptions of features that might be of value for identification, such as tattoos, piercings, hair characteristics, scars and other personal attributes. In doing this great care must be taken not to lose any trace evidence that may be trapped in hair, between fingers, in the ears, nose or mouth or adhering to the surface of the skin.

A record of the basic morphometric features of the body is an essential element of all autopsies. While measurements of a body are difficult to obtain with a high degree of precision, it is important at least to record some basic features of body size at autopsy. In routine cases this may simply take the form of measurements of height and weight. Height, or crown–heel length, is only one of a variety of morphometric values that can be determined from a body. Prior to the introduction of fingerprinting the system of 'Bertillionage', a system of human identification based on detailed measurements of the body, was used. The use of multiple anthropomorphic measurements as a technique for identification is of only historical importance today, but isolated measurements can still be of value in distinguishing among individuals within a small set. For example, shoe size may be useful.

In some autopsies additional measurements will need to be made. Autopsies of children and infants often require more detailed morphometric measurements; these may include head circumference, crown–rump length, crown–heel length, foot length, pubis–heel length, and chest and abdominal circumference. Such measurements can assist in determining whether the child's physical maturity is consistent with his or her stated age. In addition, detailed measurements of this type can assist in the identification of subtle forms of congenital abnormality involving body shape and form. Individual measurements of other structures including the ears and eyes may also be required. In some cases it may be necessary to measure the length of limbs in order to ascertain how far the individual could reach. This may be of importance in cases of alleged suicidal shooting, to assess the person's ability to pull the trigger of a particular firearm discharged at a specific range.

In the case of skeletal remains, morphometric assessment of key portions of the skeleton are relevant for anthropological assessment of race, sex, height and age. A variety of specialised anatomical equipment is available for measurement of skeletal remains and the use of such standard equipment allows consistent comparisons to be made among different bones and different skeletons.

Head

The head is usually the first external surface of the body that is examined in detail. The eyes, ears, mouth and nose are examined, together with the adjacent skin. This initial stage of the external examination of the head is very similar to the general external medical examination performed on the living; indeed, similar medical and dental equipment can be used. For example, auroscopes may be of use in examining the nose and the mouth as well as the ears, and ophthalmoscopes may be used to examine the eyes if the cornea is not opaque. The ordinary characteristics of faces with which we are all familiar should be noted. These include features such as eye and hair colour, skin pigmentation, facial hair and shape of ears, nose and lips. In addition to the appearance of hairstyle, length and colouring (both natural and artificial), the distribution and type of cosmetics on the face should be described. Evidence of previous medical treatment and injuries including scars, as well as marks such as tattoos, must also be noted, as these can assist with confirming identification as well as corroborating other information from medical records or witness statements.

In the case of a forensic autopsy where there is a suspicion of homicide, special attention is given to the classification and recording of head and facial injuries. Detailed injury descriptions are crucial if the pathologist is to assist with reconstructing the circumstances surrounding the death and effectively present such evidence in court. In this respect the use of charts, diagrams and/or photographs to record the observations and findings is essential.

During the external examination of the head, great care must be taken not to lose trace evidence that may be present in the external ears, nose and mouth, or in the hair. Such material may be foreign to the body. For example, the tissue may have come from the offender, in which case molecular biology techniques may permit their identification. Subsequent clinical examination of the offender may identify an injury from which tissue has been lost, which is complementary to the foreign tissue identified on the victim. Alternative trace evidence may comprise the body's own tissues, such as fragments of bone or teeth. Where the body is grossly decomposed, every care should be taken to ensure that easily detached structures such as teeth are not lost from the body during handling and transportation. In the case of badly burnt remains, the skeletal tissues themselves may become carbonised. In this state the bony and dental hard tissue remains may be extremely friable and brittle; as a result they may need to be stabilised with resins, glues and or waxes [1] before the body remains are handled and transported.

Trunk

The surface of the trunk includes the front, sides and back of the chest, the abdomen, the loins or sides of the abdomen, the small of the back, the region of the shoulders, and the buttocks. Identifying features such as scars or other skin characteristics may be noted on the trunk. Distortions of the chest and features such as distension of the abdomen may provide useful information regarding the possibility of internal trauma or disease. Perineal, anal and genital examination must be carefully performed, especially in cases where there is any suspicion of sexual assault. These examinations may be further assisted by the inclusion of a forensic physician in the autopsy team.

Limbs

The hands and feet may show anatomical characteristics acquired as a result of particular occupations. The loss of digits can be useful as an identifying characteristic. Examination of the nails may provide information about underlying disease as well as the level of personal care and hygiene. Injuries to the limbs may provide important information regarding the circumstances in which trauma occurred, allowing inferences to be drawn regarding whether an injury occurred accidentally, as the result of the person defending himself or herself against violence, or as the result of the person inflicting violence.

Documentation of rigor mortis (the stiffening of muscles after death) and livor mortis (the discolouration of the skin caused by the settling of the blood in dependent blood vessels after death) are also important. These features can occasionally be used to provide a very general estimation of the time of death, and in the case of livor mortis may provide information on the position of the body after death and whether it has been moved or interfered with. In the case of bodies showing advanced decomposition, however, some of these features may not easily be identified.

Many areas of the body are more difficult to examine at autopsy and may be omitted by clinical pathologists unfamiliar with forensic practice or by inexperienced forensic pathologists. Such areas can include:

- the palate and cheek mucosa;
- the tonsilar fossa and nasopharynx;
- the external auditory canals;
- the axillae (underarms);
- the skin between the fingers;
- the area beneath the female breasts;
- the skin of the umbilicus;
- the ventral aspects of the penis;
- the posterior aspect of the scrotum;
- the popliteal fossae (back of knees);
- the heels;
- the skin between the toes;
- the skin surface of the scalp (by removing or methodically parting the hair);
- the skin behind the ears;
- the back of the trunk;
- the skin between the buttocks;
- the skin of the anal canal;
- the perineum;
- the medial aspects of the labia majora; and
- the labia minora, introitus, hymen, clitoris and lower vagina.

Internal examination

On completion of the external examination, an internal examination is carried out. This part of the autopsy involves a systematic examination of the organs and tissues found within the body cavities and the solid tissues forming the musculoskeletal system. These cavities include the cranial, thoracic and abdominal cavities, but in addition areas such as the head, the face, the neck, the spine, the limbs, the pelvis and the genitalia are also examined. Not only are the major organs from these cavities examined but also the walls of the cavities themselves, which are assessed for characteristic features and signs of disease.

The visual inspection of body organs is only one part of the internal autopsy. The alterations to body tissues caused by some diseases can only be seen with a microscope. In other cases a disease will be visible first as a microscopic change to the body tissues that precedes changes to the 'naked eye' appearance of the relevant body organ. An example of the latter can be seen in the case of myocardial infarction, one of the pathological processes that can cause or constitute part of a heart attack. This pathology occurs when parts of the heart muscle die as a result of a lack of adequate blood supply. It may take several days following such an infarct for the dead areas of heart muscle to become visible to the 'naked eye'. As a result, if the patient dies at the time of the infarct or a few hours later, the macroscopic examination of the heart muscle may reveal nothing. The microscopic signs of such damage to the heart muscle are visible much earlier (in the case of electron microscopy examination, after a matter of hours), and therefore it is essential that the heart muscle be examined under the microscope. In practice the only way to ensure that these issues are covered is to perform routine microscopy on all body tissues. Of course, it is logistically impossible to examine all of each tissue microscopically, but adequate sampling can achieve the best possible pathology detection rate.

With some body organs, macroscopic examination at the time of the physical autopsy is particularly difficult. Organs such as the brain and the spinal cord are so soft and fragile that they may be damaged and distorted by the process of dissection and tissue sampling. In these cases it is often necessary to process the organs by 'fixing' them for days or weeks in a preservative solution, to make them rigid and robust enough to permit detailed dissection and examination. In the case of brain diseases or trauma to the brain, such a process is generally advisable, although there are exceptional circumstances when dissection can be performed without fixation. These considerations are also applicable to other body organs in particular circumstances of disease, and it may be necessary to retain such organs during the physical autopsy and 'fix' them for further examination.

As well as demonstrating the presence of disease or injury, the autopsy can reveal the extent and severity of disease and some of the effects of treatments that may have been provided. However, many disorders are the result of functional disturbances of body systems that involve abnormalities of vital responses. Unless these abnormal responses have caused macroscopic or microscopic structural changes in the body tissues, they will not necessarily be detected by the routine physical autopsy. The same is true of deaths due to some drugs and poisons. Although such chemicals can cause visible alterations to body organs, in many cases the changes are non-specific and particular toxicological tests will have to be performed on tissues and fluids collected from the body in order to identify the chemicals involved.

The face, head and neck

There is probably no more sensitive area of human dissection during the autopsy than the human face and head. In interacting with each other during everyday life it is faces that we see, react to and relate to. Where physical injury has occurred, the area of injury that most people fear the most is disfiguring injury to the face; as a result, there is great sensitivity about the face being interfered with during an autopsy.

The internal examination of the head and neck of a body is of particular importance in medico-legal autopsies since a number of natural diseases causing sudden death can be found within the brain. In addition, head injury is one of the major forms of fatal trauma. Assessment of head injury can provide considerable information about the circumstances in which the injury and death occurred.

The examination of the face, head and neck at autopsy may be performed in a variety of ways. In practice, the method chosen will depend to a large extent on the existence of any identification issues that need to be addressed, the nature of any suspected head and neck trauma or disease, and the state of the human remains (burnt, decomposed, traumatised, or skeletonised). For example, where there are problems with identification, the choice of autopsy technique will depend on the particular comparison that is to be employed. For dental identification, techniques such as oral photography, jaw radiography, exposure of the oral cavity, dental impressions and/or excision of the jaws might be employed; these require their own particular dissection processes.

Dissection of the face is not an uncommon procedure during autopsy. It is required in many death investigations – particularly in those where facial injury has occurred. At first glance it may be thought that dissection of the face will be associated with permanent disfigurement: change in the visible identifying characteristics of the face. In practice such a degree of disfigurement of the face is rarely the result of autopsy dissection. In situations where complaints are made that the face has been altered as a result of the autopsy, examination of the allegation usually reveals that there was prior facial damage and disfigurement before the autopsy commenced. It is often the case that the family will not have seen the body of the deceased prior to a medico-legal autopsy. As a result they can confuse the effects of the autopsy procedure with injuries that the deceased suffered prior to death.

In the clinical autopsy it may be necessary to dissect the soft tissues of the face in order to identify pathology in salivary glands, muscle and other soft tissue. Skin pathology may also need to be explored. Where skin tumours have invaded the deeper structures, facial dissection may be required in order to determine the extent of their spread. Examination of the structures within the lining of the mouth including the tongue, the nose, the nasopharynx and the oropharynx will also require a degree of facial dissection. In the forensic autopsy, soft tissue dissection of the face may be required in order to identify areas of trauma. Again oral structures may need to be dissected and the region of the lips, the nose and the eyes may require specific examination. Given the nature of forensic casework and the fact that injuries to the face are a common feature of the pattern of trauma seen in interpersonal violence, the forensic autopsy often requires an examination of the subcutaneous tissues of the face in order to identify areas of bruising that may be markers of areas of externally applied force to the head.

In addition to soft tissue dissection, examination of the bony tissues of the face may be required. Again in the clinical autopsy, pathology in the overlying soft tissues may have spread to involve the underlying bony tissues of the face.

Specific areas of the facial skeleton may need to be dissected in some detail. Bone tumours involving the skull, including the dental structures, may require removal of portions of bone in order to determine the extent of the disease. Specific structures such as the sinuses and the deeper regions of the nose and orbits require special dissection techniques. In the forensic autopsy it may be necessary to examine the bony tissues of the face in order to determine the extent and nature of trauma to the face. Fine fractures of the facial skeleton may be difficult to determine on x-ray. For this reason facial dissection should be carried out in all autopsies where the deceased has suffered a facial injury.

Gross trauma to the facial skeletal structures is a feature of many forensic autopsy subjects. Firearm injuries to the face are particularly destructive of the facial skeleton and the exploration of these injuries can involve the dissection and removal of large portions of the mandible and the maxilla.

In order to expose the facial structures adequately, it is essential that the body be opened in the correct fashion. Traditionally the opening of the head initially involves opening the scalp. This is usually accomplished by an incision that extends in the coronal plane over the top of the head just posterior to the vertex and extending down on each side of the head to just behind each external ear. Prior to making this incision in the head, it is important to ensure that the hair is first parted forwards and backwards on each side of the line of the incision. If this is done the sutures from the eventual closure of this incision will be covered by the hair of the deceased when it is combed back.

When the scalp is being dissected forwards and backwards on either side of this incision, it is important to examine the soft tissue of the scalp and the under-lying cranial vault. Haemorrhage in the deep scalp can be associated with blunt force injuries to the head, underlying skull fractures and hair avulsion trauma (particularly in infants). Following exposure of the vertex of the skull, the temporalis muscle over the temporal bone must be cleanly cut free from the surface of the skull. In a routine autopsy the cranial vault would then be opened using a handsaw or oscillating orthopaedic or plaster saw. The cuts in the bone are made over the front of the mid-forehead approximately two centimetres above the supra-orbital ridges. This saw cut in the bone is continued on either side, across the frontal bone and into the posterior portion of the temporal bone. The direction of the saw cut is then changed to a superior orientation so that the saw passes through the parietal bone on either side of the head at the posterior. The saw cut should cross the posterior of the skull vault just above the occipital bone in the midline. The removal of the brain will not be described further here. However, it should be noted that it would sometimes assist in the subsequent facial dissection if the brain has been previously removed from the cranial cavity. This opening of the cranial vault prior to facial dissection is not always appropriate, and where multiple facial fractures are present in conjunction with cranial vault fractures, it may be useful to leave the skull unopened, at least during the initial phases of the facial dissection.

It is usually not possible to dissect the face without including the neck and the region of the thoracic inlet as part of the general dissection field. There has been considerable debate regarding the skin incision needed for best exposure of the structures of the upper chest, neck and lower face. Various incisions have been suggested for this procedure. These include a single mainline incision extending from the midline of the neck in the front over the larynx down to the pubis, and a wide yoke incision that extends over the front of the shoulders crossing the midline in the upper part of the chest. Where a detailed facial dissection is to be performed, these methods of opening the trunk of the body are not suitable; instead the best incision is one that begins behind each ear and passes down the postero-lateral part of the neck on each side before moving anteriorly to pass just below the supraclavicular fossae on each side and then medially to join in the midline of the upper chest. It is important to ensure that the incision runs in the posterior part of the neck on each side and only moves to the front once it has reached the top of the shoulders where they join the neck. If this is done, the incision will not usually be apparent to family and friends who wish to view the front of the body after autopsy. However, if the incision is made too far back on the neck and extends too far onto the front of the upper chest, the amount of skin forming the neck flap will be excessive and will make the subsequent facial dissection more difficult.

In order to expose the lower part of the face, it is necessary to dissect the skin flap formed by the meeting of the incisions in the skin on each side of the neck that have originated from behind the ears. This dissection exposes the tissues at the front of the neck. If the thoracic organs have been removed prior to the neck dissection, the amount of bleeding that will occur during dissection of the anterior neck structures will be reduced. The removal of the thoracic organs in this way involves separating them from the anterior neck structures at the level of the thoracic inlet. Care should be taken in reflecting the anterior neck flap upward towards the mandible. In many forensic autopsies it is necessary to examine the structures of the anterior neck to look for signs of neck compression. This will involve examining the layers of soft tissue at the front of the neck and cutting free each of the strap muscles on either side of, and at the front of, the larynx.

Once this anterior neck dissection is complete, the neck skin flap can be dissected up over the outer surface of the mandible and the underlying neck structures, including the tongue and floor of mouth, can be removed. The removal of the tongue and the larynx at this time is not essential. However, if it is important to examine the palate prior to the upper facial dissection, removal of the tissues of the floor of the mouth will facilitate this. In order to complete the examination of the external surface of the mandible, particularly in its posterior and lateral parts, it is necessary to extend the lateral neck skin incisions so that they join with the coronal incision in the scalp over the vertex of the head. It is useful to mark where these incisions join so that the anterior and posterior skin flaps can be correctly aligned with each other during facial reconstruction.

Once the natural skin incisions in the neck have been joined with the scalp incision, it is possible to bring forward the lateral edges of the facial skin flap that has been formed. This involves cutting through the external auditory meatus on each side and dissecting the skin and muscle free from the lateral or external surface of the mandible. Again, if assessment of soft tissue injury is relevant, then it is important to carry out this dissection in layers. It must be remembered that there are no deep fascia in the face. The facial muscles insert directly into the skin; as a result, cutting the musculature free from the overlying subcutaneous tissues can be difficult.

The incision across the top of the scalp allows the two skin flaps to be made, one of which can be dissected forwards over the forehead and to the level of the roof of the orbits. If required, this skin flap can be extended across the bridge of the nose and around the lateral borders of the orbits. If this anterior dissection is accompanied by anterior dissection of the neck and face skin flap, the whole of the facial skeleton can be exposed with the facial skin held in place by the tip of the nose. Some pathologists carry out this form of complete facial dissection in most of their autopsies. Other pathologists only carry out this dissection when they wish to assess the degree and nature of facial injury or disease processes affecting the facial skeleton, the skin of the face and other associated deep soft tissue structures.

The posterior skin flap of the scalp can be dissected from behind, over the occiput at the back of the skull, and on to expose the upper part of the neck at the back. Again, if the lateral aspects of the neck flap are also dissected posteriorly, the area behind the ears can also be exposed and access to the cervical spine provided.

To gain access to the brain, the skull must be opened. This is usually performed using a vibrating saw. A horizontal saw cut is made across the midpart of the forehead region of the skull; this is extended into the temporal region on both sides. From this point, the saw cut is angled upwards on each side to pass across the top of the head in the posteriorly parietal and high occipital region. This cut across the top of the skull must be made well posterior to the skin incision across the top of the scalp.

With the skull opened, the free portion of bone often referred to as the skullcap can be lifted free from the head, exposing the dura mater, the thick fibrous membrane that adheres to the under-surface of the skull that covers the brain. Haemorrhages outside the dura are referred to as extradural haemorrhages; they are usually the result of trauma involving a fracture of the skull. It is important to assess the size of any such haemorrhages and to note their location. The upper part of the dura can now be excised along the line of the bone cut made in the skull. This exposes the arachnoid mater, the thin membrane surrounding the brain. The presence, nature and size of any subdural haemorrhages should be noted. It may be necessary to collect any subdural blood clot to assess its volume more accurately and to take portions of the blood clot for histological examination to assist in determining its age.

The brain is removed by gently lifting the frontal lobes free from the anterior fossa, or the floor of the skull at the front above the eyes. By lifting the frontal lobes, the anterior cranial nerves and internal carotid arteries can be severed, the temporal poles can then be lifted and the tentorium cerebelli severed laterally and posteriorly on both sides. Finally the upper portion of the cervical spinal cord can be cut, along with the upper part of the vertebral arteries just above the foramen magnum. This frees the brain from the floor of the skull, allowing it to be removed from the body.

The brain is examined either in its fresh state or following fixation in formalin. The examination of the brain is a specialised procedure. In the case of the fixed specimen, it may take considerable time. The blood vessels at the base of the brain are examined for any congenital defects, such as aneurysms, and to see if there are any areas of substantive blockage by atheroma. The cranial nerves are examined as they emerge from the brain and the surface of all portions of the brain is inspected. The hind brain – comprising the cerebellum, pons, and medulla – is then removed and sliced to display any internal pathology. The cerebral hemispheres are also sliced at approximately 1-centimetre intervals from front to back in the coronal plane. In the case of fixed brains, the cerebral hemispheres are often first cut in the coronal plane in their midpart, dividing them into an anterior and a posterior half prior to serial slicing. Once the external and internal surfaces of the brain have been examined, small blocks of tissue are collected from different regions of the brain for histological examination. A number of other methods of dissecting the brain are described in neuropathological texts. The exact approach taken will depend on the nature of the suspected pathology and the personal preference of the pathologist.

Once the brain has been removed from the skull, it is possible to examine the floor of the skull in detail. The pituitary gland is removed and sectioned for histological examination. The course of the internal carotid artery can be explored on each side, as can the course of cranial nerves through the floor of the skull. The venous sinuses within the dura can be opened and examined for thrombi. The middle ear cavities can be opened and examined for haemorrhage or signs of infection.

The examination of the internal structures of the neck is another area of the forensic autopsy that requires particular attention. This is because pressure on the neck can occur in circumstances of violence resulting in death. It is best to examine the internal neck structures once the brain has been removed from the cranial cavity, as this allows blood to drain more freely from the neck structures before they are dissected. The strap muscles that support the head anteriorly and laterally should be severed at their lower ends and individually dissected superiorly, so as to examine each muscle and the tissue planes between the muscles for evidence of bruising or haemorrhage. This can be performed with the anterior neck structures in situ or following their removal from the body as a discrete block of tissue that includes the tongue, the floor of the mouth, the larynx, the upper trachea, the thyroid gland, the neck vessels and the strap muscles. Following examination of the strap muscles, the thyroid gland can be removed and the structures of the larynx dissected free of soft tissue, so that any fractures or breaks in the cartilage and bone making up the laryngeal skeleton can be revealed. The thyroid gland should be sliced to determine whether there is any internal pathology within the gland and a sample collected for histological analysis. The presence of haemorrhage in soft tissue surrounding breaks in the thyroid cartilage or hyoid bone can help in determining whether the injury occurred in life rather than after death. The vascular structures, including the carotid arteries and the jugular vein on each side of the neck, should be examined for trauma and natural disease. In some autopsies it may be necessary to remove the cervical spine in order to examine the vertebral arteries that lie within the lateral parts of the cervical vertebrae. These structures can be damaged as a result of blunt trauma and rotational injuries to the neck and head, resulting in subarachnoid haemorrhage and death. Finally, the tongue should be examined for signs of injury or disease. Bite injuries to the tongue can occur in a variety of situations, including facial trauma or epileptic seizures.

The post-cranial aspect of the autopsy is covered in lesser detail here, and other texts that cover further details are given in the recommended readings at the end of the chapter.

The thorax

The thorax and abdomen are opened by a common incision that runs from the base of the neck anteriorly to just above the pubis. The upper end of the incision is divided into two at the base of the neck and then extends, as described above, either to the shoulder tips or to the area behind the ears. The skin over the chest wall is then dissected back from the midline incision to each side of the chest. The skin is dissected in the subcutaneous plane in the deepest part of the adipose tissue, the fatty layer beneath the skin. This allows any bruising that may be present in the subcutaneous fat to be revealed. Such bruising may not appear on the outer surface of the skin and, if the subcutaneous tissue is not dissected, such bruises may be missed. Following the folding back of the skin of the front of the chest, the tissue comprising the area beneath the breasts is examined for any breast pathology. The muscle layers between the skin and the chest wall – the pectoral muscles – should also be dissected back to reveal the ribs and sternum.

The front of the chest wall is then removed by cutting through the ribs on each side of the front of the chest. In young individuals, because the medial ends of the ribs are composed of cartilage, it is possible to cut through the soft cartilaginous tissue with a scalpel. In older individuals, it may be necessary to use shears or a saw to cut through the ribs. The sternum and anterior medial ribs are then removed en bloc by cutting through the diaphragm below and freeing the underside of the sternum from the soft tissues of the mediastinum.

The contents of the thoracic cavity (the heart, lungs, trachea, oesophagus and aorta) are then removed from the chest cavity to be examined in detail. If the anterior neck structures have not yet been removed, these are now removed as part of the thoracic organ block of tissue. The oesophagus is opened from the back and removed. The windpipe or trachea is then opened from the back and its lining and any contents examined. At this point it is usually convenient to open the descending thoracic aorta from behind, following which the block of organs can be turned over and examined from the front.

The pericardium or sac around the heart is then opened and any defects in the sac described. The surface of the heart is now examined and any visible abnormalities including congenital anomalies recorded. If there has been ischaemic damage of the heart, there may be scarring visible over the surface of the heart, or if the ischaemic damage is more recent and the individual has suffered a recent myocardial infarction, there may be haemorrhagic reddening of the heart muscle. Prior to removal of the heart, it is prudent for the pathologist to open the superior vena cava and the main pulmonary trunk and arteries to examine their lumena for evidence of thrombosis or foreign material. If a pulmonary thromboembolus is found within the pulmonary trunk, this would be sufficient to account for an otherwise unexpected death and would raise the possibility that the deep veins in the lower half of the body may contain thrombus.

The heart is now removed from the block of thoracic organs and its chambers opened. When all the blood has been removed from the cavities within the heart, the organ can be weighed. The coronary arteries that supply blood to the heart are examined for the presence and degree of any atherosclerosis. If significant occlusion of coronary arteries is found, this may represent significant pathology capable of causing sudden death. The area in which the occlusion of the coronary arteries is found is important, as it may indicate which regions of the heart may have been starved of blood and as a consequence may have suffered significant ischaemic damage. The lining of the cardiac chambers should be examined for the presence of any vegetations or adherent thrombus. Similarly the configuration and surfaces of the cardiac valves must be examined for any abnormalities. Vegetations on the surface of the valves or on the linings of the cardiac chambers may be found in association with cardiac abnormalities; some of these vegetations will contain clumps of bacteria, which can slowly destroy the adjacent cardiac structures, a condition known as subacute bacterial endocarditis. The thickness of the walls of the ventricles should be assessed and any abnormality of the muscle of the heart described. Fibrosis or scarring within the heart muscle can lead to problems with cardiac rhythm and be associated with sudden and unexpected death. Problems with cardiac rhythm are not always associated with macroscopic pathology within the heart muscle and it is sometimes necessary to carry out detailed microscopic examination of the areas within the heart muscle that are responsible for the generation and conduction of the electrical impulses that cause the heart to beat. In all cases, however, it is necessary to take samples of the heart muscle for examination under the microscope. Such examination can reveal the presence of previous episodes of ischaemia as well as any old or recent inflammation of the heart muscle.

The lungs are now removed from the mediastinum, weighed, and their configuration described. The outer surface of the lungs is examined and the pulmonary arteries and airways that branch throughout the lungs dissected. Finally, the parenchyma of the lung is serially sliced in order to identify whether there is any significant pathology present such as infection, infarction or tumour.

The abdomen and pelvis

Following the dissection of the subcutaneous tissue, the abdominal musculature is incised in the midline and folded back on each side. The presence of any inflammation of the lining of the abdomen (peritonitis) should now be noted and the quantity and nature of any significant collection of fluid within the abdominal cavity recorded. The position of the contents of the abdominal cavity should be noted and the presence of any surgical modifications described. The major part of the bowel comprising the jejunum, ileum and colon should now be removed. Again it is prudent to tie ligatures around the bowel prior to severing it so as to prevent leakage of bowel contents into the abdominal cavity. The removed bowel should be opened in its entirety and its lining and contents examined.

The organs in the upper part of the abdominal cavity – the liver, spleen, stomach, pancreas and duodenum – can now be removed as a block of tissue. The spleen can be removed from the block, weighed and dissected. The liver can also be dissected free from the block of tissue and the connecting structures of bile ducts and blood vessels opened and examined. The gall bladder is opened and any gallstones described. The liver is weighed and serially sliced so that its external and internal surfaces can be described. Discolourations of the liver tissue can be associated with a variety of pathological conditions including toxic damage. The stomach should be opened and any gastric contents collected for potential toxicological analysis. The lining of the stomach should be examined for the presence of ulceration or tumour. The opening in the stomach is continued into the duodenum, which is similarly examined. Finally, the pancreas is examined for the presence of any tumour, haemorrhage or inflammation.

With the removal of the organs lying within the upper part of the abdominal cavity, the retroperitoneal tissues can be examined and the kidneys and abdominal aorta removed in continuity, together with the contents of the pelvis including the bladder, the remainder of the rectum and, in the case of a female, the internal genitalia (the uterus, fallopian tubes and ovaries). The kidneys are removed, weighed and cut open so that the parenchyma of the renal cortex and medulla can be examined. The capsule of the kidneys is dissected free from the surface of the kidney, which is then examined in detail. The urine collection system of the renal pelves, including the calyces and ureters, are then opened and their linings examined. Inflammation of the lining of the ureters may indicate a urinary tract infection. The bladder is opened and its lining examined in a similar fashion to the examination of the ureters.

The genitalia

The examination of the female internal genitalia is often performed with the structures attached to the block of tissue containing the kidneys and abdominal aorta. It is important to examine the lining of the uterus macroscopically and microscopically for any evidence of a pregnancy. The ovaries and fallopian tubes should be dissected and samples taken for microscopic examination.

In the male, the prostate gland around the urethra at the base of the bladder should be removed and, if enlarged, weighed. The gland should be sliced and portions of the glands, together with any abnormal areas, sampled for histological examination.

The limbs

Detailed internal dissection of the limbs is not usually performed in a routine autopsy. However, there are a number of situations where it is appropriate to examine the subcutaneous tissues of the limbs for the presence of hidden injuries, such as bruises, not visible externally. The position of such bruises may provide valuable information regarding the circumstances in which injuries may have been inflicted. For example, bruising to the back of the knuckles may occur where the person has thrown punches, and bruising to the outer aspects of the forearms may occur where the person has attempted to defend himself or herself from physical blows to the face. It is often necessary to dissect the front of the elbows and to examine the veins in this area for evidence of recent intravenous injection sites. Where a pulmonary thromboembolism has been found during the autopsy, it is usually necessary to dissect the calf veins of the lower legs to ascertain whether any thrombus is present.

Post-autopsy procedures

At the completion of the autopsy, tissue samples should have been collected from most of the major parenchymal organs for microscopic examination. In addition, body fluids may have been collected for toxicological or microbiological analysis. The organs removed during the autopsy for detailed dissection must now be returned to the body cavities and replaced in such a way that there will be no possibility of leakage of fluids through the suture lines used to reconstruct the body. Any retention of organs should only occur where there is a specific medical or medico-legal need and permission has been obtained for this from the individuals or agencies having control of the body. This means that in medico-legal cases the coroner's approval needs to be sought.

The physical autopsy is not complete until the body of the deceased person has been restored to a state where the family as part of their funeral tradition can view it. The technical and scientific staff who are employed in assisting in this task are usually highly skilled and experienced. They are aware of the needs of the funeral industry and a number of them are also qualified embalmers. In all cases the aim is to restore the outward appearance of the deceased to that which they had before death. Where a death has resulted from severe trauma, specialised restorative techniques may be required to repair areas of the body damaged before the autopsy. Similarly, if large amounts of structurally significant tissue have been collected for investigation or for transplantation, such as the spinal column or the pelvis, more extensive restorative work will be required. In most cases relatively little restoration is required because the routine procedures employed in a standard autopsy are non-disfiguring.

Following the completion of the restoration and reconstruction of the body, it is washed, wrapped, and stored to await collection by the family's funeral director. However, even at this stage there are issues that have to be kept in mind. The body must be stored in a safe and secure environment. Unless the body is being stored for several weeks, it should not be allowed to become frozen but must be kept cold enough to delay significant decomposition. This can be more difficult to achieve than is often realised, since some deaths are associated with rapid onset and progression of decomposition even in otherwise ideal environments.

Injuries

The tissues of the body may be injured in a variety of ways. These include:
- mechanical energy effects;
- chemical energy effects;
- thermal energy effects;
- electrical energy effects; and
- ionising radiation energy effects.

These forms of energy can be applied directly to the body so as to cause injury. However, in many forensic situations, energy is applied to the body indirectly – often through everyday clothing or special protective clothing. These intervening materials may reduce the effect of a particular force on the body while allowing other forces to be transmitted completely. For example, the protective leather clothing worn by some motorcyclists can protect the surface of the body from abrasion injuries and minor penetrating injuries.

In forensic autopsies in settings of alleged homicide or major transport incidents, mechanical energy trauma is most commonly found.

Mechanical force can be applied to the whole body. The most common circumstance in which this occurs is in motor vehicle accidents where the body is subject to significant acceleration or deceleration injuries. A body that is ejected from a motor vehicle during a collision or thrown from a seat to another place within the vehicle is subject to very considerable injuries of this type. During rapid changes in acceleration, organs of the body will respond at different times and degrees. This can result in individual organs within the body being stretched beyond their elastic limits so that they become torn away from their connections to the rest of the body. Flexion and extension of the body during such acceleration and deceleration can also cause significant pressure changes within body cavities, resulting in different degrees of movement of individual organs; this can cause them to be separated or compressed together.

Mechanical forces delivered by moving blunt objects striking the body or a moving body striking a stationary blunt object will result in kinetic energy being delivered to the body tissues. The effect of such forces will depend on the nature of the object that delivers the force to the body, as well as the region of the body that is struck. A range of injuries may be caused by the application of mechanical blunt force. If the force moves across the surface of the skin at a tangent, superficial layers of skin may be scraped away, resulting in an abrasion or graze. Squeezing of skin and subcutaneous tissues by applied blunt force may rupture small blood vessels, leading to extravasation of blood and resulting in the appearance of bruising. If the blunt force is applied to the skin in a region of the body where there is closely positioned underlying bone, this skin may be squeezed between the object applying the force and the underlying bone with the result that the skin becomes torn or lacerated. A blunt object with a small contact surface that forcefully strikes the body may breach the skin and penetrate deeply into the underlying tissues, causing a laceration to the skin and irregular tears to underlying tissue.

Where the mechanical force is delivered to the surface of the skin by a sharp object such as a knife or shard of glass, the skin or underlying tissues may be severed or incised. The degree of incision damage to the body will depend on the nature of the incising object. A long, thin, sharp object delivered in a near perpendicular fashion may give rise to a deep penetrating stab wound, whereas if the object applies force to the skin in a tangential fashion across the surface a superficial incise wound may be caused.

Classification of injuries

Forensic pathologists put a considerable amount of time and effort into injury classification. Their approach may often be seen as pedantic by their clinical colleagues, who are usually more concerned with treating injuries than finding out how they were caused.

There are a variety of ways of classifying injuries, but there is a broad general agreement among forensic pathologists as to the meanings of the injury descriptions in common use. The correct classification of injuries increases the quality of communication between pathologists, so that one pathologist reading another pathologist's report understands the significance of the injuries described. The use of a limited set of terms increases certainty and reproducibility of observations. By avoiding injury terms that are often used by lay persons in an inexact fashion (for example, the word 'cut', which could mean a laceration or an incision), accuracy of examination is enhanced.

Perhaps the most important aspect of classification is the fact that different injuries imply different forms of causation – correctly describing an injury can provide a more accurate reconstruction of the events that led to the injury. Classifications are so closely linked to interpretation that pathologists may leap to an interpretation of how a wound occurred prior to classifying it. This is a dangerous course, as it is only by correctly identifying all features of a wound and arriving at an appropriate classification that an erroneous interpretation as to cause can be avoided.

There are a variety of ways of classifying wounds and the following classification is just one of many that can be found in standard forensic medical texts dealing with the interpretation of injuries in a medico-legal context [2]. It is important to remember that any classification is simply a way of drawing distinctions between different types of wounds. In practice wounds are often compound – that is, an admixture of several injury types together.

Abrasions

Abrasions are injuries that involve damage to the superficial layers of the skin. The word 'abrasion' comes from the Latin words 'ab', meaning 'from', and 'radere', meaning 'to scrape'. Strictly speaking, an abrasion should only injure the outermost layer of the skin, known as the epidermis. The epidermis consists of multiple layers of cells. These cells are produced at the base of the epidermis and migrate upwards towards the skin surface, where they die and their contents are replaced by keratin, which forms a waterproof barrier. The keratinised cells at the skin surface are continually shed from the body and replaced by cells migrating up from below. The epidermis does not contain any blood vessels, and as a result technically abrasions damaging this layer should not bleed. However, the dermis, which is situated immediately beneath the epidermis, does contain blood vessels. If the dermis is injured, bleeding will occur. The interface between the epidermis and the underlying dermis is not smooth and pegs of outward-pointing dermis interdigitate with pegs of inward-pointing epidermis. As a result, a superficial scraping injury to the epidermis may damage some of the outward-pointing dermal pegs. This can result in a particular pattern of bleeding that may be seen in deeper abrasions. This pattern features a punctate or spot-like quality in the area at the bottom of the abrasion, reflecting the small pegs of injured dermis that contain blood vessels.

Abrasions can be caused after death, when their characteristics may be somewhat different. Post-mortem abrasions rarely bleed despite their depth. Because of the loss of the waterproof layer of the skin, they rapidly dry out to give a hard, pale yellow–orange, parchment-like characteristic to the affected area. Even ante-mortem abrasions will eventually show such a parchment-like change as a result of the dermis drying out once it has been denuded of its water-resistant epidermis. Because of the surface bleeding or the underlying subcutaneous bruising that may have occurred in association with the ante-mortem injury, when the abrasion dries out after death it often takes on a purple/black appearance. From a lay perspective ante-mortem abrasions, when photographed or viewed some time after death, may take on the appearance of a more 'severe' type of injury as a result of this drying and darkening of the injured skin.

Lacerations

Lacerations are tears or splits in body tissues caused by the direct application of blunt force. They must be clearly distinguished from incisions, which are caused by the cutting action of a sharp instrument cleaving or severing the tissues. This is perhaps the best example of the importance of correctly classifying an injury, as the correct identification of a skin break as a laceration rather than an incision has particular significance in respect of causation. Unfortunately, the most common lay expression for injuries that completely breach the skin is 'a cut'. However, the word 'cut' should not be used in any forensic report, as it can be interpreted to mean either a laceration or an incision, and as a result information regarding causation is lost.

Distinguishing a linear laceration from a linear incision can be difficult in some regions of the body, particularly on the scalp. Close inspection of a laceration with the assistance of some magnification will usually reveal that the edges of the wound have a fine rim of abrasion and that what appears to the naked eye to be a clean sharp edge to the wound is in fact irregular under a low level of magnification. The mechanism causing the wound is a stretching process that exceeds the elastic limit of some of the skin tissues. However, not all of the tissues constituting the skin will necessarily break. Rigid tissues are more likely to tear than strong elastic tissues. Close inspection of the depth of a laceration will reveal a number of structures bridging the gap in the skin in its deeper parts; these are likely to be small blood vessels and nerves. Had the defect been caused by an incision of a sharp object, these fine bridging structures would have been severed as well.

Because a laceration is caused by the direct application of blunt force squeezing the skin and splitting it, any material present either on the surface of the skin or on the object applying the force can be driven into the depths of the wound. Such foreign material may include fibres from clothing, body hairs, splinters of wood, fragments of glass or paint, or fragments of plastic or metal. The examination of a laceration therefore should include detailed inspection of the depths of the wound in order to recover any such foreign material, which may be useful in identifying the object that caused the wound.

There is a subtype of laceration perhaps best described as a traction laceration. Such traction lacerations can occur within the mouth if sheer forces applied to the lips tear the frenulum connecting the back of the upper lip to the gums in the midline.

Bruises

A bruise occurs where there is any leakage of blood into the soft tissues of the body. Bruising therefore necessarily involves damage to blood vessels. Any injury to the skin that causes bleeding will cause some local bruising. As a result, incisions, lacerations and abrasions may be associated with some local bruising. The most obvious bruises occur, however, where there has been direct blunt force applied to the skin but without any direct breach in the skin surface. These bruises, sometimes referred to as contusions, represent bleeding from small blood vessels in the skin, extending into the soft tissues in the deeper layers of skin or the subcutaneous fat. Where there is considerable crushing of tissues beneath the skin, the haemorrhage may be more extensive. Cavities or tissue spaces formed by large masses of blood pushing the soft tissues of the body apart are often referred to as haematomas. As with lacerations, areas of soft tissue overlying bony prominences of the body are more prone to bruising from a given degree of force than softer areas. This is because the softer regions of the body can stretch more and absorb the force prior to the blood vessels rupturing.

Blunt injuries inflicted after death rarely cause significant bruising as there is little or no pressure within the blood vessels of a deceased person. However, pressure may be maintained in some blood vessels after death as a result of hydrostatic pressures that force blood into some blood vessels even though there is no cardiac function. A post-mortem injury in an area of hypostatic lividity may cause a degree of bleeding leading to a post-mortem bruise. Once the blood has clotted though, significant amounts of bleeding will not occur from damaged vessels and no appreciable bruising will be caused.

Bruises can move over time. The movement of a bruise from deep tissue layers to the surface of the body is one example of this, as is the movement of bruising as a result of gravitational influences where they can migrate towards the lowest aspect of the body. A good example of this is a bruise or injury to the scalp that descends over the face, leading to the development of a 'black eye' several days later.

One of the most challenging and potentially controversial aspects of bruising is determining the age of a bruise [3]. Recent fresh bruising usually has a red or purple appearance and this appearance may continue for several days. As the haemoglobin within red cells breaks down, the bruise will gradually change colour, becoming brown, green and yellow. The time that it takes for this to occur is enormously variable, with some bruises showing areas of yellowing after 18 hours and others taking many days to show the same changes. These differences may be related to the size and density of the haemorrhage in the soft tissue, as well as the capacity of the particular individual to break down and absorb the blood. Elderly persons and those with poor health may take longer to break down bruises. As a result of this extreme variability, it is very difficult to age bruises with any degree of accuracy. Any statement of the precise age of a bruise in a medical report should be treated with scepticism.

A number of bruises have particular features that can aid in the reconstruction of the circumstances in which the injury occurred. Perhaps the best recognised of these is the so-called 'tramline' bruise. This denotes a pair of parallel linear bruises with a pale area between them. This bruise represents the effects of a rod-like object or an object with a rounded edge striking the body once. The single blow causes two areas of linear bruising because the rounded edge of the object squeezes the skin as it strikes, forcing the blood to each side of the object where the skin is stretched as the object presses into the soft tissue of the body. The blood in the stretched, damaged blood vessels on either side of the object leaks out into the soft tissue on each side to cause parallel linear bruises.

Suction bruises may also occur as a result of negative pressure applied to the surface of the skin, leading to a small collection of fine petechial haemorrhages. Such an appearance may be seen in what is often called a 'love-bite', where a person's skin is sucked into a mouth. Lines of petechial bruising may also be found in areas where the skin has been pinched or squeezed which may also be part of the mechanism of bruising in a 'love-bite'. Such injuries can also occur in skin folds where the body has been forced into a compressed position or where the skin has been squeezed by traction and pulling on items of clothing.

Incisions

As mentioned above, incisions are injuries involving a cleaving or incising of the skin. They are inflicted by sharp-edged objects that sever rather than tear the skin. Many objects can cause incisions. The objects may have linear sharp edges such as are found on knives, or sharp points such as pieces of glass or jagged edges of metal. Even soft, relatively blunt-edged objects can cause incisions if their linear axis is swept along over the skin surface.

Traditional injury classifications distinguish between incised wounds, lacerated wounds and stab wounds. To distinguish between incised wounds and stab wounds, it is usually stated that incised wounds are longer than they are deep and stab wounds are deeper than they are long. This definition certainly assists in the interpretation of how a wound was caused, but it says little about the nature of the object causing the wound. It can be convenient to divide both lacerations and incisions into superficial forms of the injury and penetrating or stab-type forms. A stab wound does not necessarily have to be an incised wound, as a blunt-pointed object can cause a penetrating type of laceration. In practice, however, the majority of penetrating or stab wounds are of the incised type.

Superficial incised wounds may occur in a variety of circumstances. These include:

- glass injuries in motor accidents;
- suicidal incised wounds to the wrists and/or neck;
- accidental incised wounds to the hands and/or the limbs;
- self-defence injuries to the hands;
- surgical wounds; and
- paper cuts.

It is unusual for superficial incised wounds to result in serious physical injury of a type that might cause death. The main danger comes from wounds that are deep enough to incise vital structures beneath the skin, such as major blood vessels or the trachea. Loss of blood or gas embolism is the most dangerous physiological consequence of such wounds.

It is difficult to identify the exact nature of a weapon that may have caused an incised wound. Some knives show varying degrees of serration. Occasionally the edges of an incised wound may have irregularities or other features to suggest that a serrated sharp-edged weapon has been used.

Incised wounds of stab type are inflicted by sharp-edged implements such as knife blades, scissor blades or long shards of glass. An incised stab wound usually has an ovoid appearance with clean, regular, long edges and ends that are either sharp or blunt in appearance. The degree to which the ovoid wound gapes depends upon the orientation of the wound in the skin. Natural lines of elasticity and tension exist in the skin; these are referred to as Langer's lines. If the wound is oriented so that its long axis lies parallel to Langer's lines, then the wound will not gape. However, if the wound's axis crosses Langer's lines it may gape significantly. The appearance of incised wounds will also vary depending upon the position of the body and the orientation of the limbs. Moving the head, arms or legs stretches the skin over several regions of the body. This stretching can distort the appearance of incised wounds. This factor may be very important in reconstructing the position of the body at the time the injury occurred.

In describing these wounds in a medical report it is important to include information on:
- the number and surface length of all wounds inflicted;
- the nature of each wound, including its minimum and maximum width, shape and direction;
- the exact location of each wound, including the height of each wound from the heel or other fixed point;
- the course and depth of each wound, including the tissues and viscera penetrated;
- the presence of any foreign material along the wound tract; and
- the apparent direction of penetration and presumed force.

Stab wounds pose considerable danger because of the risk of serious injury to deep structures within the body. Where a stab wound penetrates a body cavity and damages internal organs there may be considerable haemorrhage, particularly if vascular structures are damaged. Where there are multiple stab wounds, the pattern of the wounds may be helpful in determining the circumstances in which the injuries occurred. Pattern differences are recognisable between homicidal stabbings, suicidal stabbings and accidental injuries of stab type. The location of the wounds, their orientation and number provide valuable information as to the circumstances in which the injuries occurred.

Burns

Burning of the skin can occur in a variety of circumstances. Traditionally we think of heat as being the main cause of burns, and there are a variety of clinical definitions of types and degrees of burning of the skin. These definitions are certainly of relevance in post-mortem injury interpretation. However, the length of time between the infliction of the injury and death may result in considerable differences between classical clinical descriptions and the actual appearance of the post-mortem wound.

Burning can occur via a variety of mechanisms. These different types of burns include:
- thermal burns from flame and dry heat;
- thermal burns from the passage of electricity;
- thermal burns from wet heat and fumes (scalds);
- thermal burns caused by extreme cold;
- burns caused by ionising radiation;
- burns caused by electromagnetic radiation; and
- burns caused by chemicals.

The most common burns encountered in medico-legal death investigations are those caused by flame and by the passage of electricity. House fires and motor vehicle fires are the most common examples of the former and industrial accidents and suicides the most common examples of the latter.

Compound injuries

While individual injuries may take the form of one of the types described above, in many cases the assessment of a wound will reveal it to be composed of a mixture of individual injury subtypes. This is particularly true for certain special wound types such as gunshot wounds. Where compound injuries have occurred, one injury subtype may well predominate. For example, where an individual has suffered a knife stab wound, the predominant wound will be an incised wound of stab type. However, there may be some minor abrasion around the edges of the stab wound caused by an irregularity of the surface of the side of the blade, and perhaps some bruising around the stab wound caused by the hilt of the knife being driven against the skin's surface.

Gunshot wounds

The characteristic features of gunshot injuries are determined by both the calibre of the weapon and the distance of the victim from the gun. A 'penetrating' injury is one in which the fired projectile (missile or bullet) has entered but not exited the body and a 'perforating' injury is one in which the projectile has passed through the body completely. Factors influencing the wounds produced relate to the weapon, firing distance and design of the projectile itself, some of which are designed to cause penetrating injuries and others perforating injuries with the projectile fragmenting and spinning within the soft tissues.

The typical entrance wound, that is where the initial contact of the projectile is with the body, has a round or oval shaped skin defect surrounded by a region of abrasion, often referred to as an 'abrasion collar' or a 'circumferential marginal abrasion'. The width of the marginal abrasion may give an indication of the relative angle of the projectile as it enters the skin surface. For example, if it enters perpendicularly the width of the marginal abrasion will remain relatively constant. Often the projectile passes through other objects, that is 'intermediary' or 'interposed' targets, which will affect the shape of the marginal rim.

The firing distance will affect the appearance of the entrance wound. In contact wounds over the skull, products of the discharge on firing can dissect between skin and bone in the marginal rim region producing a 'stellate' or 'sunburst' appearance. Soot and gunpowder will be present around the entrance wound if the weapon is close to but not in contact with the skin. Soot may surround the entrance wound, and gunpowder may become embedded within the wound producing a stippled effect if the range is less than approximately 30 cm. If the firing distance is 30–90 cm, gunpowder stippling, but not soot deposition, may be evident and at a range of over 90 cm gunpowder lacks the energy to result in such stipple injuries. Clothing or other interposed targets will prevent the close range changes and the range is then considered 'indeterminate'.

The appearances of exit wounds are variable and may include slit-like, comma-shaped, x-shaped or irregular. A central round or oval defect may or may not be present. Typically exit wounds lack marginal abrasions. Exit wounds produced by high-velocity projectiles are often large and destructive.

A graze wound is one in which the skin surface is struck in a tangential manner and therefore typically has an elongated oval shape. Such injuries may involve the epidermis only or involve epidermis, dermis and subcutaneous tissues.

High-velocity wounds may share features of low-velocity wounds depending on the firing range, but there are differences. Frequently there is no significant marginal abrasion, but rather marginal micro-lacerations. The wounds are often large and destructive.

Shotgun wounds share both features and differences of low-velocity gunshot wounds. At close range a single round to oval defect with smooth borders is produced, but as range increases the borders become scalloped then circumferential individual pellet wounds occur around the central defect until at distance no central defect is present. Measuring the diameter of pellet spread across the skin surface may give an indication of the range of fire.

Asphyxia

Asphyxia is the term used to describe decreased uptake of oxygen and decreased carbon dioxide elimination. Airway obstruction may be due to smothering, neck compression, foreign body aspiration, excess secretions or swelling of the airways. Chemicals produce asphyxia in several ways. Methane or carbon dioxide deplete the environment of oxygen. Carbon monoxide will interfere with oxygen uptake. Body position, for example as a result of motor vehicle accidents, may result in airway obstruction or prevention of chest expansion.

Neck compression as a result of hanging or strangulation can produce asphyxia by obstruction of the airway or occlusion of the major vessels of the neck. The features present may be difficult to interpret and rely on consideration of all aspects of the case.

Drowning is a result of inhalation of water filling the alveolar air sacs and therefore preventing gaseous oxygen exchange.

Injury interpretation

The interpretation of a wound's appearance and the reconstruction of the events of its causation by reference to wound type are among the major skills of the forensic pathologist. When a wound or a collection of wounds is being evaluated, there are a number of questions that may arise.

These include:

- Could a particular wound have caused death?
- Could the wound have caused unconsciousness?
- Did the wound occur before or after death?
- Where there are multiple wounds, which wound was caused first and what was the subsequent order?
- What weapon or object caused the wound?
- Does the weapon have some unique identifying feature?
- How much force would have been required to cause the wound?
- In what manner was the force exerted?
- What was the direction of the force?
- Will the object that caused the injury have been damaged?
- Will there be biological trace evidence on the object causing the injury?

Many of these questions require consideration of information about matters other than the wounds in order to arrive at a reasonable interpretation. In many cases the question appears to be answerable from a common-sense approach. If this is true, it may not be an issue that needs to be addressed by a forensic medical expert but one that can be left to the coroner or coronial jury to decide. However, in exploring the possible circumstances in which an injury occurred, it is probable that specialist forensic medical issues will arise at some point, and this will require appropriate forensic medical expertise.

The answer to whether a particular wound could have caused death may have important legal consequences. In an assault where multiple individuals are alleged to have inflicted injuries, they may have been armed with different weapons. If this is the case, then it may be possible by identifying one specific injury that caused the death to identify indirectly the individual responsible for the death. It is often the case, however, that a person's death is caused by more than one injury, with injuries of different type and severity acting together to cause physiological and anatomical derangement leading to death. Often a phrase such as 'all of these injuries were acting together at the time of death' is used to explain the causal relationship between the effects of multiple injuries and the death. Where multiple injuries are involved, it may well be that one of the injuries is more significant or is the cause of more serious damage to the body. It might be possible that this serious injury, on its own, would have been capable of going on to cause death at some time in the future, but the addition of other more minor injuries resulted in the person dying at an earlier stage. These more minor injuries on their own might not necessarily have been fatal, but as part of the combined injury load on the body, they contributed to the death.

In addition to the physical factors in the interpretation of the circumstances of wounding sociological, psychological and legal issues can sometimes arise and be addressed by reference to the pattern and characteristics of wounds.

These broader issues include questions such as:
- Was the wound self-inflicted or inflicted by someone else?
- Was the wound caused accidentally or intentionally?
- Does the wound or wound pattern have a cultural significance?
- Does the wound pattern imply a form of considered infliction or simply a frenzied attack?
- In what social settings of violence might this particular wound be more likely to occur?
- Does the wound pattern imply ritual abuse or torture?

Injury and cause of death

At the completion of a forensic autopsy, the medical practitioner arrives at a conclusion regarding the significance of the injuries and the other medical and pathological findings. For examinations undertaken on behalf of the coroner, the forensic pathologist is usually required to provide the coroner with information regarding the identity of the deceased, when and where the death occurred, the cause of the death, the manner and mechanism of the death, and the circumstances of the death. These are all questions that the coroner is legally obliged to determine. Autopsies will not necessarily reveal information that can answer all of these questions; however, a full and detailed pathology examination will provide some of the best evidence from which a coroner can draw such conclusions. Coming to an understanding as to how an individual died can involve an evaluation not just of the medical or pathological evidence, but also of factors associated with the environment and human behaviour. This raises the question as to how a forensic pathologist or a coroner should arrive at a cause of death. A unique feature of the English coroner's system is that the forensic pathologist can arrive at a medical cause of death based on an investigation that includes a medical evaluation of the scene of death, the autopsy findings and any background medical history. This conclusion is then passed on to a coroner, who can hear further evidence from a wide variety of witnesses at the inquest, and this can result in a modification of the conclusion as to the final cause of death. It is a particular hallmark of the coroner's death investigation that the evaluations of these complex medical issues, which have potentially significant medico-legal consequences, are evaluated by not only a medical practitioner but also by a legal practitioner. This combination of medical and legal skills has the potential to provide the community with more information and a more balanced approach to interpretation of evidence than would be obtained from a medical practitioner or lawyer alone.

References

1 Mincer HH, Berryman HE, Murray GA et al. (1990) Methods for physical stabilization of ashed teeth in incinerated remains. *Journal of Forensic Sciences* **35**, 971–974.
2 Wells DLN, Ogden EJD, Young S. (1993) Clinical forensic medicine. In: Freckelton I, Selby H (eds) *Expert Evidence,* 6 volume looseleaf service. Law Book Company, Sydney.
3 Langlois NE, Gresham GA. (1991) The ageing of bruises: A review and study of the colour changes with time. *Forensic Science International* **50**, 227–238.

Recommended reading

1 Cotton DW, Cross SS (eds) (1994) *The Hospital Autopsy*. Butterworth Heinemann, Oxford.
2 Di Maio VJM, Di Maio D. (2001) *Forensic Pathology*. 2nd edn, CRC Press, Boca Raton.
3 Dolinak D, Matshes EW. (2002) *Medicolegal Neuropathology: A Color Atlas*. CRC Press, Boca Raton.
4 Gresham GA, Turner AF. (1969) *Post-Mortem Procedures: An Illustrated Textbook*. Wolfe Medical, London.
5 Hill RB, Anderson RE. (1988) *The Autopsy: Medical Practice and Public Policy*. Butterworths, Boston.
6 Hutchins GM (ed.) (1994) *An Introduction to Autopsy Technique*. Northfield, Illinois.
7 Knight B. (1984) *The Post-Mortem Technician's Handbook: A Manual of Mortuary Practice*. Blackwell Scientific, Oxford.
8 Mann A. (1985) *The Medical Assessment of Injuries for Legal Purposes*. Butterworths, Sydney.
9 Mason JK, Purdue BN (eds) (2000) *The Pathology of Trauma*. 3rd edn, Arnold Publishing, London.
10 Vanezis P. (1989) *Pathology of Neck Injury*. Butterworths, London.

CHAPTER 5

Human identification

Stephen Knott

Queen Elizabeth Medical Centre and Faculty of Medicine, Dentistry and Health Sciences, University of Western Australia, Australia

Human identification

We have the right to our name when we die

Human societies, throughout time, have acknowledged and shown respect for the past lives of the deceased. Various forms of both private and public ritual have been, and continue to be, integral to showing this respect for the deceased. All necessitate naming of the deceased, for without this past lives cannot be linked and acknowledged. Thus, the primary humanitarian aim of human identification is to give the unidentified deceased back their name, as when we are born we are given a name, we live our lives with that name and it follows we should have the right to that name when we die.

Identification by name also has significance for human beliefs: both religious and cultural. Many religions, to a greater or lesser extent, believe life on earth is simply part of life's journey: life continues beyond death. When doubt about a deceased's identity exists, adherents may believe their loved ones will be deprived of life beyond death, and experience significant grief and anxiety. And, when human remains cannot be identified, or a person's whereabouts cannot be established, those close to them struggle to resolve similar levels of grief and anxiety. While no one can change the outcome for the deceased or likely deceased, in other words the primary victims, positive identification by name assists outcomes for those left behind. Those left behind are secondary victims and, as the living, have a strong desire to resolve their grief and anxiety.

As stated above, societies have both legal and humanitarian obligations to the deceased and those linked to them. Confirmation of identity by name of all deceased is a primary legal requirement of most judicial systems. Where such judicial systems are in place, a death certificate cannot be issued without the correct name of deceased individuals. There are many consequences for secondary victims when legal identification is not achieved; the courts will not accept many legal documents until identification has been achieved. Without formal

Forensic Odontology: Principles and Practice, First Edition. Edited by Jane A. Taylor and Jules A. Kieser.

© 2016 John Wiley & Sons, Ltd. Published 2016 by John Wiley & Sons, Ltd.

identification deliberation in the courts is considerable, resulting in delay in the burial of a person's remains and also in the settlement of their will and estate. There are similar consequences in criminal matters where a primary victim's identification cannot be confirmed, such as a homicide. Without confirmed identity of the victim, a criminal case may be aborted or an open finding declared. Of particular concern, secondary victims could be destined to years of living with the humanitarian and legal consequences.

In summary, giving a name to the deceased fulfils both the humanitarian need of the bereaved as well as the legal requirements of the judicial system of the society in which they live. Most importantly, it allows the bereaved to eventually resolve their grief and move on in their lives.

Methods of identification

The methods of identification of the deceased involve many areas of forensic investigation and scientific research. The justice systems within each country will stipulate their legislative requirements for an identification to be established. In the event of a mass disaster the criteria outlined in the Interpol Disaster Victim identification (DVI) Guidelines are used by the legal system in many countries including Australia.

The final decision on what constitutes identification is determined by a court or board within each justice system. The principle arbitrator of the court may be a coroner, medical examiner, magistrate or legally nominated official.

The method of identification can vary from a single or multiple primary identifier or if acceptable by the court, a combination of circumstantial evidence and secondary identifiers.

Primary methods for identification are:
- visual
- fingerprints
- dental data
- DNA
- medical and anthropological.

Primary identifiers are often referred to as 'stand alone' identifiers.

Secondary identifiers in themselves are not acceptable to establish identification. The secondary identifiers are many and include:
- height, sex, age
- clothes
- jewellery
- personal documents
- fragments of hair
- any object that is unique to the individual
- location of the deceased etc.

The accumulative effect of secondary identifiers is to help direct the court in their decision. Also, information gathered from secondary identifiers can narrow the search for ante-mortem data required to satisfy a primary identifier. In countries that do not have a national population database for fingerprints, DNA or dental data, any mechanism to narrow the search parameters is helpful. This narrowing of data was highlighted following the need for identification of victims from the Asian tsunami in December 2004. The retrieval and accumulation of secondary identifiers from the deceased focused the investigating teams reviewing the primary identifiers.

Human dentition

Teeth: the last tissue to disintegrate

In more recent times, the practice of forensic dentistry backed by published research and texts has led to practitioners within the dental field being recognised as specialists with the speciality title 'forensic odontologist'. The role of the forensic odontologist is to investigate and advise the justice system on issues within the field of dentistry that are of legal concern. A significant role of the forensic odontologist is to investigate the identity of deceased individuals. It is rarely required that living persons need be identified by their dentition. The education and experience required to qualify as a forensic odontologist is currently being debated worldwide as jurisdictions endeavour to secure satisfactory standards of professional conduct.

In the state of Western Australia, with a population of 2.2 million people, the caseload requiring forensic odontological investigation is approximately 100 cases per year. Of these approximately 83% are for confirmation of identification. The remainder of cases involve consultation on orofacial trauma, bite marks (both living and deceased), opinions on historic skeletal remains and occasionally age assessment. These consultation topics are covered in other chapters within this text. Mass disaster incidents are not included in this approximation.

The uniqueness and durability of the human dentition has aided human identification for many centuries. The deceased person's dentition provides investigators with two distinct characteristics that assist identification: the dentition's biological features and a record of the deceased person's past dental therapies. First, biologically, human dentition and individual teeth are specific to an individual [1, 2]. Plueckham and Cordner [3, pp. 300–301] state: '… with 32 teeth in the adult dentition and five surfaces from each tooth recorded in an oral examination, there are 160 surfaces.' Significantly, they also state: 'Combined with restorative treatment, root anatomy and surrounding oral tissues, there are 2.5 billion possibilities in producing a dental formula.' Similar quantitative analysis and research of the biological characteristics of the human dentition by

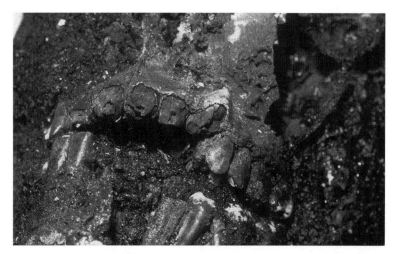

Fig. 5.1 Incinerated remains following motor vehicle crash. (*See insert for colour representation of the figure.*)

Adams [4] and Martins-de-las-heras [5] supports Plueckham and Cordner's view that each individual's dentition can be shown to be unique.

Human teeth have also been shown to be extremely durable. Studies investigating the range of temperature and the length of the exposure to heat, state that tooth structures can remain intact even up to 1600°C [6]. However, extreme temperatures and length of exposure influence the calcination of teeth, necessitating greater care in handling post-mortem dental material (Fig. 5.1). In the 2009 Black Saturday bushfires in Victoria, Australia, teeth recovered were described as being not only incinerated but cremated [7].

Additional evidence that attests to the durability of human teeth is the fact that in all states of decomposition, teeth or parts of teeth are the last part of the body to be destroyed.

Second, the status of an individual's dentition reflects both the history of dental treatment and an individual's personal characteristics, that is occlusal function, smoking habits, medical conditions that affect teeth and even cultural practices. Each individual's recorded dental data is unique and kept 'on file' making it ideal as a primary identifier. Documentation and the storage of data for the other scientific primary identifiers, fingerprints and a DNA profile, are not currently undertaken. This may occur in the future, but is currently controversial.

The examination of the deceased's dentition will record permanent changes due to human intervention such as tooth extraction, restorations and shaping of teeth. Recorded permanent changes such as missing teeth and restoration cannot be reversed. Because these changes cannot be reversed, their presence, or absence, assists in the identification process.

Cultural practices through time have changed an individual's dentition. Archaeological material has recorded tooth jewellery, restorations and tooth shaping. For example, although on the decline, the removal of a permanent central incisor continues to be a traditional practice of the Australian Aboriginal. And in Bali, Indonesia the practice of tooth grinding (Patong Gigi) through the months of July and August is a common practice to help people rid themselves of the terrible forces of evil.

Within the context of identification of skeletonised remains, dentition plays a significant role in age assessment. To a lesser extent dentition can give clues to ancestry and sex. In practice in cases of skeletal remains, particularly of the cranium, the forensic odontologist would be part of a forensic team accompanied by a physical anthropologist, forensic pathologist and DNA scientist.

Dental anthropology parameters with supporting identification characteristics by the dentition are discussed in Chapter 10.

Role of the primary identifiers

Visual

Visual identification falls into a unique category within the primary identifiers as being determined by subjective analysis.

The ability of humans to identify an individual, often in milliseconds, has been debated for years. Humans are extremely adept at recognising each other from prior contact. Unfortunately, in the identification of a deceased individual the capacity and circumstances of the observer can change. Additionally the appearance of the person to be identified may be altered by circumstances (i.e. decomposition, trauma and disfigurement).

In recent years, research has developed measurable facial parameters to reduce the subjectivity of an individual's visual evidence [8, 9].

It is for these reasons that jurisdictions are cautious about relying on visual evidence and prefer scientific data to support identification. In a mass disaster where there are multiple deceased that have been subject to a similar cause of death, identification by visual means is not acceptable [10].

Fingerprints

Fingerprint evidence in criminal cases has been used in the UK and America since the turn of the 19th century. Print evidence has been accepted by the justice system as a primary 'stand-alone' identifier. Traditionally the recording analysis and identification decisions have been the role of the police. Like many aspects of forensic science, the validity of fingerprints is under continual scrutiny.

The success of recording prints is influenced by the physical condition of the deceased. Latter stages of decomposition, incineration, submersions and fragmentation all limit or prevent the recording of a print.

Ante-mortem prints are recorded from personal items or accessed from a database. An investigation will endeavour to lift prints from surfaces in the deceased's dwelling or from known personal property. Contamination is an issue and the longer retrieval is delayed the less likely a comparative print will be obtained. This highlights the advantage of early recording of prints from personal property of a suspected missing person. Very few countries have fingerprints of their individual population recorded on a database; the majority have data from criminal offenders, members of their defence forces, security personnel both private and government and possibly prominent public officials.

DNA

The use of DNA as a primary identifier was first introduced and accepted by the courts as a valid method of identification in the Colin Pitchfork case in 1987 [11].

The post-mortem biological sample collected will vary depending on the physical condition of the deceased. The tissue samples commonly requested by the forensic biologist are blood, cortical bone, muscle and teeth. Teeth are a reliable source of DNA but techniques for obtaining samples from within a tooth are more complex. If the less-complex analyses of blood, bone and muscle samples do not provide a DNA profile then the teeth are analysed [12].

Within different laboratories the procedure for recovering DNA samples from teeth will vary; however, the laboratory techniques for the analysis are similar.

If a tooth is required as a post-mortem sample the forensic odontologist needs to decide the appropriate tooth and employ techniques to eliminate contamination. The protocols and procedures for procuring teeth are outlined in the International Commission for Missing Persons Standard Operating Procedures [13].

There needs to be close liaison between the forensic biologist and the forensic odontologist on the method of choice for extraction of sample material. The aim of the forensic odontologist is to provide the laboratory with the most uncontaminated dental sample possible.

Ante-mortem comparison profiles are obtained from the biological relatives, the deceased's personal items or government databases. The recording of ante-mortem samples from biological relatives is usually a task undertaken by the police or the forensic biologist where an intra-oral buccal swab is the common method of choice. Preferred samples taken from the deceased's dwelling are those that have been in close physical contact, such as a toothbrush, hair comb/brush or razor. Samples from items that the deceased has made contact with, such as eating and drinking utensils, clothing and bedding are more likely to be contaminated. Hence their validity may be questioned in court.

An ante-mortem profile may exist on a government database following prior police contact with the deceased. Or, as is the case with certain key personnel, their profile is on record.

Medical and anthropological

The comparison of an individual's unique medical and anatomical characteristics is a less commonly used primary identifier. Features such as bony abnormalities, healed fractures, surgical prostheses and unique tattoos may be conclusive identifiers.

During the autopsy by the forensic pathologist unique individual features may be exposed. These features are described, photographed, radiographed and specific details such as serial numbers on a prosthesis recorded. In cases of late decomposition, fragmentation and skeletonisation, consultation with a forensic physical anthropologist strengthens the findings of the autopsy.

Ante-mortem data is collected from the deceased's medical notes. Much of the recorded medical treatment in the notes may not be useful for identification, but specific treatment will be highlighted. Specific treatment can include surgical procedures for bone fractures, placement of prostheses and extensive tissue repairs. Procedures that involved radiographic analysis are particularly useful. Recordings of serial numbers on prostheses are individual specific and enable identification to be established.

Ante-mortem medical radiographs may be difficult to locate. Prior to digital radiography the traditional 'wet film' radiographs were placed in storage files or given to the patient. In both of these circumstances with the progress of time the radiographs could be discarded.

Ante-mortem dental data

Essential to the scientific primary methods of identification is access to reference material in ante-mortem data.

In most routine casework the authorities know who the deceased is or, in closed mass disasters, who they are trying to locate. Mass disasters are labelled either *open* or *closed*. A closed disaster is one where the deceased victims are known occupants, such as a plane or bus crash where passengers' names have been recorded. An open disaster is one where the names of the victims are completely unknown, for example commuter-train crash, fire in a shopping precinct, and so on. The responsibility for establishing the deceased's identity is that of the police. The retrieval of data is commonly coordinated by the police with advice from scientists. The scientists and fingerprint specialists analyse both the ante- and post-mortem data to provide evidence to the justice system.

The retrieval of the ante-mortem comparison data needs to be undertaken in a timely manner, as previously discussed with fingerprints and DNA samples. Dental ante-mortem data retrieval does not require the same urgency as compared to fingerprints and DNA, however prolonged delays run the risk of dental material being discarded or lost.

The legal requirement for the retention of dental records varies around the world. In Australia the requirement is retention for seven years since the last attendance at a clinic and for seven years after the age of 18 years. Fortunately most practitioners retain patient dental data for longer periods. The development of electronic data recording should enhance the likelihood of longer retention.

Dental records or dental data?

The term *dental record* has traditionally been used. Unfortunately this is synonymous with clinical notes. Consequently, the police when collecting dental material may only request written files and hopefully associated radiographs (Fig. 5.2). However, in more recent times dental treatment has expanded to include photographs, dental casts, mouth guards, orthodontic appliances, occlusal splints, bleaching appliances and even spare dentures as well as written notes and radiographs. Therefore the term *dental data* is preferable because it encompasses all the items listed above. Using the term dental data is more likely to encourage investigators to collect all available material from a dental clinic, a dental laboratory and the deceased's residence.

The location of a deceased's dental data relies on information provided by relatives and friends. Additionally, databases held in public dental services, defence forces or university dental schools can be reviewed. In recent years the location of the deceased's dental data held at unknown private dental clinics, in

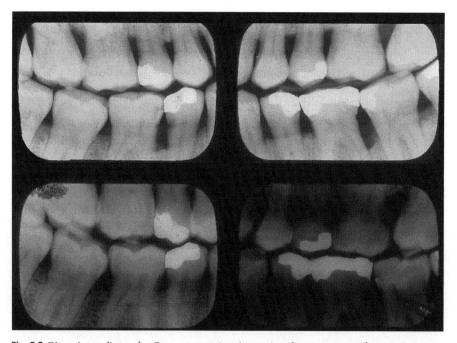

Fig. 5.2 Bite-wing radiographs. Post-mortem (top images) and ante-mortem (bottom images).

the state of Western Australia, has been successful by *e-blasts* to members of the state Australian Dental Association. The message requests practitioners scan their dental files and report to the police if they have treated the deceased. Also private health providers give a similar level of support by liaising with the authorities on reviewing their database and reporting on members' past treatments.

Close liaison with the police collecting agency will enable the forensic odontologist to review the data as quickly as possible. With many patients being referred to dental specialists it is critical that the reviewing forensic odontologist notifies the police of the presence and location of additional material. This is essential for missing persons where the missing ante-mortem dental data may not be requested and utilised for many years after an individual is reported missing.

For the Missing Persons Department, the policy of when to collect ante-mortem data for all the primary identifiers is a sensitive issue. With the collection of data the families may assume that authorities believe that their loved one is deceased. When collecting ante-mortem data, assistance from trained counsellors is recommended to reduce family anxiety.

For missing persons, once the ante-mortem data has been reviewed and dental status recorded, ideally on Interpol forms, the collated data should be made available for review by national and international investigators. Within Australia the establishment of a National and International Missing Persons dental database is currently a work in progress. The possibility of establishing a national and an international dental database for missing persons has been widely discussed but, as yet, not implemented.

Dental prostheses

Named prostheses benefit both the living and the deceased.

When providing a patient with a dental prosthesis, fixed or removable, it is logical that there is an identifier relating the prosthesis to the patient. Unfortunately this is not general practice. Insertion of the patient's name in a dental removable prosthesis or appliance not only assists in the identification of the deceased, but also in the living where it provides proof of ownership. Named dentures allow staff caring for individuals in aged care centres, particularly those suffering from medical or age-related memory loss, to quickly return the prosthesis to their rightful owner. The return of missing mouth guards and orthodontic appliances is a relief to both parents and their children.

Many identification systems for dental prosthesis have been suggested and implemented. The embedding of bar-coded devices is one of the current directions of research, with their reliability under investigation [14]. Currently few jurisdictions make it a legal requirement for the dental profession to include an identifier in the fabrication of prostheses. The insertion of a person's name to a removable prosthesis or appliance would fulfil the requirements for forensic, medical and personal needs (Fig. 5.3).

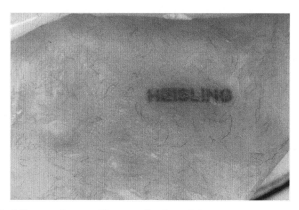

Fig. 5.3 Name in full upper denture 18 years after insertion.

Oral implants

Incorporation of a personal identifier in dental implants follows a similar history as personalising removable prostheses. Specific legislation is required to make the dental profession and manufacturers incorporate change. Current legal obligations and possible future directions have been thoroughly reviewed by Berketa [15].

Orthodontics

In children, the effect of fluoridation treatments has reduced the need for restorative care and oral radiographs. In a quest to identify juveniles, the forensic odontologist will need to rely more on orthodontic data. All phases of orthodontic treatment and referral correspondence provide unique data in the form of dental casts, radiographs, photographs and dental appliances.

As previously outlined, it is important that an early review of the dental notes of a missing person's general dentist be undertaken by an odontologist. The review will reveal referrals to dental specialists such as orthodontists, radiologists, surgeons and so on. The police who collect the ante-mortem dental data can then be made aware of the presence and location of this additional material. The review by the odontologist may also reveal information on dental appliances that are possibly at the deceased's residence.

Radiographic images: facial sinuses and anatomical features within the bone

When forensic odontologists analyse the dentition from extra- and intra-oral radiographs and scans, they need to be aware of the adjacent anatomical features. More specifically, clinical radiography and scanned images of the skull provide useful ante-mortem data for comparison of sinus, bone trabeculae patterns and nutrient canals.

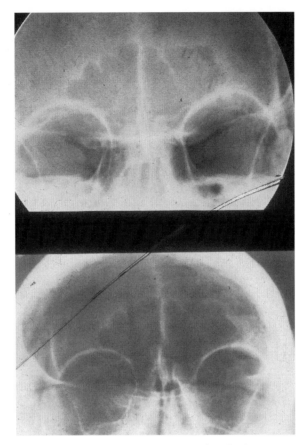

Fig. 5.4 Frontal sinus radiographs. Ante-mortem at clinical medical examination (top image) and post-mortem at autopsy (bottom image).

Frontal sinus trabeculae patterns (form, shape and size) have been shown to be individual specific with a high level of accuracy from visual comparison [16]. Besana reports that the traits of the sinus pattern, when superimposed, are a viable method of identification [17]. For example, use of ante-mortem frontal sinus radiographs has been reported as enabling identification to be established [18].

The bony outline of the maxillary sinus is evident in the dental panoramic image; sections of the floor of the sinus are evident in most maxillary posterior periapical films. In addition, the relationship between the floor of the maxillary sinus, the maxillary teeth and the height of the alveolar bony ridge are useful indicators when comparing ante-mortem and post-mortem dental data (Fig. 5.4).

Quatrehomme identified individual patterns in long bone trabeculae [19]. This suggests similar patterns within the maxilla and mandible may provide specific information for the identification of deceased at reconciliation. Further research would be required, however, to establish the specificity of maxilla and mandible bone trabeculae patterns with due consideration given to the influence of function and age. The significance of nutrient canals within the bony structures of the maxilla and mandible are also reported to be unique [20].

Superimposition

The techniques of superimposition are utilised in circumstances where the authorities suspect they know the identity of the deceased [21]. A confirmed ante-mortem photograph of the possible identity is compared to a post-mortem image of the deceased. Superimposition differs from facial approximation in that the authorities have a connection between the deceased remains and a known missing person; with facial approximation there is no link. Glaister and Brash are credited for first presenting this technique in criminal proceedings in the Ruxton Case in 1937.

The technique involves the layering of a photographic image of the deceased's post-mortem image over the photo of the suspect's ante-mortem image (Fig. 5.5). Following an analysis of the 'fit' of anatomical features to each other a decision is made on areas of concordance or difference. Traditionally the technique involved the manual layering of exact sized photographs over each other. With the advent of new video and computer technology the problems of skull orientation, magnification, angles of photographs and clarity can be significantly reduced. Access to high-definition imaging equipment and skilled operators familiar with programs such as Photoshop are vital in the comparison of images [22].

Comparison of ante-mortem and post-mortem images of anterior dentition is commonly used for comparison. The availability of ante-mortem photographs showing a broad smile with the anterior teeth showing is ideal for comparison. Often these types of photographs, taken at times of celebration, are consequently termed 'happy snappies'. This term is easily understood by the families and police when there is a request for ante-mortem photographs. Photographs from

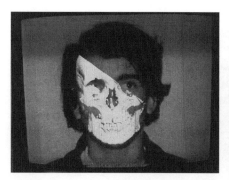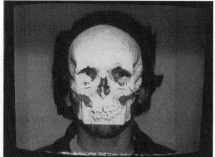

Fig. 5.5 Superimposition overlay. Image of skull overlaid over suspected long-term missing person.

personal mobile phones, in particular 'selfies', may also provide close-up images of the dentition.

The acceptance by the court in establishing an identity will depend on the comparison material available, competence of the person undertaking the comparison, and the validity and logging of how the images have been manipulated (i.e. have the images been manipulated to obtain a 'fit'?) [23, 24].

Facial reconstruction

When all methods of identification of unknown skeletal remains have been exhausted, the techniques of facial reconstruction can be employed. The ability to reconstruct an exact replica of a face is unlikely, what is more likely to occur is creation of features that trigger a possible recognition in a witness. To exactly reproduce the deceased's face is extremely unlikely, hence technically a more descriptive term for the technique is *facial approximation*. It is imperative when discussing facial approximation cases that the reason for instigating the technique is clarified. The case will either be for historic resemblance or for forensic identification.

Opinion varies on whether the technique is science or art. Having an in-depth knowledge of cranial skeletal and soft tissue anatomy combined with artistic experience in the facial form are necessary to create a face that approximates the deceased. The approximation can be achieved by a two-dimensional technique of drawing an image over a picture of the skull to specific tissue depth markers. Alternatively, a three-dimensional build-up, either manually with clay or by using a computer software program, can be used for approximation.

The father of modern-day three-dimensional facial reconstruction is Russian palaeontologist, Professor Mikhail Gerasimov (1907–1970). The creditability of using an anatomical approach is constantly under review by practitioners [25, 26]. Currently there are two main techniques employed in undertaking the approximation. One technique of facial build up uses a combination of muscle anatomy with reference to datasets of approximate tissue depths, commonly called the 'Manchester' technique [27] (Fig. 5.6). Alternatively the facial build up relies extensively on using tissue depth datasets to determine the facial form, termed the 'American' method [28]. Historical reconstructions are traditionally undertaken on the remains of individuals who have been deceased for considerable time. The identity of the deceased may be known and the final reconstruction is displayed in a museum or public thoroughfare. These reconstructions lend themselves to artistic flare (Fig. 5.7).

Forensic reconstructions are undertaken with strict adherence to anatomical features and scientifically researched interpretation of skeletal features. Additional information may be recovered at the site of the skeletal remains. This additional information such as hair, clothing and jewellery need to be clearly

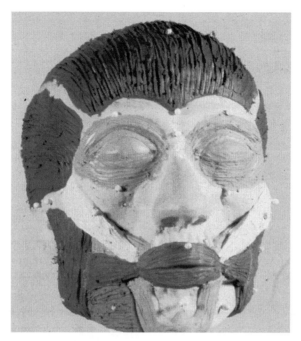

Fig. 5.6 Anatomical muscle build-up, coloured for teaching purposes. (Courtesy of Ronn Taylor.)

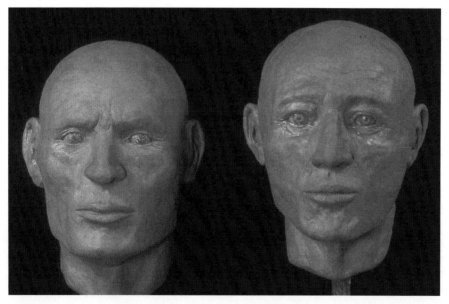

Fig. 5.7 Completed clay reconstruction of skeletal remains from Dutch shipwreck in 1629. (Courtesy of Stephen Knott.)

associated with the remains. This subjective identification can provide directions for authorities to collect ante-mortem data that may be used to satisfy identification by one of the primary identifiers. For the courts to rely solely on the establishment of an individual's identity by facial reconstruction techniques alone is highly unlikely.

On completion of the forensic reconstruction a photographic image is published in the media, that is newspapers, magazines and television. It is hoped the published image will trigger recognition in the memory of a member of the public, enabling a name to be given to the deceased. The subjective recognition of the photographic image would not be sufficient to satisfy positive identification by the courts but it gives the investigators a possible lead to collect data for biometric analysis to satisfy one of the primary identifiers.

The skeletal analysis is a team approach by a forensic anthropologist, odontologist and reconstruction practitioner. Initial analysis is to determine the critical parameters of ethnicity, sex and age. The role of the forensic odontologist is particularly significant in the determination of age and possibly information from the type of materials used in dental restorations. To have a complete postcranial skeleton is a distinct advantage in determining these parameters.

Success of establishing identification is dependent on how much skeletal material is available, the experience of the forensic team, the ability of the reconstruction practitioner to incorporate the available information in the facial form and the response from the public. Success rates to establish an exact identification tend to be low, but information provided by the public enables police with alternative directions in their investigation.

The validity in undertaking a reconstruction is that a successful identification or additional information for the investigation is better than having no identification or direction to investigate prior to the reconstruction being undertaken.

Standards for acceptance of identification

The Australian Society of Forensic Odontology (AuSFO) recommended standards for acceptance of dental identification states the following:

> The principle underlying dental comparison should be one of elimination. The comparison process must be methodical and include each tooth as well as all associated dental structures.
>
> No minimum number of concordant points is required. All apparent discrepancies in evidence (e.g. errors in recording, dental treatment subsequent to the available ante-mortem information) must be resolved. No assumptions must be made about missing information or unresolved discrepancies. In all circumstances it is better to err on the side of caution and be conservative in decisions [29].

The findings of an odontology investigation team should be based on recognised guidelines of human identification. It would be ideal if all jurisdictions used the same criteria and nomenclature both nationally and internationally. This is not the current situation, however, as differences exist in both nomenclature and criteria in different jurisdictions. Unfortunately, this may cause confusion in possible legal proceedings in a deceased's country of origin when identification of the deceased from that jurisdiction has taken place in another.

Below are two examples of the criteria currently stated for dental identification:

1 The ABFO Reference Manual by the American Board of Forensic Odontology (ABFO) states the following four criteria:
   - Positive identification
     The ante-mortem and post-mortem data match in sufficient detail to establish that they are from the same individual. In addition, there are no irreconcilable discrepancies.
   - Possible identification
     The ante-mortem and post-mortem data have consistent features, but, due to the quality of either the post-mortem remains or the ante-mortem evidence, it is not possible to positively establish dental identification.
   - Insufficient evidence
     The available information is insufficient to form the basis for a conclusion.
   - Exclusion
     The ante-mortem and post-mortem data are clearly inconsistent. However, it should be understood that identification by exclusion is a valid technique in certain circumstances [30].

2 The Interpol DVI Guide 2014 states the following five criteria:
   - Identification (absolute certainty the post-mortem and ante-mortem records are from the same person).
   - Identification probable (specific characteristics correspond between post-mortem and ante-mortem but either post-mortem or ante-mortem data or both are minimal).
   - Identification possible (there is nothing that excludes the identity but either post-mortem or ante-mortem data or both are minimal).
   - Identity excluded (post-mortem and ante-mortem records are from different persons).
   - Insufficient evidence (neither post-mortem nor ante-mortem comparison can be made) [10].

The Interpol guidelines above use four very similar criteria to the ABFO guidelines, yet include the additional criterion of *probable* identification. Both sets of guidelines add description aimed at better application of each criterion, but close comparison of the wording used suggests confusion may readily arise should identification be contested in the across-jurisdiction circumstance referred to above. For example, in the description for criterion 1, the ABFO guidelines states data should, 'match in sufficient detail … with no irreconcilable discrepancies', but the similar criterion in the Interpol guidelines states: 'There must be absolute certainty both AM and PM data are from the same person'. Both criteria are to declare identification has been achieved, yet one requires sufficient detail and the other absolute certainty. The aim of forensic odontology should be to support the judicial process not confuse it [10, p. 95, 30, p.116].

In some other jurisdictions (e.g. in jurisdictions in some of the Australian states) guidelines use words such as *confirm, conclusive, support, strongly support, consistent with, not possible, lack of information*. This nomenclature is unhelpful [31].

References

1 Pretty IA, Sweet D. (2001) A look at forensic dentistry – Part 1: The role of teeth in the determination of human identity. *British Dental Journal* **190**, 359–366.

2 Metcalf RD, Brumit PC, Schrader BA et al. On the uniqueness of human dentition. Proceedings of the International Scientific Congress of IOFOS 2013 August 29–31, Florence, Italy.

3 Plueckhahn VD, Cordner SM. (1991) *Ethics, Legal Medicine and Forensic Pathology.* 2nd edn, Melbourne University Press, Melbourne.

4 Adams BJ. (2003) Establishing personal identification based on specific patterns of missing, filled and unrestored teeth. *Journal of Forensic Sciences* **48**, 487–496.

5 Martin-de-las-Heras S, Valenzuela A, de Dios Luna J et al. (2010) The utility of dental patterns in forensic dentistry. *Forensic Science International* **195**, 166–188.

6 Clement JG. (1998) Dental identification: age changes. In: Clement JG, Ranson DL (eds) *Craniofacial identification in Forensic Medicine.* Arnold, London.

7 Lain R, Taylor J, Croker S et al. (2011) Comparative dental anatomy in Disaster Victim Identification: Lessons from the 2009 Victorian bushfires. *Forensic Science International* **205**, 36–39.

8 Ishii M, Yayama K, Motani H et al. (2011) Application of superimposition–based personal identification using skull computed tomography images. *Journal of Forensic Sciences* **56**, 960–966.

9 Van Der Meer DT, Brumit PC, Schrader BA et al. (2010) Root morphology and anatomical patterns in forensic dental identification: A comparison of computer–aided identification with traditional forensic dental identification. *Journal of Forensic Sciences* **55**, 1499–1503.

10 Interpol. Interpol DVI Guide 2014 [Internet]. Interpol; 2014 October 14. Available from: http://www.interpol.int/INTERPOL–expertise/Forensics/DVI–Pages/DVI–guide. Accessed August 2015.

11 Elvidge S. Colin Pitchfork: first exoneration through DNA [Internet]. United Kingdom: Explore Forensics; [updated 2015 February 24. Available from: http://www.exploreforensics.co.uk/forenisc–cases–colin–pitchfork–first–exoneration–through–dna.html. Accessed August 2015.

12 Higgins D, Austin JJ. (2013) Teeth as a source of DNA for forensic identification of human remains: A review. *Science and Justice* **53**, 434–441.

13 International Commission for Missing Persons (ICMP). Standard operating procedures for sampling bone and tooth specimens from human remains for DNA testing at the ICMP [Internet]. ICMP; 2013 August 19; 2015 January 1. Available from: http://www.ic–mp.org/?resources=standard–operating–procedure–for–sampling–bone–and–tooth–specimens–from–human–remains–for–dna–testing–at–the–icmp. Accessed August 2015.

14 Ragavendra TR, Mhaske S, Gouraha A et al. (2014) Quick response code in acrylic denture: Will it respond when needed? *Journal of Forensic Sciences* **59**, 514–516.

15 Berketa JW, Hirsch RS, Higgins D et al. (2009) Radiographic recognition of dental implants as an aid to identifying the deceased. *Journal of Forensic Sciences* **55**, 66–70.

16 Smith VA, Christensen AM, Myers SW. (2010) The reliability of visually comparing small frontal sinuses. *Journal of Forensic Sciences* **55**, 1413–1415.

17 Besana JL, Rogers TL. (2010) Personal identification using the frontal sinus. *Journal of Forensic Sciences* **55**, 584–589.

18 da Silva RF, Prado FB, Caputo IGC et al. (2009) The forensic importance of frontal sinus radiographs. *Journal of Forensic and Legal Medicine* **16**, 18–23.

19 Quatrehomme G, Biglia E, Padovani B et al. (2014) Positive identification by X–rays bone trabeculae comparison. *Forensic Science International* **245**, 11–14.

20 Fielding CG. (2002) Nutrient canals of the alveolar process as an anatomic feature for dental identifications. *Journal of Forensic Sciences* **47**, 381–383.

21 Al-Amad S, McCullough M, Graham J et al. (2006) Craniofacial identification by computer–mediated superimposition. *Journal of Forensic Odontostomatology* **24**, 47–52.

22 Campomanes-Alvarez B, Ibanez O, Navarro F et al. (2014) Computer vision and soft computing for automatic skull–face overlay in craniofacial superimposition. *Forensic Science International* **245**, 77–86.

23 Mallet X, Evison MP. (2013) Forensic facial comparison: Issues of admissibility in the development of novel analytical technique. *Journal of Forensic Sciences* **58**, 859–865.

24 Jayaprakash PT. (2014) Conceptual transitions in methods of skull–photo superimposition that impact the reliability of identification: A review. *Forensic Science International* **246**, 110–121.

25 Ulrich H, Stephan CN. (2011) On Gerasimov's plastic facial reconstruction technique: New insights to facilitate repeatability. *Journal of Forensic Sciences* **56**, 470–474.

26 Parks CL, Richard AH, Monson KL. (2014) Preliminary assessment of facial soft tissue thickness utilizing three–dimensional computed tomography models of living individuals. *Forensic Science International* **237**, 146–156.

27 Prag J, Neave R. (1997) *Making Faces*. British Museum Press, London.

28 Wilkinson C. (2004) *Forensic Facial Reconstruction*. Cambridge University Press, Cambridge.

29 Australian Society of Forensic Odontology. Disaster Victim Identification Forensic Odontology Guide [Internet]. 2012 February 14. Available from: http://www.ausfo.com.au/component/content/article/2–uncategorised/28–ausfo–resources. Accessed August 2015.

30 American Board of Forensic Odontolgy. ABFO Reference Manual [Internet]. ABFO; 2015 [updated 2015 March 10; cited 2015 March 26] Available from: http://www.abfo.org/wp–content/uploads/2012/08/ABFO–Reference–Manual–March–2015.pdf. Accessed August 2015.

31 Higgins D, James H. (2006) Classifications used by Australian forensic odontologists in identification reports. *Journal of Forensic Odontostomatology* **24**, 32–35.

CHAPTER 6

Mortuary techniques

Alain G. Middleton

NSW Forensic Dental Identification Unit, Westmead Hospital, Australia

The dental post-mortem

The dental post-mortem aims to gather and document information in the area of expertise of the forensic odontologist. While the dental post-mortem is most frequently an examination of a deceased person, there will be occasions where the examination will be performed on a living person or on a non-human entity. The primary aim is to produce a set of findings that can be analysed and compared to dental information available about a person in life, for comparison with information about another person (dead or alive), or to provide an opinion in relation to one's findings. The examination in some instances is performed to develop a dental or 'odontological' profile of the subject material.

It is important to think in terms of the traditional hard and soft tissues but also other anatomical features in the area of examination, coupled with the practitioner's level of expertise.

What is the purpose of the dental post-mortem?

A dental post-mortem may be performed for a number of reasons. The primary and most common reason is to gather information in relation to the possible identification of the individual.

Other reasons may be to gather information to assist in the determination of the age of the victim (especially in developing dentitions), cause of death, examine and document injury patterns in relation to physical and sexual assaults, and to examine and document racial, social and other demographic and sociographic indicators. The examination may provide indicators about aspects such as ancestry, socioeconomic status, habits, cultural and geographic indicators, genetic and medical conditions.

This process is performed not only in a dental context, but also often in an investigative, and/or legal (criminal or civil) context. The findings of the forensic odontologists will usually be presented for legal and or judicial review and possible challenge.

Forensic Odontology: Principles and Practice, First Edition. Edited by Jane A. Taylor and Jules A. Kieser.

© 2016 John Wiley & Sons, Ltd. Published 2016 by John Wiley & Sons, Ltd.

The dental post-mortem is usually one of a number of examinations that may be performed on the remains of a deceased person. The process of examination and documentation has of necessity and professionalism to be thorough and concisely documented. This documentation must be understandable to peers, often in an international context (such as in a mass casualty event). We live in an increasingly international society, so the acquiring or providing of information internationally is not uncommon. The adoption of standards and systems that meet these requirements is good practice and saves having to use different systems for different scenarios.

Components of a dental post-mortem

A number of key factors must be considered before the actual examination begins.

Location
Most examinations, and certainly routine examinations, will occur in a purpose-built facility such as a forensic or hospital mortuary. There are usually other forensic activities occurring at the same site.

During mass casualty incidents, the mortuary may be located at a site related to the event. This site may be an established facility or a green field (usually temporary) facility located in the vicinity of the mass casualty event, and often away from one's 'usual workplace'.

Facilities
A dental post-mortem conducted in an established forensic facility is a very different situation to the same activity 'in the field' in some far flung geographical location with minimal and or temporary facilities and infrastructure.

Always insist on the best facilities possible, bearing in mind that these will vary according to the site of the examination. Good facilities are important to minimise stress, errors, to maximise the information gathered, and for occupational health and safety.

In mass casualty events it is easy to forget these important issues and laudable to 'make do' in 'tough' or makeshift situations.

Do not become a 'victim' of the event. In field examinations will always be challenging. Remember that the odontologist will always be held accountable for errors or deficiencies in spite of the conditions that prevailed at the time of the examination.

Equipment – basic requirements

Ventilation
Odour is ever present at the post-mortem venue. This will often reflect the stage and or manner of decomposition, but may also represent chemicals and other manmade substances present with the deceased. Increasingly there exist bacterial,

viral and other immune system challenging materials contaminating the post-mortem material to be examined. Good ventilation will not only reduce the risk to the examining team, but will assist in productivity.

Lighting

Lighting is of paramount importance. Poor lighting will result in increased errors, tiredness and stress. In this day and age of LED, small light units that are excellent, efficient and relatively inexpensive (although perhaps not colour corrected) are readily available. Many are battery operated, which is useful in remote locations and in minimising cords and the risk of electrical faults/dangers. Units can be fixed overhead by hanging from a ceiling structure, on a vertical pole or wall beside the operator, and/or worn as headgear. In rare situations, directional lighting may need to be held by a third person.

Examination table

The physical table must be stable and at an appropriate working height, and preferably easily adjustable. There should be a specific drainage point and appropriate drainage collection. This will minimise occupational health and safety (OH&S) exposure, and help maximise the examination environment. This may be as basic as packing under one end of the table to create a slope with appropriate fluid collection at the lowest point. An examination table at an appropriate height will help minimise physical stress.

A controlled clean water supply and waste drainage and collection are essential.

Oral health and safety – personal protection

Clear demarcation between clean and 'dirty' areas should be established. These are usually colour coded as per traffic lights (red yellow and green). Appropriate personal protective clothing and equipment is mandatory. This, at the minimum, will require protection of exposed skin, eyes and face. Anyone working with human remains and or decomposing matter should be suitably vaccinated against all perceived local threats and not have any compromised immune system issues. Where possible, the infectious status of the remains by means of initial screening tests should be performed by the facility management. Basic hand washing facilities should be easily accessible and practices implemented.

Head hair

Head hair should be contained.

Face

Facial protection is mandatory with protective isolation of the eyes, nose and mouth. Full eye protection should include shatter resistant coverings.

Air quality assessment and appropriate protection should be ensured. Protection should be appropriate to the actual or perceived risks. This may range from a basic mask through to fully enclosed breathing apparatus. Training and certification either prior to or at the time may be necessary.

Hands

At the minimum, adequate supplies of vinyl or nitrile disposable gloves need to be available. These should be of adequate thickness to offer some protection from sharp objects encountered during an autopsy (such as fractured bone ends and instruments). Where the use of a scalpel is employed, then the operator should wear a 'Kevlar' type glove on the non-cutting hand to minimise self-inflicted injuries. Non-essential staff should stand clear during the use of sharp instruments such as a scalpel, and whenever bone is cut, or be also suitably protected.

Body covering

The conflict of degree of protection and the environment in which it is to be used is a constant balancing act. Full body coverage and self-contained breathing apparatus may be necessary in a highly contagious/contaminated environment, but are perhaps inappropriate when dealing with certain skeletal remains. Generally, the higher the level of protection the greater the limitation on the user's mobility and working time. An assessment (by appropriate experts) needs to be made at the time of examination of the perceived site risks associated with the examination of the remains. This will need to be further reinforced by a health assessment, by appropriately experienced personnel, of the remains and the health status of the examiner/s, at the point of examination.

The type and extent of covering will vary according to the determined risk factors and environmental conditions. The body covering material should be robust and fluid proof, but allow as much operator comfort and movement as possible. Often in routine examinations the body handler/examiner may need to wear a heavier duty fluid resistant apron.

Footwear

Suitable footwear would provide foot protection to both crush penetration type injury and fluids. Calf-height waterproof boots ending under a protective gown would be acceptable for most circumstances.

'Tools of the trade'

At a minimum a basic set of a mirror and probe is essential. A fresh set of instruments should be used for each separate specimen examination to avoid operator cross-contamination. Probes and other sharp-ended instruments should preferably not be double ended, to minimise the risk of sharps injuries. The choice of instruments would ultimately be at the examiner's behest. Regular examiners will develop a favourite set of tools.

All instruments should be procedurally removed from the specimen at the end of each examination to minimise injury risk to other handlers. Single-use material (cloth, gauze, or absorbent paper) should be available to 'clean' the examination site. All instruments should be either disposable or sterilisable. Appropriate disposal, cleaning and sterilising protocols need to be in place.

A mouth prop will also prove useful in many examination scenarios. These may be of a fixed variety, such as wedge-shaped rubber props, or may be of a mechanical nature that enables the 'forced' opening of the oral cavity using mechanical advantage where rigor mortis, heat (carbonisation), or refrigeration has fixed the musculature.

Photography

This is not a discourse on 'how to' but rather an overview of factors important in producing good images in this specific role and setting.

Good photography certainly ranks in importance with radiography and 'notes' in documenting a case. Photographs are not only objective, and capture specific subject matter in the examiner's eye at the time, but also capture surrounding information that may be useful later. As noted in the 'Radiographic' section, adopt a rigid, effective and workable routine, including strict save and backup protocols. As with all information management, thought should be given to the process of managing and using the images produced.

Capture device (camera and lens/es) and media
There is little argument for not using digital photography/cameras for routine and mass casualty work situations. Smaller, cheaper devices generally compromise on factors such as image resolution, add 'noise' on data capture and offer no or a reduced choice of lens. Smaller cameras also have smaller image capture screens. Most data collection will be 'normal' and 'close up' photography, similar to clinical photography.

Producing and processing images
If using digital recording devices, ensure images are saved at a high-quality setting. This allows for better quality images and manipulation of images (e.g. magnification), if needed, particularly during reconciliation.

Settings should be selected on the basis of producing the highest quality and most detailed images. On quality cameras the image quality should be set on 'fine'. 'JPEG compression' should be set to optimise the image rather than reduce size. Image size should be 'medium' or 'large'. Where possible a JPEG and a RAW image should be collected.

An ideal image will be a balance of:

- ISO: the speed of capturing the image. ISO sets the recording sensor's reaction to the light collected during the exposure. Increased ISO settings result in more noise in the image, thereby reducing quality.
- Shutter speed: longer shutter speeds are more affected by movement.
- Aperture: the size of the opening of the lens when capturing the image, or the amount of light that reaches the sensor during the shot. Aperture size dramatically affects the depth of field.

A high-quality image will enable useful manipulation (e.g. magnification) of the image, particularly during reconciliation.

Remember, manipulated working views can always be saved as lower quality and size images if required.

Organising images

All images should be identified with 'Body identifier', time and date, as well as some useful identifier as to specific subject matter. To minimise risks of incorrect allocation of evidence in multiple case examinations, use separate memory cards or a new roll of film for each separate case. Always ensure the memory card is 'cleared' once the images have been downloaded and appropriately archived. An identical backup procedure as used for radiographs should be adopted, if only for simplicity of procedure and familiarity. RAW images where taken and the first generation JPEG should be saved and backed up. Any manipulation of an image should be done on a copy and stored in the working file.

Using images

Always use a copy of the original so as to avoid inadvertent damage or alteration of the image and to ensure that you retain the best backup possible.

Backup

Backup protocols need to be in place. One suggested protocol is to store the RAW image (i.e. natural state – not yet processed, in effect a digital 'negative' of the subject material recorded) as the original along with a JPEG image. Working images are taken from the JPEG version, with the RAW image available should the JPEG image corrupt or degrade with use. The same is applicable to all the usual formats (TIFF, GIFF etc.).

Archiving

When archiving all the material ensure that the original RAW, JPEG and copies of any altered images used for reporting are stored separately from the case file. This ideally would be on another system or appropriate storage media off site. Ensure metadata is intact.

Use a set routine for the examination. Start with a photograph of both the photographer's identification (to record who is responsible for the photography), and the identification number or label of the subject material. The photographic examination and record should start with an overview image of the whole subject matter and then progressively document the detail of the subject matter. Ensure each view is 'relatable' back to the overview of the subject matter. This enables relationships to be maintained later when reviewing or demonstrating/explaining one's findings.

An accurate (certified) scale should be used. An example of an acceptable scale would be the ABFO No 2 scale. This is not only a certified 'ruler' but has colour correction bars and circles to help demonstrate any distortion in the photographic image.

When photographing (especially) complete skull specimens, be mindful of the type of clinical views that might be available from ante-mortem sources, for example profile views and face on views that may be compared to ante-mortem 'smiling' subject photographs.

'Auto focus' may result in out of focus subject material if not set to spot focusing. Check each image after taking the view or revert to manual focus.

Be aware of distortions due to angulation between lens and subject material. Always try and keep the area of interest at or as close to 90 degrees to the lens.

Dark subject material (such as carbonised remains) presents particular challenges in relation to contrast and recording of detail.

Ensure each photographic view is adequately identified with the specimen identifier code, or able to be easily related to other photographs suitably identified.

Audit trails are always part of 'best practice' but are particularly relevant in any subsequent legal process. Again, having a routine procedure will minimise omissions (particularly when tired, stressed or distracted).

Depth of field

This can be quite demanding for an operator who is not proficient, or a regular specimen photographer. Often with close-up photography and 'macroscopic' photography, film speeds and consequently aperture size influence the depth of field, which can be very limited. Ensure complete 'in focus' views of each tooth are obtained either as individual views or in-group views of the teeth, as well as any specific area detail.

Fragments and single teeth

Ensure that images of fragments or fragmented pieces are able to be correctly (anatomically) visualised, especially at a later date. Views that are obvious at the time can later be difficult to localise.

If using the services of a police or other professional photographer, the author's experience is that the photographer produces an excellent image, but often misses the specific 'mind's eye' required by the odontologist. It may be necessary to train the photographer to produce the best images that are appropriate from an odontologist's viewpoint.

Radiographic equipment

Not unlike photography, radiography has been/is moving into the digital age. This results in a range of systems for capturing, sorting, transferring, storing and viewing the information. The same problems as in the clinical environment pervade this activity. Sensors can be of the phosphor plate type film ranging through to expensive sensors of various size and thickness with and without an attached cord. Consideration must be given to 'holding' the recording media in situ 'on' the specimen while capturing the image in relation to optimal data collection and minimising operator radiation exposure.

All equipment coming into contact with specimens needs to be suitably protected (barrier protection). Methods will vary according to the situation and the ingenuity of the examiner. Most methods involve disposable plastic coverings (as available in clinical situations), or the use of materials such as cling wrap-type of plastic coverings as used for foods.

Likewise, methods for holding capturing sensors and to a lesser extent analogue film vary from one examiner to the next. The author's experience with most commercial devices (invariably developed for clinical situations) is problematic. Pieces of absorbent sponge material (as used in kitchens) cut into appropriate sizes to support the sensor can be useful. Often absorbent paper moistened and/or crumpled up will suffice.

CT scanning equipment

Increasingly CT tomography is being utilised in the examination of post-mortem remains. The use of CT scanning allows overview examinations and detailed reconstructions of areas of interest without needing to directly examine the remains. This results not only in rapid examination of the remains, but allows more focused traditional examinations, and the location of odontological material of interest in fragmented collections of remains. CT scanning also removes the need for direct contact with the remains. This is particularly relevant when dealing with dangerously contaminated remains (be they biological, chemical or radiological).

Teeth for DNA analysis

It is increasingly being recognised that teeth can provide viable material for DNA analysis as well as or instead of traditional sources such as muscle and oral swabs. The effects of the various post-mortem parameters affecting teeth and the choice of tooth for selection for DNA source material is an evolving and poorly understood area [1].

Tooth selection is best left to those experts in the field of DNA analysis; however, it is important that consultation with the forensic odontologist occurs. Removal of selected teeth should be carried out preferably by the forensic odontologist or certainly under their supervision. Removal of any tooth should only occur after the completion of the forensic odontologist's examination, documentation and a thorough discussion with the DNA expert as to the selection of the tooth or teeth. This should include full photographic and radiographic records, relationships with adjacent and opposing teeth, periodontal and anatomical positioning, as well as any lifestyle indicators.

The removal of any anterior teeth may have implications for any subsequent photographic or video superimposition studies and in terms of viewing of the remains by family and so on. Removal of posterior teeth may have implications in the determination of occlusal relationships with the opposing arch. Multi-rooted teeth require greater expertise to successfully remove intact and with minimal bony destruction than single-rooted teeth, as well the risk of damage to adjacent teeth requires that the person responsible for such an activity is suitably trained. The condition of the tooth to be removed is also important. Eroded, carious or previously restored teeth, age of the tooth, periodontal status, as well as post-mortem conditions are all factors to be considered in the selection of the tooth or teeth for DNA sampling. A thorough consultation with the relevant expertise is important. Appropriate permissions, consents and documentation need to be completed.

The 'what and how'

Organisation

As stated a number of times: have a procedural routine. NEVER have in your work area material relating to another case past or impending. This applies both to traditional paperwork or files open on a computer monitor. Stress and interruptions to the work schedule will almost guarantee confusion. Figures 6.1 and 6.2 are examples of a basic work flow sheet and report sheet.

Permissions

Any post-mortem is an invasive examination and potentially destructive. Consent is required to perform any examination on the living and equally applies to the deceased even when the consenting authority is more distant from the victim. Consents may relate to the investigative authority, family members of the deceased, and the examinee in living cases such as sexual assault cases. The scope of such consents may also be influenced by moral, religious and social mores. This is particularly true in multi-casualty events where international and national factors of the victim's origin may differ from those that the forensic odontologist has most commonly confronted.

DENTAL IDENTIFICATION CHECKLIST

Body #: .... / .... Trolley #: ....

Day Book Entry: ☐   Request on DVI System: ☐   AM ☐ PM ☐

Postmortem

P79A   . ☐ Filed   Date .... Sig ....

PM '600' pages   ☐ Yes   ☐ Entered   ☐ Reconciled   Date .... Sig ....

Radiographs   ☐ Taken   ☐ Entered   ☐ Reconciled   Date .... Sig ....

Photographs   ☐ Taken   ☐ Entered   ☐ Reconciled   Date .... Sig ....

Other   ☐ Yes   ☐ Entered   ☐ Reconciled   Date .... Sig ....

Antemortem

Name of Deceased: ....

Name of Contact Dentist: .... T: ....

          Address: .... E: ....

                   .... P/CODE: ....

AM '600' pages   ☐ Yes   ☐ Entered   ☐ Reconciled   Date..................... Sig ....

Radiographs   ☐ Receipt ☐ Entered   ☐ Reconciled   Date..................... Sig ....

Photographs   ☐ Receipt ☐ Entered   ☐ Reconciled   Date..................... Sig ....

Other   ☐ Yes   ☐ Entered   ☐ Reconciled   Date..................... Sig ....

Reconciliation   ☐ Positive   ☐ Consistent   ☐ Exclusion

Non-Visual report   ☐ Yes   Date .... Sig ....

Peer review   ☐ Yes   Date .... Sig ....

Report to Coroner   ☐ Yes   Date .... Sig ....

'Thank you' Letter/s   ☐ Yes   Date .... Sig ....

Date: Notes: Continued over the page

Fig. 6.1 Dental identification checklist.

NON-VISUAL IDENTIFICATION REPORT				
DATE:				
ACCESSION NUMBER:				
HAS BEEN IDENTIFIED AS:	NAME: .... AGE: .... SEX: .... ADDRESS:			
IDENTIFICATION BY:	ANTHROPOLOGY ☐ DENTAL ☐ DNA ☐ FINGERPRINT ☐		MEDICAL ☐ PROPERTY ☐ OTHER ☐	
COPIES TO:	ADMINISTRATION ☐ CORONER'S SGT ☐ GRIEF COUNSELLOR ☐ MORTUARY MANAGER ☐ PATHOLOGIST ☐ MOLECULAR BIOLOGIST ☐			
SIGNATURE IDENTIFICATION SECTION:	....			

Fig. 6.2 Non-visual identification report.

Examples of permissions relate not only to the actual examination, but also to the retention of human remains, the manner of the examination and the removal and handling of teeth for DNA analysis.

Examination and recording of the findings

Determine the purpose of the examination. The circumstances necessitating the examination may be unclear or incomplete at the time of examination. An examination for comparison and identification purposes is a vastly different examination to one for investigative purposes. The purpose of the examination will often evolve while being performed, either because of evolving investigative requirements or as a result of one's own findings.

The investigative examination

The investigative type of examination (less usual) will involve the gathering of as much information from observations as possible. This will need to consist of non-judgemental observations, and likely not be primarily for comparative (identification) purposes.

The identification examination

The examination activities for the purposes of identification are essentially no different to those that would be performed in a clinical setting on a live person. The challenge is that the 'patient' is not cooperative, and often not physically present, as we would expect in a normal clinical dental setting. The types of examinations and techniques involved will be dictated by the extent and condition of the material available for examination. This will often require some creativity and lateral thinking on the part of the forensic odontologist.

The reality has also to be faced that re-examination, especially in a mass casualty event, may be impossible or extremely difficult (for reasons such as operational, legal, jurisdictional, social, religious and ethical). It is thus very important that maximal information is gathered at the time of the examination, especially in the context of radiography and photography. The post-mortem examination is often performed without knowing the full extent and quality of ante-mortem information available. In a mass casualty scenario, the post-mortem examiner may never access the ante-mortem information. Where there are numerous deceased, it may not be known whether the remains being examined are those of a 'critical' person in the investigation (such as the driver of the vehicle, or the suspected perpetrator of the event).

Detail

There is a continuing debate (particularly regarding computerised sorting systems), in relation to basic information versus detailed information. Nothing can be truer than a 'picture paints a thousand words'. In this age of digital radiography and especially photography the production of comprehensive and informative records is easier than before. The results of the images are seen almost instantly and they can easily be retaken, reproduced and manipulated. Record images using an acceptable format such as JPEG (Graphics file type/extension-Joint Expert Photographic Group).

These are also records that one can consult later under more ideal conditions (both personal and physical) to add quality to the visual observations. Good radiographic and photographic records (particularly in relation to investigative types of reports) allows for the expansion of detail as specific requirements evolve. Never hesitate to produce 'too many' images.

Written observations and charting

In principle, the more detail the better: the quality and accuracy of the descriptive detail is more important than the quantum or particular interpretation. Very often 'in the field examination detail' may be limited for any number of reasons, some of which are noted below. Obtain only that information (particularly in identifications) that is reasonable to expect to be available in ante-mortem health records, particularly dental records. Inaccurate recording or interpretation of findings will be misleading. Underestimating is more helpful and less misleading than over enthusiastic observations, particularly in relation to restorative surfaces. Where doubt exists do not hesitate to attach a note to that effect. Recording a restoration as a mesial, occlusal, distal (MOD) restoration with an examiner decision to add, say, lingual surface because of a perceived encroachment onto that surface, will be misleading if the creator of the restoration only recorded it as a MOD. For matching purposes when reconciling the ante- and post-mortem records, the lesser detail will usually be more comparatively useful.

While all this may contradict earlier statements in relation to recording as much detail as possible due to limitations in revisiting the remains, these written observations will hopefully be backed up with good radiographic and photographic records, which, as discussed earlier, may be referred to.

Finally, always have a template for recording your findings, so that stress, distractions and tiredness do not result in incomplete records.

Recording of the findings

The forensic odontologist (particularly in relation to ongoing legal issues, further or new findings), may need to consult their records some time, even years, later.

Stress

The examination and recording of observations is often performed outside of a routine time or scenario. Any change to routine is a stressor and errors can occur. It is important to have a routine.

Legibility

It should go without saying, but all recording of findings must be legible. In the digital scenario this is less of a problem. Where hand recording is being used, either appoint a capable scribe, or ensure that the recordings are legible and meaningful. Always record in an indelible format.

Language

In some cases (particularly mass casualty events) the forensic odontologist/s, whose working language is not English, may examine your findings at another time and/or place. Use precise and clear language.

Errors

Particularly during the initial examination, the first observations may need refining as more evidence is obtained. Clearly mark any corrections while leaving visible the errors. Particularly in multi-user and multi-input documents, initial the changes so that an auditable trail is established. In mass casualty events there may frequently be additions or alterations to the initial findings by others.

Abbreviations

Where abbreviations are used, include an explanation with the documentation. This explanation should preferably be present as an addendum, and not noted as one uses them.

Transcription

Any transcription of information will risk errors. Minimise the necessity of transcribing. This can be achieved with the use of well-recognised (especially international) computer programs, with the ability to 'cut and paste'.

Charting

State the charting system being used. There are a myriad of different charting systems in use around the world. In Australia it is not uncommon to regularly see in use charting systems such as the Fédération Dentaire Internationale (FDI) system, the American Universal system and the older Palmer notation. It is preferable to use a well-known charting system.

Clearly indicate the left- and right-side convention being used. Not all charting systems use the same left and right convention. Ensure that any photographic and radiographic images are clearly marked using the same convention.

Where colours are used to indicate types of dental materials (particularly in restorations), note the protocol used (preferably as an addendum).

When 'colouring in' odontograms, adopt a consistency in relation to whether you are diagrammatic or trying to record the actual shape of the restoration. The author prefers the use of diagrammatic recordings, with annotated notes in the records for unusual surface distributions.

Clinical notes

Ensure that these are clear and concise. State facts and flag assumptions. There is no shame in ambiguity as long as it is flagged. Very often there will be ambiguity in initial examinations, especially if working in less than ideal situations or conditions. Opinions and or conjecture should also be noted as such.

Any note should be clearly related to a particular tooth or anatomical area. Support the findings with either radiographic or photographic evidence. Opinions or conjecture should also be fully explained with reasons and supporting evidence. Always remember that there may never be another chance to re-examine the post-mortem remains.

Dentally significant findings may have been recorded in a medical rather than a dental context. These should be flagged for follow up in medical ante-mortem records. An example might be frontal sinus patterns.

Radiographic

Use a set routine for the examination and account for each tooth/area. (By example, start with the 18 area (FDI) notation and proceed through all 32 tooth areas, then 'bite-wing' type radiographs, followed by any special examination). Having a routine procedure will minimise omissions, especially if tired, stressed or distracted. Ensure each radiographic view is adequately identified with the specimen identifier code. If using digital storage of images, ensure appropriate backup protocols.

There may be a need to experiment with exposure times in relation to tissue thicknesses and presenting the condition of the remains. When taking radiographs through doubled-over reflected tissues, exposure times will by necessity increase, whilst skeletal subject matter will result in decreased exposure times.

Ensure all teeth and tooth bearing areas are recorded and complete views of each tooth (root apex to crown tip) are obtained as well as any specific area detail. Where possible record 'bite-wing' angled views of posterior teeth in each quadrant.

If using digital recording devices, ensure images are saved at a high-quality setting. This allows for better quality images and manipulation of images (e.g. magnification), if needed.

Tissue thicknesses

Greater thought must be employed in selecting exposure settings compared to clinical in vivo settings. Teeth and bone with no soft tissue covering require less exposure than obtaining images taken through a double layer of tissue where the soft tissues have been reflected for examination.

Fragments and single teeth

Articulate fragments and single teeth in the normal anatomical manner, so that they may be radiographed from the usual ante-mortem aspect. NEVER radiograph a tooth from the 'inside', or lingual aspect.

Radiation safety

Observe all legal, moral and professional requirements for proper protection for all present while taking radiographs.

Photographic

Use a routine as previously stated. Photography is very useful to document an auditable trail. Photograph the subject material before the commencement of the examination. Provide overview photographs. Provide visual evidence of specific observations, notes or comments if possible

Impressions

While not performed routinely, impressions may be appropriate, particularly in bite mark analysis. Impressions of non-living tissues will be noticeably affected by the specimens' lower temperature, resulting in extended setting times. While the use of alginate-type impression materials is cheaper and usually more readily available, the use of poly vinyl siloxane type products is preferable as the resultant impressions are usually more accurate and stable over time. Factors that may become relevant in relation to the production of impressions are:

- Time taken from impression to producing the model.
- Need to duplicate models.
- Degree of accuracy required.

Age estimation

An estimate of age is often requested. Age estimation is not assessment. While with developing dentitions the age range can be narrowed significantly, adult dentitions can vary considerably. Adult age assessments or estimations can be misleading and result in delayed identification and consequent legal action. Always endeavour to use several different methods and state those used. The literature contains a plethora of ageing systems of varying complexity and using different components of the tooth structure. The choice of system/s adopted may be dictated by the dental evidence available.

Condition of the remains

Probably the most influential element of the post-mortem examination will be the condition of the remains to be examined.

Complete body or a partial set of remains?

Probably the most visually impacting element will be that of confronting an often incomplete (human) corpse versus an intact corpse. This can be unsettling even for the experienced forensic odontologist. As their role is primarily identification, they tend to see the less-complete or less well-preserved set of human remains. While the area of interest lies around the oral cavity, a rapid determination of the completeness of the area of interest needs to be made. Where fragmentation has occurred to the area of interest, try to collect all the relevant material and determine the effectiveness of the field recovery to date, and assess the benefit of any revisit of the collection site.

Once the subject material is collected, attempt to assemble it as anatomically closely as possible. This will simplify the mind's eye assessment and examination process.

Incomplete and/or fragmented?

A differentiation needs to be made between 'intact but incomplete', as in missing teeth or mandible, versus 'fragmented'. This fragmentation could take place either peri- or post-mortem and often occurs at the time of death or due to carnivore predation or human intervention. Individual teeth, particularly single-rooted teeth, will often fall from their respective bony sockets once the soft tissues have sufficiently decomposed. Teeth may fall into other body part areas or be transported from the area by (for example) animal, human or meteorological activity. Care must be exercised when working with fragmented skeletal remains, as the areas of fracture can be quite sharp and capable of piercing gloves and penetrating the examiner's fingers or hand.

Are all the teeth and bone sections present?

If teeth are missing, determine which missing teeth are the results of pre-, peri- and post-mortem activity. In relation to peri- and post-mortem loss, determine whether the teeth have been displaced into other non-anatomically correct areas of the remains. Are missing elements recoverable from the scene, and if so has this been actioned?

Usually, non-dentally trained persons have performed the recovery of the remains from the scene. Specific instructions and perhaps guidance needs to be offered to maximise the chance of recovery of such remains.

Commonly the mandible will have fractured, distal to the second or third molar, around the premolar/canine area and/or in the midline. The maxilla will often be fractured from the skull, or often along suture lines.

Skeletal remains

These are invariably the easiest remains to examine. After arranging the remains in some anatomical order the examination may begin. The fragility of skeletal remains will depend largely on the time since death to discovery and the environmental conditions of the 'burial' site. Highly acidic soil or water run off will produce harsher conditions for the longevity of skeletal material, especially thinner and less-calcified material. Burial of the skeletal material will produce both positive and negative effects on the rate of change of the state of the bones and teeth.

Incinerated remains

These can be some of the most challenging remains. Incineration can range from partial soft tissue destruction to cremains. Often severity of incineration will vary across the specimen dependent on the location and position of the body and the duration and intensity of the incineration process. As a guide most bone will incinerate from 500°C to 650°C, amalgam mercury from approximately 100°C, gold alloys from approximately 870°C, porcelains from as low as approximately 760 °C and cobalt chrome alloy from approximately 1370°C.

Handling

From the initial manner of discovery and subsequent recovery of incinerated remains the material remains extremely fragile, with extreme risk of degradation or even loss of the subject material if inappropriately handled. In situations where the remains are severely incinerated they may need to be stabilised prior to removal from the incident site. A number of methods have been proposed over the years (ranging from hair spray through to the use of glues such as cyano-acrylate-based glues). The author commonly uses the latter and then wraps the remains in padding material (such as bubble-wrap) for transport. The materials are reasonably easily procurable at short notice.

Vulnerability

Incinerated remains will vary considerably in their vulnerability. Often the burning process has not penetrated beyond the soft tissues, and associated muscle contraction has served to protect the dental arches, particularly in the posterior segments of the mouth and the lingual surfaces of the dentition. The lips, being thinnest, will often succumb to the incineration process first, exposing the incisor teeth to further destruction due to the incineration effects. In more severe cases teeth may appear in situ but be severely 'heat affected' with fracturing of the tooth structure with and without tooth integrity (especially dependent on care in discovery and recovery). Restorations will often have been destroyed in association with tooth loss. In severe cases total coronal tooth loss may have occurred with root fragments contained 'intact' within the bone. Bone, not unlike tooth structure, will also suffer the effects of the incineration process.

Soft tissues

Skin and thin facial muscles succumb quickly to the effects of fire and heat. Larger muscles resist longer and the higher moisture content and thickness serve to counter the effects of incineration and protect underlying (tooth) structures. Tetany, or the involuntary contraction of muscles associated with incinerated materials, may make oral access difficult, but will also serve to drive the tongue against the lingual surfaces of the teeth providing a negative image of the tooth surfaces as well as protecting them.

General

In general with incinerated remains, it is necessary to complete the initial photographic and radiographic examination as early as possible in case the remains 'collapse'.

Decomposed remains

Whilst not technically correct, as all degradation of remains is part of the decomposition process, the term is used to refer to the process where remains decompose in normal surroundings due primarily to time. The attendant environmental conditions impose their own specific effects on the process. The rate of changes in decomposition will relate to the manner of death, environmental conditions and time since death.

Early decomposition usually results in the discolouration of the body surfaces and some 'bloating' of the remains. From an odontological perspective, the tissues are largely intact apart from related trauma at time of death and the effects of animal/insect predation. The latter will occur very soon after death in most circumstances with the establishment of larvae colonies and subsequent maggot infestation. Entomologists can glean important information from such effects.

Odour and liquifaction aside, these remains are usually anatomically intact and relatively easy with which to work. From an odontology perspective the hard tissues are largely unaffected by the process and any remaining soft tissue and muscle is easily removed for examination. Early post-mortem tooth loss (as previously discussed) may occur from this stage.

The latter stages of these changes in decomposition will be the final loss of non-calcified body structures leaving exposed skeletal material.

Mummification

This is a condition where the remains have been desiccated or dried out. This may occur where temperature and/or moisture are low, slowing or stopping the usual changes in decomposition. These remains are usually quite resilient and relatively easy to work with.

Immersion

Very little data is available in relation to the changes in decomposition of human remains in water. Remains are similarly exposed to a variety of environmental factors and predation. Remains may be scattered over a wide area as a result of currents and when washed ashore skeletal remains may be damaged by forceful contact with rocks and the abrasive nature of sand. It is not uncommon from an odontological perspective to recover only one jaw, or for the other jaw to be recovered in a different location at a different time. Similar dynamics will be evident in floods and fast flowing rivers. (See Chapter 11 – Forensic microbial aquatic taphonomy.)

Procedure – putting it all together

Initial examination

Having read any notes or history in relation to the subject material (especially circumstances of death, place of death, environment of the death scene, presumed time since death, recovery procedure and any previous examinations to date), approach the remains mentally and physically with a 'hands off' attitude. Observe the material with a questioning mindset, deciding on one's initial approach and order of examination. Initially document the overview with both photographic views and written notes. Remember to assess not only hard tissues but also soft tissues including, if appropriate, soft tissue (such as rugae patterns). Assess the impact of one's examination on the remains and decide on the order of examination. Where 'bite mark' or 'pattern' injuries may be present, then documentation of these should take precedence (see below).

Photographic and radiographic examination

Where the remains are particularly fragile (such as with incineration), then the use of photographic documentation (close-up views) and any minimally invasive radiology examination is mandatory. Resection and/or dissection should only then commence.

While the condition of the remains may be far removed from their living state, they are still representative (usually) of a human life, and as such deserve the respect and dignity expected. The forensic odontologist must also be mindful that the family may wish to view the remains, subsequent to the examination. Resection and dissection should thus be minimised in relation to an adequate and thorough examination. The community is today more questioning of the necessity of an autopsy and, if necessary, the procedures performed during the autopsy.

Access and reflection

The primary requirement for any examination is the need to be able to access the area/s to be examined (usually and primarily the teeth). This will of course be dependent on the presenting condition of the remains. The aim is to gain maximum access for examination purposes with minimal interference with the tissues.

Intact skulls and mandible

Access requirements will be primarily dictated by the amount and condition of the soft tissues covering the underlying hard tissues. If these tissues are fresh then normal dissection activity will be necessary (see later).

Where the soft tissues are more decomposed, then the dissection techniques will need to be modified to achieve the primary aim of adequate access. In some conditions (often with advanced soft tissue decomposition and immersion cases), the soft tissues may even be peeled off the underlying hard tissues.

In lightly incinerated cases, the soft tissues will appear burnt but 'normal' tissue lies underneath the surface and normal dissection is possible. Advanced incineration will result in the drying out of the soft tissue, often resulting in dried-out soft tissue through to quite leathery soft tissue. Dissection in these cases will often result in the loss of soft tissue integrity.

One of the more challenging environments is where one is dealing with heavily incinerated material with fragmenting or crumbling hard tissue material, but is partly supported by soft tissue material that needs to be removed for access. Often here the use of cyano-acrylate-type glues to stabilise the subject material before dissection is necessary.

Fragmented skulls and mandible

The forensic odontologist is often presented with fragmentation of the hard tissues that are all contained by the covering soft tissues. This is common in those cases where bodies have suffered impact with, for example, motor vehicles or trains, or falling from a height onto a hard surface. In such situations the body may appear intact while there is multiple fragmentation of the skeletal structure, or conversely the body has been torn apart on impact with multiple body fragments containing skeletal material still attached to soft tissues.

In all these cases the examiner must be mindful to the principle of a minimally invasive examination out of respect for the victim, and the possible need for reconstruction of the remains for viewing by family. This may at times seem unlikely, but one never ceases to be amazed by expectations, requests and the abilities of those who do facial reconstruction.

Reflection technique

The reflection technique used must, as previously stated, allow for maximal access and the ability to subsequently reconstruct the victim for possible viewing and minimising the visual effects of our examination. Frequently, muscle tetany/rigidity requires the release of muscle attachments to gain adequate access.

Over the recent past, there has been a move away from the retention of body parts, including jaws, except under special circumstances that usually need permission and documentation by the relevant authorities.

The removal and separation of the mandible from the rest of the remains is no longer considered routinely acceptable in many jurisdictions. This does not, of course, preclude the need to dissect the muscle and tissue attachments around the condylar heads and rami to allow fuller access to the oral cavity, and in some cases to resect completely the mandible from the remains.

The technique favoured is one that enables maximal access, conforms with common body autopsy techniques (if performed prior to the dental autopsy) and minimises any disfigurement). Any technique used will need to be flexible in relation to the amount of tissue present and the condition of the tissue.

Floor of the mouth and tongue

Many head and neck autopsy techniques result in the tongue and floor of the mouth being displaced downwards at the time of the medical autopsy, such that any further lingual access to the mandibular teeth is minimal. Further access may require minimal removal of soft tissue from over the inner posterior surfaces of the mandible, and the freeing of the muscle attachments of the muscle attachments around the ramus and coronoid process. This autopsy technique will not usually impact on any access to the maxilla or to accessing the oral cavity via the mouth.

Access the maxilla and the oral cavity

Often the medical autopsy technique will allow for the reflection of the soft tissues from below the chin to the infra-orbital margin. Additional elevating of the soft tissues from the underlying bone may be necessary over the maxilla and zygomatic arch areas. Where such a dissection has not been already performed, then one technique is to start an incision of the skin behind the ears, descending along and behind the distal border of the ramus and then along and immediately inside the lower border of the body of the mandible. This cut should be such that the incision line under the mandible lies underneath so that the soft tissues over the lower border of the mandible are intact. The tissue above this incision is then bluntly elevated off the underlying bone and progressively reflected to below the infra-orbital margins. It is important to reflect these tissues high enough that the tissues are out of the range of the alignment of the x-ray cone when taking periodical views (particularly of the maxillary molars). If not, then correct angulation and alignment of the x-ray beam is much more difficult and exposure times have to be increased to compensate for possible increased tissue thicknesses due to the doubling over of the reflected tissues. This also allows a clear view of the maxillary teeth and the overlying bone, enabling a view of any bony defects.

Any reflection technique achieving the previously stated aims will be acceptable and will always need to be adapted to the condition of the remains being examined. Appropriate care needs to be exercised when using sharps, including a 'cut proof' glove on the non-dominant hand, or on the hands of any assistant.

Resection

As previously stated, many jurisdictions question the need to resect a jaw/s. The process is less-frequently performed today and, where needed, requires specific approval from the appropriate authorities. Locating the resected material away from the rest of the remains is not to be recommended, and where such a situation arises, should be well documented. Any protocol for such a procedure should include procedures for the reunification of the body parts after examination.

Bite mark and other pattern recording

This section is not an outline on bite mark and pattern analysis. Bite marks, or other pattern injuries, may be present on the subject material to be examined. The forensic odontologist may commence the examination aware of these features or may find them during the course of the examination. It is thus important before commencing any invasive procedure to carry out an 'external' or 'overview' examination of the subject material for any indications of bite marks or other pattern marks. Examination and recording of such marks should be carried out early in the examination to eliminate any further contamination of the mark.

If a bite mark is suspected then swabbing the site for evidence of body fluids for DNA analysis would be one of the first data collection activities. More often this will provide more useful evidence than analysis of the bite mark. Collection should be carried out using a standard testing/collection procedure and kit as provided either by the investigators or mortuary facility. The subject material should be photographed with and without a scale. The usefulness of photographs will depend on the correct angulation of the view. Impressions and other recordings may or may not be deemed necessary (refer to more detailed subject material). When taking any impressions, be mindful that all impression recording materials will set far more slowly than in vivo due to the lack of body heat. It is also important to ensure that nothing causes unnatural distortion of the tissues being examined. Again, appropriate permissions, consents and documentation need to be completed.

Reporting recording of results

There will principally be two sets of documents.
- Working notes, observations and records (including written, radiographic, photographic and any others deemed necessary).
- Report/s.

Reports
These have to be prepared in relation to the target audience, and will largely fall into two categories.
- First, those to peers. These can be written in professional terminology.
- Second, those to 'lay' persons. This audience will want facts stated simply, clearly, and understandably. This does not imply that proper and detailed explanation is not necessary.

The layout of a report will vary from person to person, jurisdiction and situation. The checklist given does not attempt to be prescriptive other than to indicate the general content.
- personal details
- name
- points of contact
- telephone
- email
- postal address
- qualifications
- position held relative to the report being generated
- present and past relative to the report
- timetable/sequence and place/s of examination/s
- co-examiners and others present

- any limitations as a result of the place/s, co-examiners or others present
- circumstance or reason for being present/performing the examination
- examination report to be detailed, concise and scientific
- note of any further tests and unreported results
- detail of the types of records generated
- written, photographic, radiographic evidence etc.
- any specimens/body parts retained
- explanation of the reason and note any authorities obtained to retain such material
- methodologies used.

Summary

This is probably the most important part of the report. In some cases it can be placed at the beginning of the report for convenience. It should be accurate and concise, usually written in 'lay' terms with appropriate reference to the more detailed portions of the report.

Finally, remember that one may need to defend this report and it would be inappropriate to need to call on data not presented within the report.

Reference

1 Higgins D, Austin JJ. (2013) Teeth as a source of DNA for forensic identification of human remains: a review. *Science and Justice* **53**, 433–441.

CHAPTER 7

Age assessment

Richard Bassed[1], Jeremy Graham[2] and Jane A. Taylor[3]

[1] Victorian Institute of Forensic Medicine, Victoria; and Monash University, Australia
[2] School of Dentistry and Oral Health, La Trobe University, Australia
[3] Faculty of Health and Medicine, University of Newcastle, Australia

Introduction

The ability to assign accurate age estimates to human remains and living individuals is an important element of forensic practice. Age estimation can contribute to a routine forensic dental identification and be a vital component in the investigation of anthropological/archaeological specimens [1]. In mass fatality events, where many people lose their lives and are often unable to be visually identified, being able to separate individuals based on their age as determined by skeletal and/or dental development is an integral part of the Disaster Victim Identification (DVI) process [2]. In the tragic bushfire disaster that struck Victoria in February 2009, for example, of the 164 victims who lost their lives and were subject to the DVI process, 25 were under the age of 20 years, and many of these were located in commingled circumstances. Due to the severity of the fires and the condition of many of the remains, it was only possible to identify a number of these by incorporating an assessment of their age using dental and skeletal development [3].

Age estimation of living individuals of unknown age also plays an important role in the assessment of those who have entered a foreign jurisdiction without identification papers or with suspect personal documents. It is necessary to be able to determine the age status of these individuals for a number of reasons, including school entry and year level age requirements, and also for assessment of legal adulthood or childhood. Determination of an individual's age status as either an adult or a child is important in terms of how that person will be treated by the law in criminal prosecutions, immigration hearings, licensing applications and, increasingly important, determination of refugee status [4–10].

As an example, approximately 65% of the Sub-Saharan African and South East Asian populations do not have their births registered in any legally verifiable way. For many individuals, it is not possible to determine objectively whether or not legal adulthood has been reached. This has major implications for criminal prosecutions of people suspected of recruiting child soldiers, and those accused of

Forensic Odontology: Principles and Practice, First Edition. Edited by Jane A. Taylor and Jules A. Kieser.
© 2016 John Wiley & Sons, Ltd. Published 2016 by John Wiley & Sons, Ltd.

sexual offences against children. A recent trial conducted by the International Criminal Court (ICC) arising from events in the Democratic Republic of Congo (ICC vs Thomas Lubanga, accused of conscripting child soldiers) demonstrated the issues that may arise when age cannot be properly determined [11].

Current age-estimation methods used across the world have been shown to be out-dated and are suspected to be inaccurate [12–16]. The reasons for this are many, but essentially the data used to develop the ageing systems currently in use were gathered from European and North American populations many decades ago. The evidence that such data are applicable to current populations of interest (e.g. African, who are of interest to the ICC; and Indonesian, who are of interest to the Australian immigration authorities and the Australian criminal justice system) is completely lacking. Also, most of the methods in use, such as the Greulich and Pyle hand/wrist atlas [17] and the Schour and Massler dental charts [18], were not designed to determine the age of unknown age individuals, but were a tool constructed for a different purpose: to assess the normality or otherwise of the skeletal/dental development of known-age individuals. Most dental ageing methods currently in use were initially developed as indicators of a child's dental maturity rather than for use in the estimation of dental age. However, Moorrees, Fanning and Hunt [19] in their introduction did state that their method could be used for such purposes.

Some techniques, such as histological analysis of teeth and development of foetal and immature salivary glands, are known to be more sensitive than radiographic methodologies, but require dissection of the organ or sacrifice and destruction of a tooth, and as such are rarely used today. A good summary of these techniques can be found in Blenkin [15].

Consideration must also be given to the issue of developmental variation between present-day populations and the effect of these on age estimations. Some authors state that there is little or no difference, while others state that developmental differences between populations are an important consideration [14, 20–23]. The debate will only be resolved by further research.

In Australia, forensic odontologists and anthropologists have been using age-estimation methods for many decades. As previously stated, these methods were developed from earlier research conducted on populations that geographically, environmentally and nutritionally do not accurately reflect current Australian population demographics. For the very young, that is those individuals under the age of 15 years, these tables – especially those describing dental development – have been assumed to be quite adequate and have served the profession well. Recent research [2, 4, 12–16, 24–26], however, would suggest that these older tables may not be as accurate as was once thought for young individuals, and it is suspected that they may be substantially more inaccurate for individuals older than 15 years of age.

It is recognised that dental development is able to provide a more reliable indicator for chronological age than skeletal development, and that dental maturation is less affected by environmental insults and systemic illness. This being said, it is also well recognised that current tables and charts need to be updated with modern population data.

Some history of age assessment

At the time of burgeoning steam powered industrialisation, from the 1770s in Victorian England, Edwin Saunders, a Fellow of the Medico-Botanical Society, addressed the Houses of Parliament with a pressing concern. It was common practice in this era to employ very young children in newly emerging large-scale factories, and in coal mines that produced the fuel to power these industries. These children, often as young as seven, were forced to work for 12–14 hours a day, six and sometimes seven days a week. Legislation was enacted in 1815, which limited the age of employment to no younger than nine years and the hours of employment to ten hours per day. This legislation was, however, almost universally flouted by the owners of industrial concerns, often with the blessings of the families of these children, as they were often the sole income earners in poverty-stricken English cities. There was no real coordinated birth registry in existence at the time, and so the age of the child had to be given by a parent, or more often by a subjective estimation. The ease with which factory owners avoided these legislated requirements was due in large measure to the inaccuracy and subjective nature of age-estimation methods utilised at the time.

Prevailing age-estimation methods relied on judging the age of a child by measurement of height and a subjective assessment of strength and development. The capacity for deception, practised by both factory owners and parents who wished to put their children to work, was extensive. It became common practice to falsify birth dates and to dress children in such a fashion that they appeared to be far older than they actually were. This practice, combined with a lackadaisical and unscientific approach to age estimation, ensured that countless young children were subjected to labour conditions that would be testing for most adults [27].

It was plain to Saunders and others that a more accurate method to assess the age of children, and one not reliant on the inherently variable height and strength criteria, was desperately needed. Saunders described in his address to the British Parliament in 1837 [27] how inaccurate this method could be, and postulated the use of dental eruption as a more reliable method for ageing children between seven and 14 years of age. He developed tables of tooth eruption based on examination of 1046 children, the majority of whom were from the lower socio-economic classes: a deliberate choice, as these children were most often those being exploited. This parliamentary address, and the research results contained within, was the first time legislative recognition had been accorded scientific age estimation based on dental development.

The use of tooth eruption/emergence as a tool for estimating the age of children became the standard method due to the ease with which it could be applied, requiring only a simple intra-oral examination to gather the appropriate data. It was recognised that there was some variability in the emergence of teeth between individuals and consequently, as the method matured with time, the concept of age ranges was developed to cater for this variability.

The overwhelming majority of the early studies focused on the emergence of the teeth through the gingiva as opposed to the chronological timing of the development of the dental structures themselves, with the work published by Legros and Magitot in 1880 [28] being a notable exception. This research involved the dissection and examination of human cadaveric material taken from both children and adults, and resulted in the production of a tooth formation table that was shown in almost unchanged form in the literature up until the 1930s.

Studying eruption of teeth is a somewhat misleading method for age determination, as the moment a tooth emerges into the oral cavity is a fleeting incident that will, in all probability, never be observed. Tooth eruption may also be delayed or advanced by external environmental influences such as dental caries, systemic illness, premature loss of deciduous teeth and crowding [19, 29–31]. In comparison, the mineralisation of tooth crowns and roots offers the opportunity to observe development as a continuous process throughout the early life of an individual. It has been noted on numerous occasions that tooth calcification is not only less variable than skeletal maturation, but is also less affected by environmental influences than is tooth eruption [32–35].

A brief review of dental development

Human dentition develops continuously from early foetal life right through until the early part of the third decade of life, and while a considerable amount of data has been accumulated regarding the timing of emergence of teeth for a wide variety of populations, far less is known about the chronology of tooth formation among differing populations, and there are relatively few major studies. This discrepancy is due to the fact that radiography or dissection is required to perform research into mineralisation, while emergence/eruption can be investigated by simply looking into the mouth.

The human dentition can be described as being diphyodont, that is two 'growths' of teeth [36]. The deciduous teeth start to form in the 16th week of intra-uterine life, with the first of the permanent dentition starting to calcify in the month just prior to birth and the last teeth, the third molars, erupting at approximately 18 years of age (see Tables 7.1 and 7.2).

The formation of teeth is sequential and to a certain extent, synchronous – it is through the relative formative stages of the developing teeth, be they deciduous or permanent, that the opportunity for dental age to be estimated exists. The

Table 7.1 Showing the approximate ages of attainment of landmarks of deciduous tooth development and exfoliation.

Tooth#	Calcification	Crown	Emergence	Exfoliation
A	3–5 miu*	4 months	6–8 months	6–7 years
B	4–5 miu*	4–5 months	7–9 months	7–8 years
C	5–6 miu*	9 months	16–20 months	9–12 years
D	5 miu*	6 months	12–16 months	9–11 years
E	6 miu*	10–12 months	20–24 months	10–12 years

Palmer–Zsigmondy system dental nomenclature for both maxillary and mandibular deciduous teeth (from *Practical Forensic Odontology* (Clark 1992)).
miu* months in utero

Table 7.2 Showing the approximate ages of attainment of landmarks of development of permanent teeth.

Tooth§	Calcification	Crown complete	Emergence	Root complete
11,21	3–4 months	4–5 years	7–8 years	10 years
12,22	10–12 months	4–5 years	8–9 years	11 years
13,23	4–5 months	6–7 years	11–12 years	13–15 years
14,24	1–1.75 years	5–6 years	10–11 years	12–14 years
15,25	2–2.5 years	6–7 years	10–12 years	12–14 years
16,26	Birth	2–3 years	6–7 years	9–10 years
17,27	2.5–3 years	7–8 years	12–13 years	14–16 years
18,28	7–9 years	12–16 years	17–21 years	18–25 years
31,41	3–4 months	4–5 years	6–7 years	9 years
32,42	3–4 months	4–5 years	7–8 years	10 years
33,43	4–5 months	6–7 years	9–10 years	12–13 years
34,44	1–2 years	5–6 years	10–12 years	12–13 years
35,45	2–2.5 years	6–7 years	11–12 years	13–14 years
36,46	Birth	2–3 years	6–7 years	9–10 years
37,47	2.5–3 years	7–8 years	11–13 years	14–15 years
38,48	8–10 years	12–16 years	17–21 years	18–25 years

§ Fédération Dentaire Internationale (FDI) dental nomenclature (from *Practical Forensic Odontology* (Clark 1992)).

lack of extraneous factors affecting the formation of teeth makes their development a better indicator and a stronger tool to ascertain chronological age than bone, which is subject to calcium metabolism and hence is more affected by local factors [5, 37].

Tooth shape is determined by an interaction between the embryological ectoderm, which gives rise to the enamel, and the mesoderm, which gives rise to the other tissues of the tooth: dentine, dental pulp, cementum, periodontal ligament and alveolar bone. The teeth start forming at the incisal edge for incisors, and at the cusp tips for canines, premolars and molars. The outermost cells of the mesodermal dental papilla differentiate into odontoblasts, laying down dentine at the cusp tip or incisal edge. Dentine formation signals the innermost cells of the enamel organ to develop into ameloblasts, which lay down the enamel superficially to the newly developed dentine. Once the occlusal surface or incisal edge is complete, the enamel continues to form down the smooth surfaces, with the dentine forming within the enamel crown form. Once the anatomical crown formation is complete, the dentine continues to form the root of the tooth. Cementoblasts originate from the surrounding dental follicle, laying down cementum on the surface of the developing radicular dentine, as do fibroblasts which form the developing periodontal ligament, and osteoblasts which continue to form the alveolar bone around the developing teeth [38].

When the root is approximately half to three-quarters formed, the tooth erupts (or emerges) into the oral cavity [39, 40]. A further two to three years are required following eruption for root completion. Once apexification of the root occurs, development is considered to be complete [38].

As the deciduous teeth are smaller and are exfoliated [41], the formation of deciduous enamel is quicker than that of permanent enamel and exhibits a different microstructure. In addition, the development of the whole deciduous tooth shape differs from that of permanent teeth, in that the coronal enamel forms a complete template within which the rest of the coronal dentine forms and the root dentine forms to the apex first, which then thickens towards the pulp with further development. This is in distinction to permanent teeth where the enamel and dentine form synchronously at and to the same level, and the root forms as a wave of dentine forming down the tooth root [38].

Developments in dental-age assessment

The discovery of ionising radiation in 1895 by Röentgen, and its subsequent development as a dental diagnostic tool by such innovative practitioners as C. Edmond Kells, revolutionised the practice of medicine and dentistry and opened up new territories for those researching human development. The introduction of dental radiography allowed researchers to directly observe the formation of the dentition in living people, and so ushered in the modern period of tooth development research.

Research on dental ageing in the modern era can be divided into general dental development, and development of the third molar as a separate issue. The third molar has received considerable attention as it is the last tooth to develop, and is therefore one of the few structures which can be used for age estimation in the late teens and early 20s.

The early modern period of research pertaining to dental development was characterised by a lack of reporting of sample sizes, which were often quite small, and many in fact did not report the source of their data at all. Later studies, from the early 1930s, would often contain small sample sizes, and would then incorporate data from other small studies in order to arrive at some sort of table or chart of tooth development. A study of some note was that performed by Logan and Kronfeld in 1933 [42] in which a combination of dissection and histology was used to construct a development table. The sample size consisted of a mere 25 individuals, 19 of whom were under the age of two years. A certain amount of guesswork was evident in this work, as the table specified development stages *in utero*, although, according to Lunt and Law in their 1974 review [43], no foetal samples were part of the study. This early Kronfeld table was printed and utilised widely through the years, and was often reprinted by other researchers with certain alterations, but without citation, and was widely attributed as belonging to work done by Schour and Massler [18]. Garn et al., in their 1958 [40] study on the variability of tooth formation, identified many instances of use of the Logan and Kronfeld table by numerous different authors without citation, and with alterations that had little scientific validity.

Once large numbers of radiographs of children began to be taken in the late 1930s, and the data collected were subjected to attempts at statistical analysis, major studies began to appear. Many of these early modern researchers read thousands of films, divided tooth development into stages, and so formulated their tables, many of which are still in use today.

Current age-estimation methods

Of the relatively modern studies, several have become so widely used that they are considered to be seminal articles in their own right. Demirjian et al. [23], in their 1973 paper with a sample size of almost 3000 radiographs of children, developed a series of formation stages, which are widely utilised today in forensic settings, and which have been adapted for use with third molar development even though the original work only charted development up to and including the second molar. Demirjian's stages are popular because they do not rely on an arbitrary length measurement to determine the developmental stage, but utilise anatomically recognisable features, such as root length equal to crown length [34, 44–50]. Both inter- and intra-examiner reliability are enhanced as a result. This makes reading radiographs simple, reproducible and independent of any distortion or magnification that may be present.

A later study by Demirjian and co-workers [50], published in 1985 and expanding on previous work of others, examined the relationship between somatic, sexual, skeletal and dental maturity, and found that tooth development seems to be independent of hormonal and nutritional factors, which means that as an age-estimation tool tooth development could be considered a more reliable method than any other, and more applicable across a wider section of any given population.

Due to the precision, reliability and ease of use of this technique, considerable research using the Demirjian methodology to determine geographic reliability of data has been undertaken, which has been comprehensively summarised by Taylor and Blenkin [6].

Another system of staging that is widely used is that developed by Moorrees, Fanning and Hunt in 1963 [19] consisting of a longitudinal study of 134 children, plus radiographs taken of 246 children derived from the Fels Institute, Philadelphia, where they developed a system with a greater number of stages than Demirjian – although some arbitrary measurement was required, such as 'R ¾' or three-quarters of root completion. This arbitrary measurement is satisfactory in longitudinal studies where the completed root length is anticipated and assists in determining what three-quarters of that root length would be. However, for forensic case work or cross-sectional study, the determination of such arbitrary lengths is subject to error and inter-examiner variation. Again, several researchers have used this methodology to develop updated datasets [2, 51, 52]. Notwithstanding this perceived fault, Moorrees, Fanning and Hunt developed one chart for the deciduous lower canine and molars, one chart for the permanent incisors, and another for the permanent canines, premolars and molars, including the third molar. Thus this method can be utilised to estimate the age of infants and very young children whereas the method of Demirjian, Goldstein and Tanner cannot, as it is only of use in children aged three and over.

The dental development chart created by Ubelaker in 1989 [53] has also become something of a recognised world standard. This chart is based heavily on the work of Schour and Massler, with some alterations to some of the standard deviation ranges to compensate for differing populations, thus making the chart applicable to a wider target group, but with considerably wider age ranges for each developmental stage. The pictorial nature of this chart, similar to the original Schour and Massler chart, is convenient and easy to interpret, hence its widespread usage in dental surgeries today. There does not seem to be any empirical testing of Ubelaker's chart in the literature, unlike Demirjian's method, and so its veracity is yet to be scientifically established.

One further system developed by Gustafson and Koch [32] for studying tooth development, involved the construction of a 'tooth development diagram' in schematic fashion, via a series of triangles placed upon a line for each tooth, the base of each triangle representing the range of ages found in their literature search and the apex the mean age found. This diagram was developed by utilising data from 20 previous studies available at that time (1973), and the diagram was tested against the actual ages of 41 children. This system has also seen wide use in forensic applications over the years, but it is limited in that most or all of a dentition is required in order to come to a conclusion, and third molars are omitted from the system. There is no separate diagram for boys and girls and once a stage is reached, some extrapolation is required, rendering the method difficult to use [54]. On the positive side, however, the deciduous dentition is also included.

Ageing of infants and toddlers can be difficult; ageing of foetuses and neonates is even more so. This is partially due to the lack of verified reference data available. Kraus and Jordan's work [55] may be regarded as the definitive reference in relation to foetal dental development.

Australasian specific research in dental age estimation

While Australasian researchers have always shown an interest in age-estimation studies [56–67], in more recent times considerable research has been undertaken to generate current and more reliable population specific data.

Blenkin [13, 68] used a modified Demirjian methodology on a large Australian sample to generate new curves that more accurately reflected current growth and development patterns. This methodology readily allows for the generation of regression formulae and regression curves from samples originating from any population. Subsequently these data have been used to generate Schour and Massler-type tables suitable for the Australian population [26].

Another study from Australia uses computed tomography (CT) imaging as the modality of choice for viewing dental development. This study used the dental ageing method developed by Moorrees, Fanning and Hunt, and reported that there is underestimation in age of some 10% when this method is applied to the modern Australian population [2], which indicates that the established age-estimation tables require modern population data.

The advent of CT has revolutionised how anatomical information can be viewed. It has the capability of producing three-dimensional images of the individual in a variety of algorithms (see Chapter 14 on imaging modalities). For example, it enables the skeletal system of the individual to be viewed, including the erupted and unerupted teeth and the status of the cranial vault, through three-dimensional surface shaded displays of the reconstructed images (Fig. 7.1). CT data may also be manipulated to produce images that resemble panoramic dental radiographs, suitable for an ageing analysis. Views of the dentition also include the axial view or occlusal view, hitherto unseen with conventional radiography (Fig. 7.2).

Notwithstanding the perceived shortcomings of the Moorrees, Fanning and Hunt assignment of stages previously referred to, the method is still used. It is easy to use with practice, it can be applied to any number or kind of developing permanent or deciduous teeth, it can be used in very young children and it has separate charts for boys and girls [19, 69]. This renders the method more adaptable and practical for use in children of all ages. In the study by Graham [2], two independent raters, blinded to the ages of 96 deceased children aged up to 15 years, viewed the reformatted CT images and used the relevant charts of Moorrees, Fanning and Hunt to estimate the dental age. One rater was an experienced dentist, the other an English dental student. These estimates were then

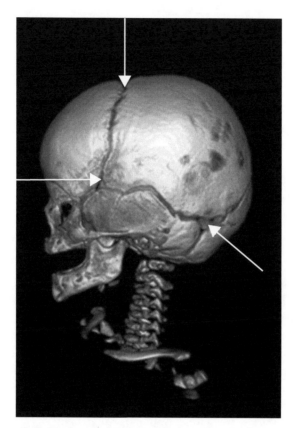

Fig. 7.1 Showing a shaded surface display view of the lateral aspect of a two-month-old child's head. The arrows indicate the fontanelles, which close at different ages: the sphenoid closes at approximately three months, the mastoid begins to close at one to two months and is complete by approximately 12 months and the frontal which closes by 18–24 months. The occipital (not pictured) closes at approximately two months. (Reproduced with permission of the Victorian Institute of Forensic Medicine.)

compared to the known chronological age. The results were statistically analysed in a one-sample t-test, using the mean log-ratio of the estimated age to the chronological age. As it is the relative error in the estimated age, not the absolute error, that is of interest, the analysis was performed using the ratio of estimated age to chronological age. This was converted to a logarithmic scale, yielding log (Estimated Age/Real Age) or 'log-ratio' as the variable of interest. This was then converted to the mean ratio (Table 7.3).

It was found that the use of reformatted CT images to perform an ageing estimate using Moorrees, Fanning and Hunt's method systematically underestimated the chronological age by 10% by both raters ($p = 0.784$), with a mean ratio of 0.908.

This underestimation could be due to a number of factors: the Moorrees, Fanning and Hunt method itself, which had been found previously to underestimate chronological age [33, 54]; secular changes within the population, even though dental development is affected less by environmental and nutritional

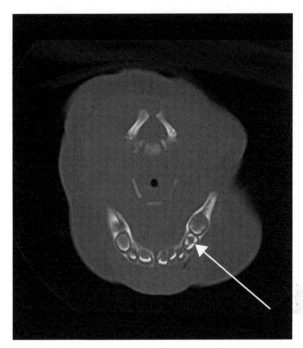

Fig. 7.2 An axial or occlusal view of the developing deciduous dentition in the mandible of a one-month-old child, obtained by CT. Note the occlusal surface of #74 (arrowed) is not complete. (Reproduced with permission of the Victorian Institute of Forensic Medicine.)

Table 7.3 Demonstrating the mean ratios, confidence intervals (CI) and p-values of age estimation values by age and by the charts produced by Moorees, Fanning and Hunt (MFH).

	Mean ratio	95% CI	p-value‡
By age cohort			
1–60 months	0.880	0.771–1.004	0.0564
61–120 months	0.982	0.882–0.977	0.0084
121–180 months	0.900	0.855–0.948	0.0004
By MFH chart			
Deciduous	1.108	0.920–1.115	0.720
Incisors	1.107	1.055–1.159	0.0014
Permanent	0.882	0.813–0.995	0.0026

factors than other parameters [70]; a different population from that used to create the Moorees, Fanning and Hunt database; the shortcomings of CT in viewing the dental tissues in the very young; and, in the younger cases, the interval of six to eight weeks between the actual mineralisation and its appearance on the CT reconstructions.

The ability to use any developing tooth visible, any number of teeth and any kind of teeth, renders this method more adaptable to use than other available methods, particularly in those aged three and younger. This was demonstrated by the results found when using the 'deciduous' Moorrees, Fanning and Hunt chart in the youngest cohort.

Interestingly, the study also tested the accuracy of estimation based on the two raters' dental experience, viewing the surface shaded displays as shown in Fig. 7.1 as well as the radiograph-like images without any documentation to hand, prior to using the Moorrees, Fanning and Hunt charts. The estimation of age using clinical dental experience by the experienced dentist showed a mean ratio of 1.017 of the chronological age (p = 0.719) compared to 1.525 for the student (p = 0.0001), with a 95% Confidence Interval (CI) of 0.925 to 1.120 for the experienced dentist and 1.333 to 1.76 for the student. Thus the Moorrees, Fanning and Hunt method systematically underestimated the chronological age when using CT, but provided more reliable findings than experience alone. When using CT, the use of experiential estimates may prove useful in the screening process following a mass disaster, though with a degree of caution if the rater is inexperienced. Both approaches may be useful in estimating ages of deceased children following mass disasters, but experience with CT may provide additional benefits.

Recent analysis of third molar development using CT, as part of a larger multifactorial study including assessment of the medial clavicular epiphysis, has been conducted in an attempt to provide better age estimates for individuals for whom an assessment of their legal status as an adult or a child is required [24]. This research has shown that for third molar development alone, age ranges are considerable and therefore of limited forensic use, but also that if the third molar root is complete there is a very high likelihood of an individual being older than 18 years.

With the inclusion of the medial clavicular epiphysis into the equation and the utilisation of multiple regression statistical modelling, more precise age estimates can be achieved (Table 7.4) [25]. This research demonstrated that a considerable reduction in the width of age ranges could be achieved with the inclusion of both skeletal and dental development sites into the same statistical model, thus producing more useful conclusions and allowing a greater number of individuals to be classified as either adults or children. This research supports recent recommendations that age estimations should use more than one technique, and ideally be completed on more than one tissue system [5, 19, 34, 50, 71].

A further issue highlighted by this research was the realisation that there is a demonstrable degree of left/right asymmetry in development of the third molar and medial clavicle, which implies that both sides require assessment in order to come to an accurate measure of the state of development of a particular individual (Figs. 7.3 and 7.4) [72].

Although confidence intervals using these methods are still too wide to provide a definitive answer in all cases, the improvements in precision and the availability of robust age ranges allow greater certainty for courts assessing the legal status of people such as asylum seekers, child soldiers and sexual assault victims [73].

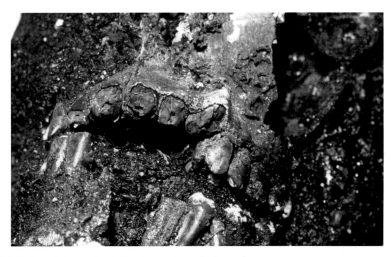

Fig. 5.1 Incinerated remains following motor vehicle crash.

Forensic Odontology: Principles and Practice, First Edition. Edited by Jane A. Taylor and Jules A. Kieser.
© 2016 John Wiley & Sons, Ltd. Published 2016 by John Wiley & Sons, Ltd.

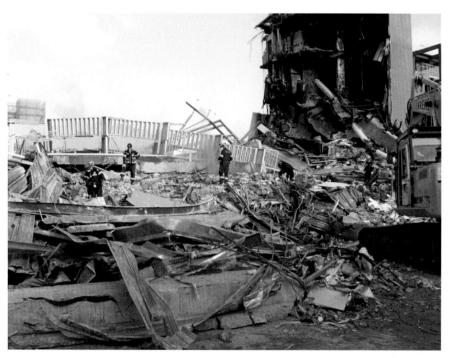

Fig. 9.2 Canterbury Television (CTV) building collapse following the Christchurch earthquake (2011).

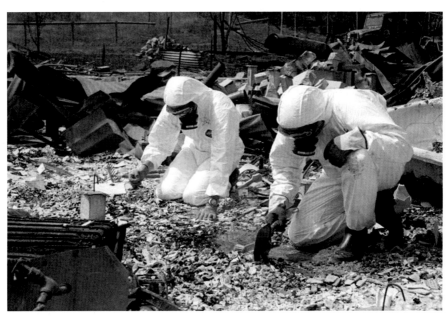

Fig. 9.6 Detailed searching is required to recover the human remains from a scene. (Courtesy of Karl Wilson.)

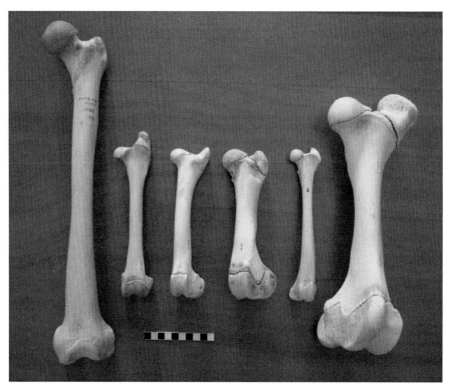

Fig. 10.4 Human, kangaroo, sheep, pig, dog, cow femora (from left to right). (Reproduced with permission from Dr S Croker.)

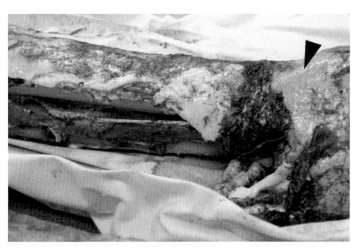

Fig. 11.2 Marine bacterial growth visible on the skin of a human cadaver recovered from coastal waters of New Zealand. (Photograph courtesy of G Dickson.)

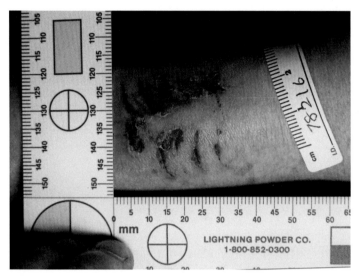

Fig. 12.8 Arm abrasions.

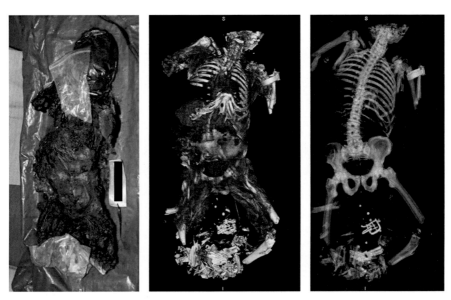

Fig. 14.1 Example of CT 'dissection'. (Reproduced with permission of the Victorian Institute of Forensic Medicine.)

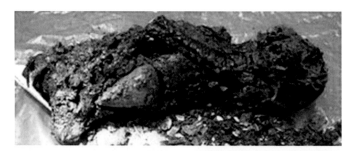

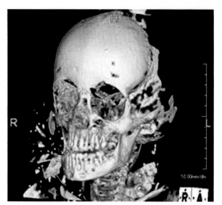 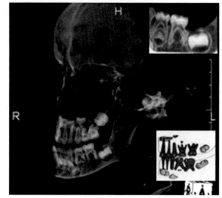

Fig. 14.7 Age estimation using CT images can identify an individual if no other people in that age range died in the incident. It also serves as an elimination tool – therefore saving investigation resources. (Reproduced with permission of the Victorian Institute of Forensic Medicine.)

Table 7.4 Demonstrating the way age ranges can be considerably reduced when a multi–factorial approach is used (M3 and medial clavicle). This allows a higher proportion of the population to be classified as either adult or child with greater certainty than using individual age markers on their own.

Case	Sex	Development score molar/calvicle		Age range using 3rd molar only	Predicted age range M.F.A*	Actual age (yrs)
1	M	4	1	13.4–19.4	14.1–16.9	15.6
2	F	3	2	14.2–16.2	14.9–18.3	15.1
3	M	7	1	14.5–22.8	16.2–19.9	15.9
4	F	4	2	13.8–19.5	15.3–19.0	16.1
5	M	5	2	14.2–19.7	16.0–19.3	16.8
6	M	4	2	13.4–19.4	15.2–18.3	17.1
7	F	4	1	13.8–19.5	13.8–17.1	16.0
8	F	6	2	14.0–23.1	16.0–20.3	17.2
9	F	5	2	14.1–21.9	15.7–19.7	18.1
10	F	5	3	14.1–21.9	17.2–21.5	18.8
11	F	7	1	14.3–24.7	14.9–19.2	18.7
12	M	7	3	14.5–22.8	18.7–22.7	19.2
13	M	8	2	17.8–	18.2–22.3	20.3
14	F	7	5	14.3–24.7	20.9–26.5	21.6
15	F	8	4	17.6–	19.7–25.4	21.8
16	M	8	4	17.8–	20.6–25.7	21.5
17	M	7	4	14.5–22.8	19.8–24.1	21.9
18	M	8	5	17.8–	21.8–	23.2
19	M	8	3	17.8–	19.4–23.7	23.3
20	F	8	5	17.6–	21.2–	23.5

* MFA = Multi–Factorial Approach (M3 and medial clavicle development in one formula)
General multiple regression formula applied to M# and Clavicle: Age = C+(ß×m3)+(ß[1]×clav)±E
Specific formula developed for each gender for the Victorian population – used to calculate the age ranges in the table above.
Males: Lower age limit = 9.91 + (0.74 × molar score) + (1.19 × clavicle score)
Upper age limit = 11.55 + (0.99 × molar score) + (1.41 × clavicle score)
Females: Lower age limit = 10.90 + (0.35 × molar score) + (1.51 × clavicle score)
Upper age limit = 12.62 + (0.67 × molar score) + (1.85 × clavicle score)
Note: Numbers for C and for ß only apply to the Victorian population.

Concluding remarks

Age assessment of living individuals is conducted by using various medical imaging modalities, such as conventional radiography and CT scanning, in order to capture images of the developing skeleton and the dentition. The anatomical sites most commonly imaged are the hand/wrist region for assessment of skeletal development, the dentition for assessment of dental age, and more recently the use of CT scanning to capture images of the developing clavicle and the dentition. This imaging necessarily involves the use of ionising radiation with concomitant exposure to various tissues. This

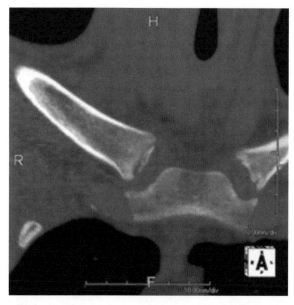

Fig. 7.3 CT image showing medial clavicular epiphysis and asymmetrical development. The left side is at stage 3 whilst the right side is a stage 2. (Reproduced with permission of the Victorian Institute of Forensic Medicine.)

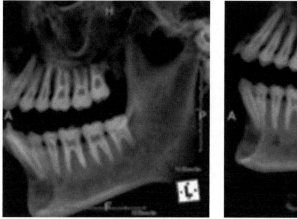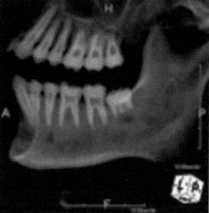

Fig. 7.4 CT images of left and right third molars in the same individual – the left third molar is at Demirjian stage G, while the right third molar is at Demirjian stage E. Two stage differences in development within the same individual, illustrating the developmental variability of the third molar and the need to assess both sides when attempting to estimate age. (Reproduced with permission of the Victorian Institute of Forensic Medicine.)

exposure is not at a level sufficient to cause immediate harm, but does raise the total lifetime dose of radiation experienced by the individual concerned. There are medical, ethical and legal considerations involved in conducting radiological procedures on living people, with no definite medical need, that are yet to be properly addressed.

In recent years, partially as a result of the production of the report into the state of forensic science in the USA, the National Academy of Science [74] reports that there have been increasing calls for forensic science to improve on the evidence basis of its conclusions. For forensic anthropologists and odontologists, this includes improving age-estimation methods, especially with regards to applicability of reference standards to a particular population. A more precise definition of the error in our age estimations is required, along with a more robust approach in assigning an age range to an estimate.

Recent research [7, 10, 25, 50, 75–78] has focused on the development of various multi-factorial approaches to age estimation. A multi-factorial system involves using a combination of developing anatomical features in concert in order to arrive at an estimate that will offer increased accuracy and precision over an estimate that uses each development site individually.

Recent advances in age-estimation research have been facilitated by the development of CT imaging. This modality allows excellent visualisation of both dental and skeletal development, and is becoming more widely employed regularly in forensic institutes around the world for age assessment of the deceased. With large sample sizes for research becoming more accessible, robust population based studies of skeletal and dental development will increase.

Historically forensic anthropologists and odontologists have worked in isolation, often independently, on the same case. They thus provide age estimations based on their own discipline's guidelines in an independent way. This can result in different age estimates being constructed for the same individual, based on separate skeletal and dental growth markers. These results may then be presented to courts and result in confusion. This is somewhat illogical, as in order to gain the most complete picture regarding an individual's developmental status, it is apparent that both dental and skeletal age markers need to be examined together. For the living, an appreciation of the overall phenotypic expression of development status via physical examination is also mandatory. Age estimation is therefore best practised as a multi-disciplinary specialty, in that practitioners engaging in this activity should be familiar with the theory and practice of forensic anthropology, forensic odontology, medical imaging, human growth and development, and anatomy. In order to achieve this, and to obtain the most accurate age estimates, it is evident that practitioners from different disciplines need to work together on both casework and research. Furthermore, researchers and practitioners in the field require a sound grounding in epidemiological techniques as related to population-based study of development. It is apparent that in order to gain the most accurate appreciation of an individual's age, multiple developmental age markers need to be assessed in conjunction. Forensic age estimation is no longer simply a matter of specialists restricting themselves to their own traditional fields. Instead, especially with the increase in undocumented international migration, mass fatality events and the advent of advanced imaging techniques, it needs to be a speciality that requires expertise in many fields of endeavour. At the very least, it is incumbent upon practitioners to not only be age-estimation experts in their own particular field, but to be familiar with the principles of related disciplines.

References

1 Bonogofsky M, Graham JP. (2011) Melanesian modeled skulls, mortuary ritual, and dental x-rays. In: Bonogofsky M (ed.) *The Bioarchaeology of the Human Head: Decapitation, Decoration and Deformation.* University Press of Florida, Gainesville, pp. 67–96.

2 Graham JP, O'Donnell CJ, Craig PJG et al. (2010) The application of computerized tomography (CT) to the dental ageing of children and adolescents. *Forensic Science International* **195**, 58–62.

3 Bassed RB, Hill AJ. (2011) The use of computed tomograpjhy (CT) to estimate age in the 2009 Victorian Bushfire victims: A case report. *Forensic Science International* **205**, 48–51.

4 Bassed RB, Ranson D. (2012) Age determination of asylum seekers and alleged people smugglers. *Journal of Law and Medicine* **20**, 261–265.

5 Solheim T, Vonen A. (2006) Dental age estimation, quality assurance and age estimation of asylum seekers in Norway. *Forensic Science International* **159S**, S56–S60.

6 Taylor J, Blenkin M. (2010) Age evaluation and odontology in the living. In: Black S, Aggrawal A, Payne–James J (eds) *Age Estimation in the Living: The Practitioners Guide.* John Wiley and Sons Ltd, Chichester, pp. 176–201.

7 Schmeling A, Reisinger W, Geserick G et al. (2006) Age estimation of unaccompanied minors. Part I. General considerations. *Forensic Science International* **159**, (Suppl 1)S61–64.

8 Olze A, Reisinger W, Geserick G et al. (2006) Age estimation of unaccompanied minors. Part II. Dental aspects. *Forensic Science International* **159**, Suppl 1: S65–67.

9 Schmeling A, Geserick G, Reisinger W et al. (2007) Age estimation. *Forensic Science International* **165**, 178–181.

10 Schmeling A, Grundmann C, Fuhrmann C et al. (2008) Criteria for age estimation in living individuals. *International Journal of Legal Medicine* **122**, 457–460.

11 International Criminal Court. (2014) ICC–01/04–01/06. Situation in the Democratic Republic of the Congo in the Case of the Prosecutor v. Thomas Lubanga Dyilo. Judgement pursuant to Article 74 of the Statute.

12 Willems G, Van Olmen A, Spiessens B et al. (2001) Dental age estimation in Belgian children; Demirjian's technique revisited. *Journal of Forensic Sciences* **46**, 893–895.

13 Liversidge HM, Lyons F, Hector MP. (2003) The accuracy of three methods of age estimation using radiographic measurements of developing teeth. *Forensic Science International* **131**, 22–29.

14 Liversidge HM, Chaillet N, Mörnstad H et al. (2006) Timing of Demirjian's tooth formation stages. *Annals of Human Biology* **33**, 454–470.

15 Blenkin M. (2009) *Forensic Odontology and Age Estimation – An Introduction to Concepts and Methods.* Verlag, Saarbrucken.

16 Thevissen P, Fieuws S, Willems G. (2010) Human third molars development: Comparison of 9 country specific populations. *Forensic Science International* **201**, 102–105.

17 Greulich WW, Pyle S. (1959) *Radiographic Atlas of Skeletal Development of the Hand and Wrist.* Stanford University Press, Stanford.

18 Schour I, Massler M. (1941) The development of the human dentition. *Journal of the American Dental Association* **28**, 1153–1160.

19 Moorrees CFA, Fanning EA, Hunt EE. (1963) Age variation of formation Stages for ten permanent teeth. *Journal of Dental Research* **42**, 1490–1502.

20 Liversidge HM, Speechly T. (2001) Growth of permanent mandibular teeth of British children aged 4 to 9 years. *Annals of Human Biology* **28**, 256–262.

21 Braga J, Heuze Y, Chabedel O et al. (2005) Non–adult dental age assessment: Correspondence analysis and linear regression versus Bayesian predictions. *International Journal of Legal Medicine* **119**, 260–274.

22 Maber M, Liversidge HM, Hector MP. (2006) Accuracy of age estimation of radiographic methods using developing teeth. *Forensic Science International* **159S**, S68–S73.

23 Demirjian A, Goldstein H, Tanner JM. (1973) A new system of dental age assessment. *Annals of Human Biology* **45**, 211–227.

24 Bassed RB, Briggs C, Drummer OH. (2011) Age estimation and the developing third molar tooth: an analysis of an Australian population using computed tomography. *Journal of Forensic Sciences* **56**, 1185–1191.

25 Bassed RB, Briggs C, Drummer OH. (2011) Age estimation using CT imaging of the third molar tooth, clavicular epiphysis and the spheno–occitpial synchondrosis: a multi–factorial approach. *Forensic Science International* **212**, 273:e1–273:e5.

26 Blenkin M, Taylor J. (2012) Age estimation charts for a modern Australian population. *Forensic Science International* **221**, 106–112.

27 Gustafson G. (1950) Age determinations on teeth. *Journal of the American Dental Association* **41**, 45–54.

28 Legros C, Magitot E. (1880) *The Origin and Formation of the Dental Follicle.* (Translated from the French by MS Dean). Jansen, McClurg and Co, Chicago.

29 Fanning E. (1961) A longitudinal study of tooth formation and root resorption. *New Zealand Dental Journal* **57**, 202–217.

30 Hägg U, Taranger J. (1985) Dental development, dental age and tooth counts. *Angle Orthodontist* **55**, 93–107.

31 Suri L, Gagari E, Vastardis H. (2004) Delayed tooth eruption: Pathogenesis, diagnosis and treatment. A literature review. *American Journal of Orthodontics and Dentofacial Orthopedics* **126**, 432–445.

32 Gustafson G, Koch G. (1974) Age estimation up to 16 years of age based on dental development. *Odontologisk Revy* **25**, 297–306.

33 Smith BH. (1991) Standards of human tooth formation and dental age assessment in dental age assessment. In: Kelly MA, Larsen CS (eds) *Advances in Dental Anthropology*, Wiley-Liss Inc, New York, pp. 143–168.

34 Liversidge HM, Herdeg B, Rösing FW. (1998) Dental age estimation of non–adults. A review of methods and principles. In: Alt WK, Rösing FW, Teschler–Nicolain M (eds) *Dental Anthropology. Fundamentals, Limits and Prospects*, Springer, New York, pp. 419–442.

35 Heuzé Y, Cardoso FV. (2008) Testing the quality of nonadult Bayesian dental age assessment methods to juvenile skeletal remains: The Lisbon Collection children and secular trend effects. *American Journal of Physical Anthropology* **135**, 275–283.

36 Scott JM, Symons NBB. (1961) *Introduction to Dental Anatomy.* E. & S. Livingstone Ltd, Edinburgh, pp. 5, 372.

37 Hall RK. (1989) The prevalence of developmental defects of tooth enamel (DDE) in a Pediatric hospital department of dentistry population. *Advances in Dental Research* **3**, 114–119.

38 Berkovitz BKB, Holland GR, Moxham BJ. (2005) *Oral Anatomy, Histology and Embryology.* Mosby International, pp. 456–456.

39 Demirjian A, Levesque GY. (1980) Sexual differences in dental development and prediction of emergence. *Journal of Dental Research* **59**, 1110–1122.

40 Garn SM, Lewis AB, Koski K et al. (1958) The sex difference in Tooth calcification. *Journal of Dental Research* **37**, 561–567.

41 Liversidge HM, Molleson T. (2004) Variation in crown and root formation and eruption of human deciduous teeth. *American Journal of Physical Anthropology* **123**, 172–180.

42 Logan WHG, Kronfeld R. (1933) Development of the human jaws and surrounding structures from birth to the age of fifteen years. *Journal of the American Dental Association* **20**, 379–427.

43 Lunt RC, Law DB. (1974) A review of the chronology of calcification of human teeth. *Journal of the American Dental Association* **89**, 599–606.

44 Hagg U, Matsson L. (1985) Dental maturity as an indicator of chronological age. The accuracy and precision of three methods. *European Journal of Orthodontics* **7**, 25–34.

45 Nyström M. (1988) Comparisons of dental maturity between the rural community of Kuhmo in northeastern Finland and the city of Helsinki. *Community Dentistry and Oral Epidemiology* **16**, 215–217.

46 Staaf V, Mörnstad H, Welander U. (1991) Age estimation based on tooth development: a test of reliability and validity. *Scandinavian Journal of Dental Research* **99**, 281–286.

47 Kullman L, Tronje G, Teivens A et al. (1996) Methods of reducing observer variation in age estimation from panoramic radiographs. *Dento–Maxillo–Facial Radiology* **25**, 173–178.

48 Frucht S, Schnegelsberg C, Schulte-Mönting J et al. (2000) Dental age in southwest Germany. A radiographic study. *Journal of Orofacial Orthopedics* **61**, 318–329.

49 Chaillet N, Nyström M, Kataja M et al. (2004) Dental maturity curves in Finnish children. Demirjians method revisited and polynomial functions for age estimation. *Journal of Forensic Sciences* **49**(6), 1324–1331.

50 Demirjian A, Buschang PH, Tanguay R, Kingnorth-Patterson D. (1985) Interrelationships among measures of somatic, skeletal, dental, and sexual maturity. *American Journal of Orthodontics* **88**, 433–438.

51 Anderson DL, Thompson GW, Popovich F. (1976) Age of attainment of mineralization stages of the permanent dentition. *Journal of Forensic Sciences* **21**, 191–200.

52 Ciapparelli L. (1992) The chronology of dental development and age assessment. In: Clark DH (ed.) *Practical Forensic Odontology*, Wright, Oxford, Boston, pp. 23–42.

53 Ubelaker DH. (1989) *Human Skeletal Remains*. Taraxacum, Washington.

54 Liversidge HM. (1994) Accuracy of age estimation from developing teeth of a population of known age (0–5.4 years). *International Journal of Osteoarchaeology* **4**, 37–45.

55 Kraus BS, Jordan RE. (1965) *The Human Dentition Before Birth*. Lea and Febiger, Philadelphia.

56 Lin NH, Ranjitkar S, Macdonald AR et al. (2006) New growth references for assessment of stature and skeltal maturation in Australians. *Australian Orthodontic Journal* **22**, 1–10.

57 Liversidge HM, Chaillet N, Mornstad H et al. (2006) A Timing of the Demirjian's tooth formation stages. *Annals of Human Biology* **33**, 454–470.

58 Ranjitkar S, Lin NH, Macdonald R et al. (2006) Stature and skeletal maturation in two cohorts of Australian children and young adults over the past two decades. *Australian Orthodontic Journal* **22**, 47–58.

59 McKenna CJ, James H, Taylor JA et al. (2002) Tooth development standards for South Australia. *Australian Dental Journal* **47**, 223–227.

60 Abd Rahman R, MacDonald R, Townsend G et al. (1999) Growth trends in South Australian children and adolescents. *Australian Dental Journal ADRF Special Research Supplement* **44**, 4.

61 Farah CS, Booth DR, Knott SC. (1999) Dental maturity of children in Perth, Western Australia, and its application in forensic age estimation. *Journal of Clinical Forensic Medicine* **6**, 14–18.

62 Bazen JJ, Booth DR, Knott SJ. (1995) Age estimation of adult persons using extracted teeth. *Australian Dental Journal* **40**, 255.

63 TeMoananui R, Kieser JA, Herbison P et al. (2008) Advanced dental maturation n New Zealand Maori and Pacific Island children. *American Journal of Human Biology* **20**, 43–50.

64 TeMoananui R, Kieser JA, Herbison P et al. (2008) Estimating age in Maori, Pacific Island and European children from New Zealand. *Journal of Forensic Sciences* **53**, 401–404.

65 Kieser JA, DeFreiter J, TeMoananui R. (2008) Automated dentalaging for child victims of disasters. *American Journal of Disaster Medicine* **3**, 109–112.

66 Timmins K, Herbison P, Farella M et al. (2012) The usefuless of dental and cervical maturation stages in New Zealand children for Disaster Victim Identification. *Forensic Science Medicine and Pathology* **8**, 101–108.

67 McGettigan A, Timmins K, Herbison P et al. (2011) Wisdom tooth formation as a method of age estimation in New Zealand. *Dentalal Anthropogy*, **24**, 33–41.

68 Blenkin MRB, Evans W. (2010) Age estimation from the teeth using a modified Demirjian system. *Journal of Forensic Sciences* **55**, 1504–1508.

69 Moorrees CFA, Fanning EA, Hunt EE. (1963) Formation and resorption of three deciduous teeth in children. *American Journal of Physical Anthropology* **21**, 205–213.

70 Demirjian A. (1978) Dentition. In: Faulkner F, Tanner JM (eds) *Human Growth – Postnatal Growth*, Plenum Press, New York.

71 Tanner JM. (1962) *Growth at Adolescence*. Blackwell Scientific, London.

72 Bassed RB, Briggs C, Drummer OH. (2012) The incidence of asymmetrical left/right skeletal and dental development in an Australian population and the effect of this on forensic age estimations. *International Journal of Legal Medicine* **126**, 251–257.

73 Bassed RB. (2011) Advances in forensic age estimation. *Forensic Science, Medicine and Pathology* **8**, 194–196.

74 Committee on Identifying the Needs of the Forensic Sciences Community, National Research Council. (2009) *Strengthening Forensic Science in the United States: A Path Forward.*

75 Ritz-Timme S, Cattaneo C, Collins MJ et al. (2000) Age estimation: the state of the art in relation to the specific demands of forensic practise. *International Journal of Legal Medicine* **113**, 129–136.

76 Bedford ME, Russell KF, Lovejoy CO et al. (1993) Test of the multifactorial aging methid using skeletons with known ages–at–death from the Grant collection. *American Journal of Physical Anthropology* **91**, 287–297.

77 Martrille L, Ubelaker DH, Cattaneo C et al. (2007) Comparison of four skeletal methods for the estimation of age at death on white and black adults. *Journal of Forensic Sciences* **52**, 302–307.

78 Schmeling A, Olze A, Reisinger W et al. (2001) Age estimation of living people undergoing criminal proceedings. *The Lancet* **358**, 89–90.

CHAPTER 8

Bite marks

Alex Forrest[1] and Alistair Soon[2]

[1] School of Natural Sciences, Griffith University Nathan Campus and Health Support Queensland, Australia
[2] Health Support Queensland, Australia

Introduction

In recent times, the terms 'bitemark', 'bite mark' and 'bite mark' have enjoyed widespread use. All these terms are acceptable and mean the same thing. The American Board of Forensic Odontology defines a bite mark in skin as being 'a physical alteration in a medium caused by the contact of teeth', and specifically as 'a representative pattern left in an object or tissue by the dental structures of an animal or human' [1, p. 116]. In this chapter, we will use the term 'bite mark' and define it as a mark, impression or injury inflicted by the act of biting with the teeth.

We will limit ourselves to discussing bite marks of human origin. While bites by animals of many different sorts occur and occasionally lead to legal proceedings, examination of these injuries falls outside the scope of this chapter. The principles discussed here also apply to the examination of non-human bite marks, however.

David Senn gives a general history of bite mark evidence, primarily from an American perspective [2], but does not cover Australian cases well and is limited by the date of publication.

It is necessary to recognise from the outset that bite marks almost always comprise circumstantial evidence in a case, unless the charge is one of biting. The probative value of such evidence depends crucially on the context in which it is found. For example, the fact that a bite mark has been found on a deceased person at a murder scene does not necessarily indicate that the biter was the murderer (as is also true of other circumstantial evidence including DNA and fingerprints), only that they bit the victim in the recent past. For this reason, one must understand that forensic evidence of this nature does not provide a substitute for a proper, thorough police investigation in the majority of cases.

Historically, the value of bite mark evidence in the courtroom has often been overstated. Bite mark comparison is primarily a pattern-matching exercise, and

Forensic Odontology: Principles and Practice, First Edition. Edited by Jane A. Taylor and Jules A. Kieser.
© 2016 John Wiley & Sons, Ltd. Published 2016 by John Wiley & Sons, Ltd.

because of the many factors that may affect the outcome, there are clear limitations to the extent to it can support a conclusion. This chapter attempts to demonstrate some of the limitations of the techniques, and to place bite mark evidence in its proper context.

The aim of this chapter is therefore to discuss the terminology associated with bite mark examination and the mechanics, pathology and morphology of bite mark injuries, and to provide some guidelines against which injuries may be judged as to whether they are likely to be bite marks or not. It will go on to examine some of the techniques and limitations of evidence collection, present and critique evidence analysis and comparison techniques, and will conclude with a section discussing the limitations of the evidence and the possible conclusions that we believe may legitimately be reached from bite mark injury examinations.

Describing bite marks

Bite marks are physical evidence

Bite marks are part of a class of injury referred to as 'patterned injuries'. This means that the injury observed reflects the physical shape and characteristics of the implement that caused it.

Bite mark examination uses the same tools and terminology as analysis of other physical evidence, which is usually the province of specially trained forensic police officers. We refer, as they do, to 'class characteristics' and to 'individual characteristics'.

Class characteristics are those that permit us to express confidence that a given type of tool (in our case, a human dentition) caused an impression. This determination on its own can be important – the fact that a bite mark is present can be of value in a criminal case, even if insufficient individual characteristics are present to enable a comparison with the dentition of suspect biters.

Individual characteristics are those that permit us to express confidence that a specific dentition, which we can clearly differentiate from all others, caused the injury.

'Clear differentiation' is the issue here. The problem is that the forensic odontologist cannot declare the chance of a random match without determining the extent to which individual dentitions are recognisably unique. This information is currently unavailable. We therefore need to state this as a limitation of our analysis. It has a profound effect on the conclusions we can legitimately reach as well as on their probative value.

In a specific incident, it is unlikely that every person alive could potentially have had access to the victim to inflict the injury, and the task is therefore to compare it with the dentitions of a 'closed population' of suspects, rather than everyone in the world (an 'open population').

Class characteristics

The class characteristics associated with human bite marks are:

- A circular or ovoid-shaped injury comprising two opposing arches, which are usually separate from each other. Sometimes these circles or ovoids may be partial, which indicates that the forensic odontologist should exercise caution in their interpretation.
- Each arch should feature a pattern of smaller injuries that represent the individual teeth in each arch that contacted the bitten surface.
- Arches should be of an appropriate size.
- Linear contusions or abrasions may be associated with each arch as the teeth drag across the bitten surface to reach their final positions.
- A central contusion (or bruise) may be present.
- Impressions of contusions representing detail of the palatal surfaces of upper incisor teeth and the embrasures between the teeth may be present.
- Multiple injuries may be present at different sites, and sometimes may be seen in the same site overlapping or superimposed on each other.
- We have also observed during the analysis phase of examination that the midlines of each dental arch, if projected along the direction of any scrape marks on the tissue that may be present, should meet within an area more-or-less centrally within the bounds of the arch. The angle between the two lines is indicative of the angle between the dentition and the bitten surface at the time of biting, and we have observed it to be greater on surfaces with greater curvature. Usually, the meeting point is closer to the lower arch than the upper because the teeth of the lower arch move less across the tissue surface compared to those of the upper arch. If this general feature is not observed, then we may question whether the injury is actually a bite mark. We should also consider this as a class characteristic of a bite mark.

Individual characteristics

The individual characteristics associated with human bite marks are those that characterise the specific dentition that inflicted the injury. They may include:

- The approximate sizes of the arches in the injury (with caveats, see below under 'Accuracy of transfer of dental features to bitten tissues', and 'Distortions due to tissue properties and movement of a bitten body part').
- The pattern resulting from the specific arrangement of teeth in an assailant's dental arches.
- Missing teeth leaving gaps in an arch of the injury.
- One or more diastemata may leave recognisable gaps in an arch injury.
- Over-erupted or misplaced teeth leaving evidence in the pattern of the injury.
- Chips, notches, or surface features in teeth that leave evidence in the pattern of the injury.

- 'Scrape marks' or abraded drag marks across a tissue surface resulting from the specific features of teeth in each arch that form a type of 'bar code' likely to be specific to a given dentition.
- The pattern produced by the bite favouring one or other side of the dentition. If this is not due to the position of the biter and victim, it may indicate a habitual biting pattern resulting from an open bite where the anterior teeth simply cannot occlude.
- Any other specific attribute of a dentition reflected in the patterned injury.

We should note that the Australian Society of Forensic Odontology (AuSFO) in its Guidelines for the Conduct of Bitemark Analysis in Australia [3] refers not only to 'class characteristics' and 'individual characteristics', but also includes 'sub-class characteristics' between the two. It defines these as being 'represented by discrete portions of the injury that could reasonably be ascribed as having been made by individual teeth. It is mainly on the comparison of sub-class characteristics, such as position and degree of rotation, that associations are made between a dentition and a bite mark in human skin.'

It goes on to define 'individual characteristics' as:

> even more discrete details that reveal information about individual teeth, such as areas attributable to notching and differential wear of teeth, are considered individual characteristics. It is doubtful that individual characteristics are represented with any accuracy on a cutaneous bite mark injury due to the nature of human skin, however, individual characteristics may be represented in bite marks on inanimate objects. [3, pp. 7–8].

Anatomical locations of bite marks

There are cases involving bite marks on the breast, arms, hands, face, torso and legs among other locations and the frequency of their locations of bite marks on different sites on the body have been well documented by Pretty and Sweet [4].

Types of bite marks

Bite marks are found on various substrates.

Bite marks on inanimate objects and materials

Inanimate objects may receive impressions of teeth from biting. Examples reported in the literature include impressions in cheese [5–7], chocolate [8], an apple [9], a sandwich [10] and in chewing gum [11]. Such materials may sometimes record impressions of dentitions more accurately than human soft tissues. Nevertheless, we need to express appropriate caution in any conclusions drawn from a comparison between the impression and a suspect's dentition because we can't quantify the chance of a random match.

Injuries in soft tissues

- Contusion (bruising) (Fig. 8.1);
- laceration/puncture (Fig. 8.2);

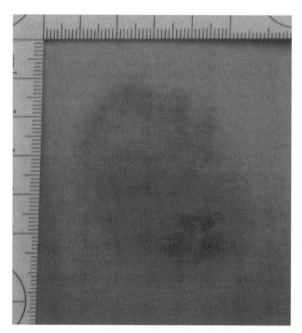

Fig. 8.1 Bruised bite mark injury, which also features a central contusion. (Image supplied by Queensland Police Service.)

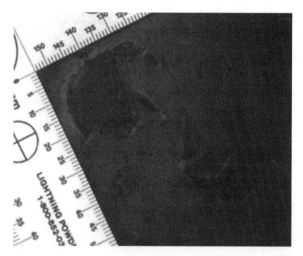

Fig. 8.2 Lacerated bite marks injury. (Image supplied by Queensland Police Service.)

- abrasion;
- imprinting (Fig. 8.3);
- avulsion (Fig. 8.4);
- in addition, bite injuries may also feature an area of central contusion;

Fig. 8.3 Bruised multiple bite mark injury. (Image supplied by Queensland Police Service.)

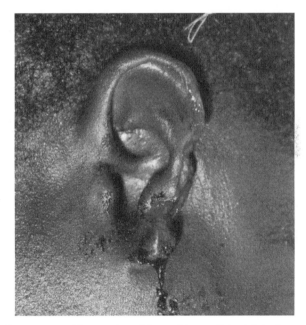

Fig. 8.4 An avulsion injury with a portion of the ear bitten off. Such injuries are usually poor candidates for bite mark comparison. (Image supplied by Queensland Police Service.)

- any combination of the above;
- multiple bite marks in a single injury site may also be present; these may indicate repeated attempts to get a grip with the teeth when the living victim attempts to pull away from the assailant (Fig. 8.3).

There have been several published attempts to classify bite mark injuries. These include the Pretty Severity Scale [12], Souviron [13] and more recently a proposed Human Bitemark Classification by Dorion [14], however they have not been established successfully and are therefore of limited forensic value.

Not everything is a bite mark

Gold et al. [15] reported several dermatological lesions that can simulate a bite mark and which should be considered in the differential diagnosis:
- fixed drug eruptions;
- subacute cutaneous lupus erythematosus;
- pityriasis rosea;
- dermatophytosis: tinea corporis;
- granuloma annulare.

Examples of other injuries that can simulate a bite mark include:
- injuries from contact with shoe soles;
- injuries from contact with belt buckles;
- injuries from contact with a domestic iron;
- injuries from application of defibrillators [16];
- injury from a saw [17];
- tattoos [18].

Conclusions based on the description of the injury

The American Board of Forensic Odontology (ABFO) Bitemark Terminology Guidelines [1, p. 117] refer to three categories into which suspected bite marks may fall on the basis of matching their features to class characteristics:

1 Human Bite Mark: Human teeth created the pattern; other possibilities were considered and excluded. Criteria: The injury pattern displays features that reflect the class and individual characteristics of human teeth.

2 Suggestive: The pattern is suggestive of a human bite mark, but there is insufficient evidence to reach a definitive conclusion at this time. Criteria: General shape and size are present but distinctive features such as individual tooth marks are missing, incomplete or distorted or a few marks resembling tooth marks are present but the arch configuration is missing.

3 Not a Human Bite Mark: Human teeth did not create the injury.

While there is some merit to these categories, we feel there is insufficient certainty in some cases to merit such clear-cut definitions. We prefer the following classification:

1 The injury satisfies the class characteristics of a human bite mark and there is sufficient detail present to proceed.

2 The injury satisfies the class characteristics of a human bite mark but there is insufficient detail present in the injury, and/or the supplied images are not of a satisfactory quality to allow us to proceed.

3 The injury does not satisfy the class characteristics of a human bite mark. It is not likely to have resulted from contact with human dental arches.

4 There is insufficient information in the injury for us to make a decision to continue.

The majority of partial bite marks and defensive injuries resulting from possible contact with an assailant's teeth where only one or two single marks are present fall into categories 2 or 4.

The process of biting and how it relates to bite marks

Much of the literature on biting covers the final part of the closing cycle, which is of pathological interest. The concern in biting associated with injury is that the jaws tend to be open wide, and we will refer to this as 'wide biting'.

The incisal profiles of lower anterior teeth tend to be smaller and narrower than the upper incisors, and this reflects their function in the wide bite, which is to stabilise the material being bitten. The upper teeth close on the object and the palatal surfaces are often the first to contact the bitten material (Fig. 8.5). They have a greater surface area than the lower incisor edges, and therefore the pressure they exert is correspondingly less, depending on the mechanics of the specific situation. This may seem counter-intuitive because we understand that it is the mandible that moves, but in this case, the lesser friction generated by the upper teeth results in the upper arch moving more across the substrate towards the closing position than the lower arch. It is therefore not unusual to find more diffuse bruising associated with teeth of an upper arch as opposed to more defined marks from the lower teeth. If the bite has not fully closed, we can sometimes recognise impressions or bruises corresponding to the anatomy of the palatal surfaces of the upper incisors in the injury. Sperber [19] attributed them

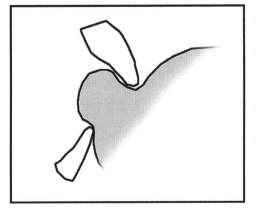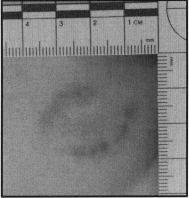

Fig. 8.5 The incisal edges of the lower teeth impact against the tissue while the palatal surfaces of the upper incisors press against the tissue in the early stages of the wide bite. This also explains the central bruising seen in some bite injuries. (Right image supplied by Queensland Police Service.)

to the pressing of skin by lower teeth against the lingual surfaces of overlapping upper teeth when bites were inflicted in a centric relationship. This fact highlights a major flaw in many of the current methods of comparison, which rely on creating a bite mark template by mapping only the incisal edges of incisor teeth. As the arches continue to move together, they trap tissue between them, and forces on the trapped tissue may cause capillary damage producing a central area of bruising. This has been verified experimentally as a viable mechanism [20, 21]; however, other contributing causes including suction and tongue-thrusting probably cannot be ruled out as contributory causes in individual cases.

As the bite continues to close, the upper incisors drag across the object until the inner incisal edges begin to come into register.

Usually the amount of drag associated with the lower arch is less than that associated with the upper arch because the upper teeth tend to move further and with reduced relative pressure. However, because the teeth of an arch move as a unit, they sometimes leave distinctive 'scrape' marks across the tissue surface. Frequently, we observe that these are better defined and more distinct with the lower arch due to the greater pressure and smaller amount of movement, and the pattern of scrapes left is in many ways comparable with a barcode, which appears to be distinctive for a given dentition. The marks produced by the lower dental arch are an invaluable source of information.

The individuality of the dentition and its transfer to the bite mark

Bite mark comparison rests on two simple assumptions. The first is that the anterior teeth of different dentitions vary sufficiently for there to be recognisable differences between them. The second is that features from the teeth will transfer to the injury with sufficient detail and accuracy for the forensic odontologist to be able to certify the set of teeth responsible by comparing the features of the injury with the features of the teeth. Both assumptions need to be true to support the contention that bite mark comparison can identify the assailant. On examination, we find that published research supports neither of them well.

The individuality of the human dentition

The issue of individuality of the dentition in relation to bite marks has been the subject of several studies in the last three decades including a famous but flawed 1984 study by Rawson [22], none of which clarified the issue. In 2007, Kieser et al. [23] reported a morphometric study in which they stated that the incisal surfaces of the anterior dentition were unique.

Bush et al. [24] revisited the work of Rawson and examined their data for similarity of dentitions rather than differences with a resolution of ±1 mm and with a rotation of ±5 degrees to simulate comparison with a bite injury where transfer of dental features has not been perfect (see next section). They concluded that:

> The number of matches increases geometrically with database size as the number of possible comparisons of n specimens increases with the square of n as the number of possible comparisons is $n(n-1)/2$. In a closed population when comparing a small number of dentitions, the likelihood of a match is low, but still possible. The implication of this study is that given a large enough population the next dentition compared to the database will be highly likely to match an existing sample. [24, p. 122]

These results suggest a limit on the degree to which we can make claims of a reliable match between dentition and injury, even with the best possible apparent match, unless we have observed the injury occurring and we know its cause. By way of example, Thompson and Phillips report a case in which they felt that neither of two suspects could be excluded as the biter, but the actual assailant was shown to be a different person [25]. This will resonate with all forensic odontologists who have undertaken bite mark comparison.

Accuracy of transfer of dental features to bitten tissues

Miller et al. [26] conducted a cadaver study and showed that, using a population of 100 dental models they determined to be unique, they had difficulty in distinguishing the biting cast from other casts with similarly aligned dentitions. They also stated that in some cases, an incorrect biting cast appeared better correlated to the injury than the correct one.

Bush et al. [27] took a critical look at this issue. They examined distortions resulting from the biomechanical properties of the skin and underlying tissues in different anatomical locations, and considered the role of skin tension lines (also known as Langer lines [28, 29]), which alter the properties of the skin depending on the direction in which forces are applied. Considered together, these variations can affect the various component parts of an injury, including their relative sizes and positions as well at the overall shape of the injury. They thus linked anatomic location, skin tension and movement in their study, although it was conducted using unembalmed cadavers rather than living subjects.

They concluded that bites inflicted perpendicular to Langer lines showed the least distortion, suggesting that familiarity with these lines should be a matter of underlying knowledge for anyone involved in bite mark analysis and comparison. Further, they noted a general widening of the bite mark as compared to the size of the dentition that caused it, which resulted in a flattening of the arch shape in the injury. They also noted that bites in thin skin tended to exhibit palatal detail from teeth in the upper arch, an observation we have also made, although they state that this varies and seems to depend on the degree of firmness of the tissue. They further examined the distortions caused by movement of body parts after the bite had occurred.

They found that bites oriented parallel to Langer lines showed a greater 'dragging' of the upper arch, again something we have noted in observation.

Such bites tended to exhibit constriction of the arches in the injury, resulting in smaller arch widths and emphasised curvature in comparison with the causative dentition – except where there was extensive subcutaneous fat, in which event the injuries appeared similar to those perpendicular to the Langer lines.

The clear implication is that accurate transfer of dental features to tissue is infrequent at best, and it is possible that the dentition of incorrect suspects will correlate with the resulting injury as well as or better than the dentition of the actual assailant. Clearly, this should limit the degree of certainty expressed in any bite mark comparison, and it should trigger similar analyses for other patterned injuries.

Imaging in bite mark cases

We recommend that a police officer trained in photography should take all the images of the injuries intended for use in the analysis and comparison stages for probity.

It is important to secure initial 'context images' that show the entire region of a body and illustrate the relative locations and distribution of the injuries that are present as this permits easy visualisation of their location and orientation.

Each injury should then be imaged separately both with appropriate forensic scales (the ABFO No 2 scale is considered the standard instrument for this purpose) and without scales, to demonstrate that the scale is not inadvertently concealing any aspect of the injury. We illustrate this in Fig. 8.6.

We suggest that images be recorded images in 8-bit colour (RGB), preferably using an Adobe RGB 1998 colour space because this has a sufficiently wide gamut to record the necessary range of colours visible on the best monitors. There is no value in using a 16-bit colour image as successive filters will not be applied and rounding errors will therefore not cumulate to a destructive level.

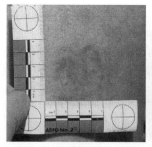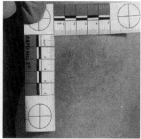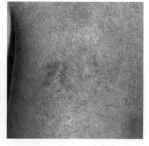

Fig. 8.6 Take photos with the scale in the upper-right corner, lower=left corner, and without the scale to demonstrate that it is not hiding any feature of the injury. (Image supplied by Queensland Police Service.)

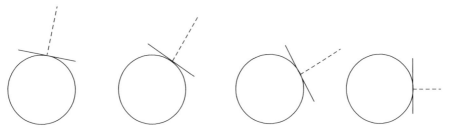

Fig. 8.7 If the injury extends around a curved tissue surface, image each part of the wound separately with the scale perpendicular to each area of forensic interest and to the scale. The scale should lie tangential to the tissue surface but not compress it. It must lie in the plane of current forensic interest. A straight, unbroken line represents the plane of the forensic scale, and the broken line depicts the long axis of the lens.

There is no value in recording monochrome images with a digital camera, because converting an image to monochrome simply means that two of the three colour channels are lost, and the remaining channel records only the luminance information. This process removes information but adds none, and so reveals nothing new. In the past it was recommended in chemical photography, because monochrome films used to be sensitive to colours in a way that could show detail that was not present in colour images recorded with colour film.

The various surfaces of the human body are rarely flat and most commonly comprise compound curves (curves in more than one direction). If the injury lies on a curved surface such as a limb, then we need to image each section of the injury separately with the scale placed adjacent to the region of forensic interest (Fig. 8.7) to ensure that each section can be scaled. The long axis of the camera lens needs to be perpendicular to the plane of the scale, which in turn needs to be placed in the plane of the injury at each point, touching but not compressing the tissue. This ensures that we can accurately scale each portion of the injury.

Avoiding distortions due to perspective

Errors due to perspective occur when the camera lens is too close to the tissue surface. Perspective in this context is the property that makes distant objects appear smaller. If the camera lens is too close to a curved surface, the distance between the lens and the nearest point on the surface can be comparable to the distance between the nearest and the most distant parts of the surface. This causes artificial enlargement of the nearest part, as shown with a face in Fig. 8.8. In the case of a face, the nose becomes wider and more prominent, and the face 'balloons' to make the eyes move to the side of the head. This causes the proportions of the subject to change in the image.

The solution is to use a telephoto lens with a focal length of between 100 mm and 150 mm, and to ensure that the distance between the lens and the subject

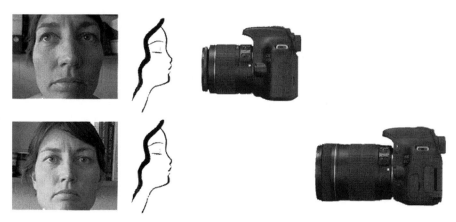

Fig. 8.8 The effect of perspective. The only factor affecting perspective is the vantage point of the camera relative to the photographic subject – how close or far it is from the item being imaged. Using a zoom lens does *not* affect perspective, so it is a good way to fill the viewfinder without incurring this type of distortion. (Image courtesy of K Wright.)

is large in comparison to the distance between the nearest and most distant parts of the subject. For imaging curved surfaces on the human body, we recommend taking the image from a distance between 1.5 m and 2.0 m from the subject. This ensures that we represent the proportions of all the items in the image accurately. We can zoom in to ensure that the region of forensic interest fills the image, because zooming does not affect the perspective, which depends solely on our vantage point in relation to the subject. Note that this advice contradicts the requirement of the AuSFO Guidelines for the Conduct of Bitemark Analysis in Australia [3, p. 4], which recommend that 'close-up' photographs be taken.

A different perspective error with respect to the forensic scale can occur if we position it at an angle to the camera lens, even if the lens itself is correctly positioned perpendicular to the plane of forensic interest. This is also known as a Type II error [30, p. 33]. In this case, the lens is perpendicular to the plane of the injury, but the scale is not parallel to that plane.

This leads to an apparent compression of the length of the scale depending on the angles involved. We can assess the extent of the error by measuring the angle between the two limbs of the scale (Fig. 8.9). If the angle is not 90 degrees, then the plane of the forensic scale is at an angle to the lens. An obtuse (divergent) angle between the limbs (as shown) means that the junction of the two limbs is too close to the camera. An acute (convergent) angle results if it is too far. It is better to use measurement of the angle between the limbs of the scale to determine this rather than the circular shapes on the scale, as the magnitude of the limbs is much greater and therefore provides more sensitivity. Once again, attempts to correct this type of scaling error digitally result in an outcome similar to that shown in Fig. 8.10, and we advise against this.

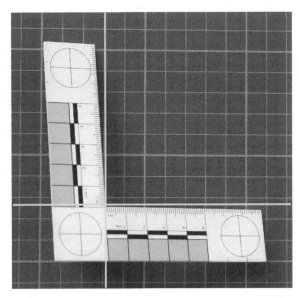

Fig. 8.9 An ABFO No 2 scale at an angle to the long axis of the camera lens. We have imaged the background correctly. We can illustrate the extent of this error by comparing the angle between the two limbs of the scale with a 90-degree angle (crossed guide lines). This demonstrates that the angle between the limbs of the scale is not 90 degrees. It is up to the odontologist to determine if the degree of error is sufficiently large to affect the outcome of a comparison or not. We should not apply this type of digital correction.

Avoiding distortions due to parallax

Parallax errors occur when the lens is not positioned perpendicular to the plane of forensic interest (which should also be parallel to the plane of the forensic scale). These are also known as Type I distortions, and can result in uncorrectable errors. Trying to correct this type of error digitally results in a geometric distortion in which the error in scaling becomes worse further from the centre line of the lens (Fig. 8.11).

Note that this advice contradicts recommendation 4.2.3.1 of the AuSFO Guidelines for the Conduct of Bitemark Analysis in Australia [3], which subscribes to the method popularised by Bowers and Johansen [30] suggesting that this type of error can and should be corrected. They recommended correction with the outcome shown in Fig. 8.11. Following their instructions introduces a new and avoidable distortion into the process and therefore we cannot condone it.

The forensic odontologist undertaking the analysis should examine their images for all these errors and use their judgement to determine if any difference from ideal is large enough to have a significant effect on the validity of a comparison. If, in their view, it is, then they should reject the image.

Photographic lighting

The area we are imaging needs to be lit to ensure correct colour, minimise specular reflection and shadow and obtain a light intensity that is as even as possible over the whole field of view.

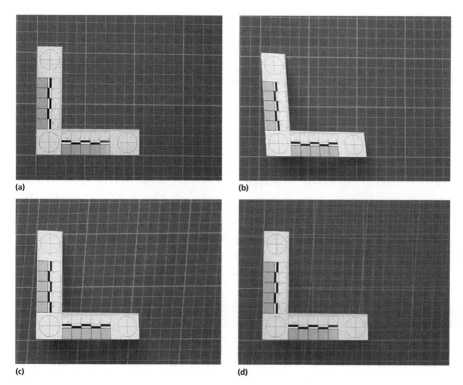

(a)　　　　　　　　　　　　　　　　　(b)

(c)　　　　　　　　　　　　　　　　　(d)

Fig. 8.10 Digital 'correction' of the perspective error in the forensic scale shown in Fig. 8.9.
(a) Correctly imaged scale and background. (b) Scale with corner too close to camera. (c) The
scale shown in (b) has been digitally 'corrected' to match that shown in (a). We can see the
consequence of attempting to correct this error in (d) where the backgrounds from (b) and
(c) have been superimposed. We can illustrate the geometric distortion we have introduced to
the background by the 'correction' by viewing the mismatch in the background grid lines.
This type of 'correction' should not be undertaken as it introduces a new (and uncontrolled)
distortion into the process.

Correct colour can be achieved by using daylight flash (about 5500 K) to
ensure that the light does not have a colour cast (for example the green colour
due to fluorescent lighting). Flashes also serve to provide fill lighting on curved
surfaces and help to eliminate lighting gradients (where there is a variation in
light intensity from one side of an image to the other).

Specular reflection is the reflection (generally of a of a point light source such as
an internal flash pointing at the surface from close to the vantage point) that creates
highlights or 'burns out' and obscures detail in the surface being imaged (Fig. 8.12).
It is a particular problem when a surface is glossy or wet, so it is recommended that
the surface be dried prior to asking a police officer to photograph it. This is especially
important in the post-mortem situation where condensation may occur on the
skin. Ring flashes generally do not help to minimise specular reflection.

Commonly, small point sources of light create sharp shadows and large ones
create more diffuse ones (Fig. 8.13). It is therefore better to maximise the size of

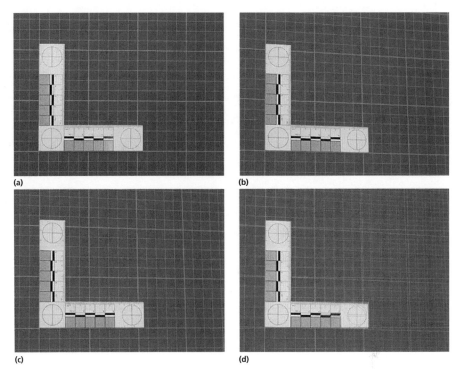

(a) (b) (c) (d)

Fig. 8.11 Digital 'correction' of a parallax error. (a) ABFO No 2 bite mark scale photographed with the long axis of the camera lens perpendicular to the centre of the area enclosed by the scale. (b) The same scale photographed with the long axis of the lens at an angle and offset from the centre of the area enclosed by the scale. (c) Shows the effect of digitally 'correcting' the scale in (b) until the limbs of the scale match as nearly as possible. (d) Shows the distortion introduced where the semitransparent correction is superimposed over the correctly photographed image shown in (a). By examining the grid in the background, one can see that we have introduced a geometric error, meaning its magnitude becomes greater the further one moves from the centre angle of the scale. This image demonstrates why it is not appropriate to perform such parallax corrections in forensic images, because the process introduces a further uncontrolled distortion into the image being 'corrected'.

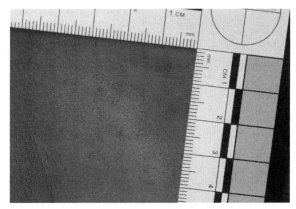

Fig. 8.12 Specular reflection can obscure important detail in the image. (Image supplied by Queensland Police Service.)

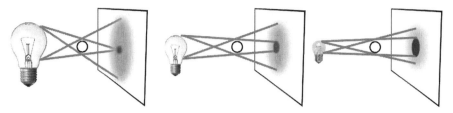

Fig. 8.13 Large light sources create more diffuse shadows than smaller ones (grey = penumbra, black = umbra).

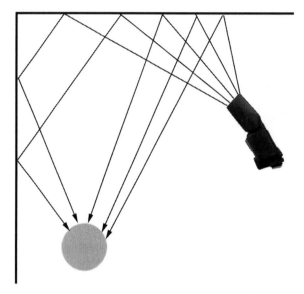

Fig. 8.14 Bounce flash used to light an object using the ceiling as a diffuser. Multiple flash units help reduce the lighting gradient that would occur in this case by adding fill lighting. Beware a coloured ceiling as this may introduce an unwanted colour cast.

the source of the light. This can be done by using 'bounce flash' where reflection from the ceiling acts as a diffuse light source (Fig. 8.14).

We can improve this technique by fitting a diffuser to the flash unit first, or by the simple expedient of using a white paper bag or plastic bag to cover the flash unit if a dedicated diffuser is not available. It is preferable not to use the inbuilt camera flash for this purpose, but rather a top-mounted single flash with a rotating head. Multiple light sources are better if they are available (for example in a studio, or with remotely triggered slave units if photographing in the field) to reduce or eliminate lighting intensity gradients. Brackets are available for fitting multiple flash units to DSLR cameras and these are valuable because the light sources are not close to the vantage point of the lens. They assist in reducing specular reflection and lighting gradients when properly diffused.

Lighting from one side is likely to create a light intensity gradient across the image, and should be avoided wherever possible unless counterbalanced by an additional light source from the opposite side.

File format for image files

The preferred format of image storage is camera RAW. The RAW file is not a viewable image and therefore acts as a digital 'negative' to ensure the probity of any image used in bite mark comparison. If this is not feasible, a lossless format such as TIFF is acceptable. A lossy compressed format such as JPEG is not suitable for primary images. Unfortunately, in the authors' experience, most images supplied by authorities come to us as JPEG images with varying levels of compression. Further saving of such images using JPEG compression will introduce additional compression artefact, progressively degrading the quality of the images.

We need to recognise this and state it in our reports, because we must then rely on the chain of custody to ensure the probity of such an image and account for any loss in quality from an original.

Using alternative light sources

Some authorities recommend taking images using a reflective ultraviolet light source. They report that this method makes an injury visible long after it has faded in visible light [31–33]. Golden [34] advocated using it contemporaneously with visible light photography while the injury was still visible. The recommended technique is to use light with a wavelength of 360–400 nm [35, p. 97]. Infrared light has also been proposed as an alternative light source because it penetrates the skin to a greater depth than ultraviolet light.

Generally, caution should be taken with alternate light imaging until longitudinal studies documenting injuries metrically demonstrate the value of these techniques.

Imaging the dental casts for comparison
Perspective, parallax and lighting

All of the dental models needed in the comparison process should be photographed. The same considerations apply to the photography of dental casts as apply to the imaging of injuries. The models should be photographed using a lens of at least 100 mm focal length from a minimum distance of 1.5–2 m. Zooming in so that the model occupies a large amount of the field of view is permissible because this does not affect perspective. Avoid parallax issues that will introduce new geometric scaling errors.

Scaling the models accurately is important because the probity of the comparison process depends on all of the items we compare conforming to precisely the same scale. Hence, a forensic scale should be placed in the field of view at the approximate level of the occlusal plane, located it so that it is most representative of the plane in the region of the teeth involved in biting. Most commonly, this will involve the six anterior teeth.

Lighting the models under controlled conditions is quite different from photographing injuries in the field. Soft lighting is appropriate (large light sources), and inappropriate shadows and light gradients need to be avoided by using multiple lights. Correct lighting can be crucial to being able to observe all the necessary detail in a dental cast.

Avoid using flatbed scanners

Flatbed scanners should not be used in any circumstance to capture images of three-dimensional objects such as dental study models. The result depends on where we place the item on the scanner platen, and therefore the image is not likely to be reproducible. Figure 8.15 shows a dental model that has been scanned from the right side of the platen, and the same model scanned from the left side. Note that even though the dot on the incisal surface of tooth 21 stays in the same place, the perspective caused by the extremely short focal length of the scanner causes problematic results.

Flatbed scanners may introduce additional errors because they can also alter the length dimensions of the scanned original. They are therefore problematic when scanning two-dimensional printed images into a digital format. Images

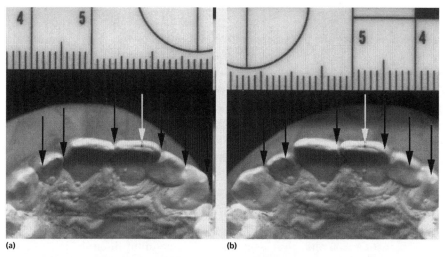

(a)   (b)

Fig. 8.15 Images resulting when we have used a flatbed scanner to scan a dental model may look reasonable, but may have hidden problems. (a) Shows the image when the same dental model is placed on the left side of the scanner platen. The white arrow shows the position of a fiduciary dot on tooth 21, which does not move between (a) and (b). The black arrows indicate positions of some features of importance in bite mark comparison. (b) Shows the result when the dental model is placed on the right side of the scanner platen without moving the arrows. This technique introduces a further uncontrolled error into the process. Clearly (a) and (b) would give a different result with many bite mark template techniques. (Image courtesy of J Garner.)

printed from photographic negatives are becoming less common, but in older matters police may still supply them.

The stepper motors in flatbed scanners are not always accurately calibrated, and this can result in stretching of the image in one dimension, most often along the long axis of the scanner platen. The range of stretching we have observed lies between 0.1% and as much as 5%, and does not seem to relate to the cost of the scanner. It is good practice to measure the amount of stretching/compression for each individual scanner and to tape an easy-to-see label stating the percentage error to it for reference. We recommend re-measuring every month to maintain currency and including a mention of it in a statement in any case where we have corrected such an error in the scanned image.

With such a distorted image, we recommend that one should correct it by shortening the longer axis of the image rather than stretching the shorter axis (Fig. 8.16) to avoid a potential accusation of 'manufacturing' evidence by an unknown process. We have also observed similar length-distortion issues in

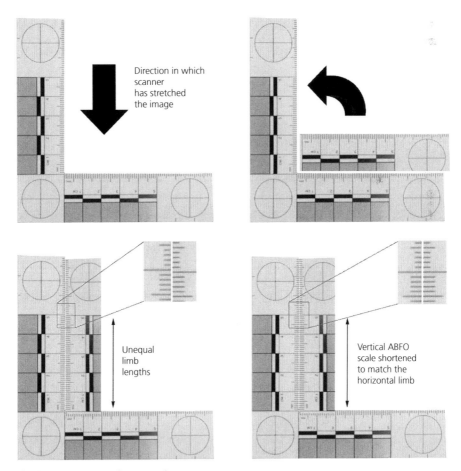

Fig. 8.16 Correction of scanner distortion.

images printed with a computer printer. However, with such images, it is very difficult to determine if unequal lengths of the forensic scale are due to printing, a past scanning process or poor photography. It is good practice to avoid using such printed images and request digital copies instead.

If police provide images printed from photographic negatives, it is possible that they have printed the negatives first and scanned the print to a digital format before they supply them as digital images. We may have no knowledge of this, and therefore may believe that they were captured as original digital images. The forensic odontologist should not assume that just because an image has been supplied in a digital format other than RAW that it comes from a digital camera.

We recommend that this test be applied to all digitally supplied images if they are in any format other that RAW, as it is possible that they are scanned copies of printed photographs with the errors inherent to the scanning process.

When there is the opportunity to request, always ask that the police provide images in an uncompressed format at the highest possible resolution, and preferably in RAW format. Regrettably, the majority of images supplied to the authors continue to be in compressed formats, commonly as JPEG images included in PDF documents. Compression artefacts in these images are another issue with which the forensic odontologist must contend.

A note on the use of the ABFO No 2 bite mark scale

We recommend the use of the ABFO No 2 bite mark scale, if for no other reason than that it is the most commonly used forensic scale for documenting small injuries. There are issues with this scale, however.

First, not all brands accurate. Figure 8.17 shows a comparison between the graduations on the vertical and the horizontal limbs of the scale. While the correlation of the overall measurement between the 0 cm and 5 cm marks is good, it becomes less so from place to place along the length of the limbs, and is poor towards the free end of the limbs. While the magnitude of the errors between the 0 cm and 5 cm is small, we should recognise the issue nonetheless and state it in our legal reports to comply with Uniform Civil Procedure Rules in jurisdictions where they apply, and for probity elsewhere.

Second, the scale features some grey patches along the length of both limbs (Fig. 8.17). These patches should ideally be a perfect 50% grey (also known as 18% neutral grey because 18% of the incident white light is reflected) for use in colour correction of images in which they appear. In fact, we have determined that the best available ABFO No 2 scales have grey patches substantially different from this, and we recommend gluing a correct grey patch to the scale prior to photography or including a colour reference card in the field of view prior to image capture if colour accuracy is an issue. One brand of ABFO No 2 scale with which we are familiar features grey patches that appear to have been printed by an ink-jet printer and show individual dots of varying shades. These are useless for colour correction and they should be avoided in forensic work.

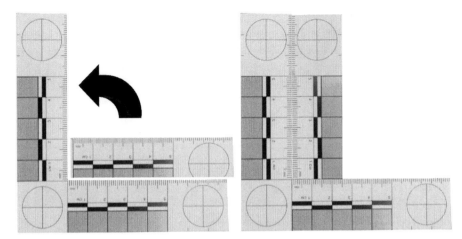

Fig. 8.17 Comparison between the horizontal and vertical limbs of an ABFO No 2 bite mark scale. We have copied and rotated the horizontal limb to lie against the vertical limb for comparison. Note the minor differences in the positions of the graduations in the length between 0 cm and 5 cm. We have found substantial variation in the magnitudes of errors in the scales available from different suppliers. Note the grey patches towards the outer edges of the limbs. These are present to provide a reference grey for colour correction, but the grey is commonly inaccurate.

Finally, the scales are not rigid and may be bent, or may bend if stored incorrectly, especially in high-temperature environments. They also fade over time and exposure to light. It is recommended that bent or faded scales be replaced prior to use, and at regular intervals regardless.

Place the scale level with the plane of forensic interest to avoid scaling errors in the final image. In the case of a dental model, this would be coincident with the occlusal plane, or parallel with it and at the correct level for a tooth that was substantially above or below the occlusal plane. The use of the scale in bite mark imaging is discussed below (Selection and preparation of working images).

Undertaking the case

A full bite mark examination comprises two stages. The first is bite mark analysis, in which the alleged injury thought to be a bite mark (or images thereof) is examined to determine if it is indeed a human bite mark, and if enough information is present to permit a valid comparison between it and possible suspect dentitions. At the analysis stage, the quality of the available evidence relating to the alleged injury is scrupulously assessed. If it is considered that there is insufficient evidence to move forward, then the case stops at this point.

If the forensic odontologist believes that there is sufficient information, then the second phase, bite mark comparison, is undertaken. This is the stage where the alleged injury is compared with the suspect dentition or dentitions (or representations of this), and conclusions are reached.

We will examine the entire process by considering:

- case selection;
- clinical appointment with the victim;
- clinical appointment with the suspect(s);
- bite mark analysis; and
- bite mark comparison.

Case selection

As with many other areas of dentistry, case selection is a crucial step in determining success. The factors on which the decision to proceed will turn include:

- Injuries must clearly meet the class characteristics of a bite mark, and contain sufficient detail to permit comparison with dentitions.
- Adequate images of the injuries must be available if the forensic odontologist cannot direct the imaging personally. They must be undistorted and contain appropriate and correctly used scaling aids.
- The lighting of the injury must be good and with no specular reflection and no shadows that obscure detail. There should be no lighting gradient in the field of interest.
- Images must be of sufficiently high resolution to show all the detail needed for comparison, and there should be access to them in an uncompressed format if they are digital.
- Dental casts and bite records of suspects must be available and adequate if the forensic odontologist cannot take them personally. If it is physically possible for the victim to have self-inflicted the injury, they are considered a suspect for the purposes of elimination.

Some of these factors will be under the control of the forensic odontologist but some may not. We provide a protocol for imaging in the section on imaging.

The clinical appointments
1.   The appointment with the victim
History

If the victim is deceased, then the less known about the incident leading to the injury, the less the forensic odontologist is likely to suffer from (and can defend against an accusation of) possible confirmation bias, which is where we unconsciously seek a particular outcome in the light of information that the police or others have given to us [36].

If the victim is living and conscious, taking the history can be an emotional experience. Apart from the physical and emotional state of the victim, other injuries may be present and these may be severe. This can have an effect on us, and can again lead to a potential allegation of confirmation bias in court.

For this reason, as well as to gain the maximum possible amount of information with which to work, it is necessary to take a careful and objective history from the victim. This history should include details (to the best of the victim's memory) about their body position and reactions during the biting process. We also seek clarification about the assailant's position, including the position of their teeth at the time of injury. It should include any recollection the victim may have about the appearance and distinctive features of their assailant's teeth.

If it is anatomically possible, there is always the possibility that the victim is the biter and careful observation will reveal whether the injuries are in positions that the victim could reach with their own teeth.

The forensic odontologist should compare the victim's information for consistency with the positions and features of the injuries observed.

It is also important to determine what, if any, clothing the victim was wearing at the time of injury. We sometimes observe a pattern from clothing material impressed on the skin during the bite, and it may obfuscate some of the detail of the individual characteristics of the biting dentition. Information from the history may help us explain these patterns.

The expert is able to refer to contemporaneous notes (those made at the time of examination) in court as an aid to memory, so these should be written in objective and unemotional language.

Physical examination

The physical examination of the victim includes a thorough examination of the relevant parts of the victim's body and clear and careful recording of all the injuries that the forensic odontologist considers could be potential bite marks.

In the case of a deceased victim, it is not sufficient to take advice from police, forensic pathologists or others as to the numbers and locations of any injuries. The examining forensic odontologist has responsibility to conduct their own examination and to verify that they have considered all possible injuries.

In the case of a living, conscious victim, the examination is undertaken in light of information from the police, doctors and the victim. During the examination, a third person must always be present, such as a police officer and/or a nurse.

The forensic odontologist should record the following information in writing:
- Time, date and place of examination.
- Names and job descriptions of others present at the examination.
     For each injury observed:
- Location of the injury.
- Class characteristics observed, including:
  ○ type of injury (contusion, laceration, avulsion or any combination of these);
  ○ presence of multiple bites in the same location;

- ○ size of the complete injury (length and breadth);
- ○ size of each arch;
- ○ distance between the arches;
- ○ form of the arches;
- ○ number of discrete points in each arch;
- ○ presence or absence of a central contusion;
- ○ presence, number and direction of any scrape marks from an arch;
- ○ skin patterns from overlying fabric;
- ○ presence of distinctive features (such as gaps in the arch); and
- ○ any other relevant observations.
- Sketches of each injury can be useful as an aid to recording these observations.
- If the injury lies in an area in which body movement may change the measurements (for instance, an upper arm), consider measuring and recording the changes in injury dimensions you observe from moving the relevant joints or body parts.
- Record details of any images taken, including the name and job description of the person taking each. Police officers should take the images for probity, advised by the forensic odontologist.

Remember that the notes recorded at this appointment may be taken into court for reference if a court appearance is required. The clearer and more comprehensive the notes, the more use they may be.

If the victim is a potential suspect, then a complete dental examination will also be needed. This will include clinical recording of the dentition, imaging, impressions for pouring dental casts for use in bite mark comparison, bite registration, and written records of any distinguishing features of the teeth.

Avulsion of the tissue bearing the bite mark (in post-mortem cases) is commonly practised on deceased victims in the United States. McNamee and Sweet reported in 2003 that 87.5% of the diplomates of the American Board of Forensic Odontology (ABFO) practised excision of the site bearing the injury [37]. Dorion, for example [38, p. 170], describes the ring techniques he has developed (versions I–V). The purpose of the technique appears to include the prevention of distortions due to shrinkage of the skin and to permit transillumination of the tissue, but fails to address the maintenance of the original skin contour (for example, the rise in tissue contour on a breast or buttock). Further, fixation of the excised tissue also resulted in some shrinkage, which increased over time (p. 179). Dorion maintains that the technique is contraindicated in only a few circumstances.

It is disfiguring to the deceased when a large area of skin is excised and it may require a special application to the coroner justifying the procedure. On the grounds of disfigurement alone, we should question the need for the procedure, but since it has the potential to introduce yet another uncontrolled distortion into the process, we cannot justify it. Indeed, the AuSFO Guideline states that:

> Despite several techniques being described, the potential for distortion in this process currently outweighs any advantages it may have for forensic comparison. While research continues in this area, and practitioners in the US are particularly noted for this technique, it remains unsupported by any advantages over the use of good digital photographic records for comparison, and cannot be reasonably endorsed as a method of bite mark evidence collection in Australia. [3, p. 3]

Images of the victim

We recommend that you ask for as many images as you wish. It is also good practice to check the images the police officer is recording to ensure that they are the images you expect.

Initial images should be 'context shots', showing the locations of injuries relative to the whole region on the body.

For closer shots, the use of a zoom lens with a focal length of 100–150 mm from a distance of a minimum of 1 m and preferably 1.5–2.0 m is required to obtain a good image size in the viewfinder. This reduces distortion caused by perspective when the lens is close to the photographic subject. Zooming in does not change perspective and permits taking a high-resolution image that occupies a large portion of the image area.

Such images of injuries both with and without a forensic scale should be taken. The absence of a scale demonstrates that no image has any important aspect of the injury hidden by the device. Scales should be L-shaped, and positioned both above and to the left, and again below and to the right, in different images. The plane of the scale should be in the plane of forensic interest and the long axis of the lens should be perpendicular to this plane.

We discuss the imaging of injuries in detail above in Imaging in bite mark cases.

2.   The appointment with the suspect(s)

Multiple suspects and multiple injuries

If multiple bite marks are present, even if there is only one suspect, it is important for the examining odontologist not to assume that this suspect is responsible for all the injuries observed. It is always possible that further suspects will be implicated if any bite mark can be excluded as having been caused by the current suspect. Therefore each injury must be compared against all suspects' dentitions. This protects against a possible allegation of confirmation bias, where one unconsciously seeks a predetermined outcome.·

Legal requirements

The forensic odontologist recording the dentition of a suspect must be aware of the legal requirements for the process. In Australia, a court order for the forensic procedure may be required. The court order must be sighted prior to beginning any work with the suspect, otherwise there is potential for the suspect to bring an assault charge against the clinician. If the suspect does consent, it is advisable to record this on their dental record and get them to countersign. The forensic odontologist should ensure that they take a copy of the order document and keep it with the suspect's dental record. If the document is not available, then the odontologist should refuse to perform the procedure until it is.

In New Zealand, the safe way to proceed is by examination after gaining informed consent (nature, reason and possible consequences) from the suspect. The only examinations or sampling that can be compelled in New Zealand are the recording of fingerprints and the taking of blood for purposes of evidential blood alcohol analysis. It is unlikely that a court order to compel a suspect to comply with an examination or sampling would be sought or obtained in this jurisdiction.

A forensic odontologist recording the dentition of a suspect may be required to attend court and provide details of the matter.

Police officers will probably accompany the suspect to the dental office and the suspect may be handcuffed. The examination may be recorded on audio and sometimes on video. A police photographer will take any images requested by the clinician. Any or all of these things may be used in evidence later.

Because of the potentially intrusive nature of these appointments, adequate time should be allocated in the appointment book, and scheduling them as the last appointment of the day avoids concern in the waiting room.

Clinical examination of the suspect

The forensic odontologist needs to record the dentitions of all of possible suspects for comparison with the bite mark injury. This should also include the victim if it is anatomically possible for them to have self-inflicted the injury.

Thorough examination of the dentition of the suspect and complete dental charting must be undertaken in the event that some features become important at a later stage. The relationship between the bony jaws, the occlusal relationship (both molar and canine relationships) and the position of the dental midline should be recorded, as well as an estimate of the maximal opening of the mouth (distance between the incisal edges of the upper- and lower-central incisors, measured in millimetres). Excellent impressions of the upper and lower teeth are required.

A bite registration must be obtained. The AuSFO Guidelines for the Conduct of Bitemark Analysis in Australia [3] also recommend taking a 'bite sample' during the examination (Guideline 3.6, p. 12) by asking the suspect to bite into polyvinyl siloxane putty in the same way they would normally chew without complete closure of the jaws.

Images of the suspect

A police photographer should take all of the images of the suspect for probity, advised by the forensic odontologist. A context photograph of the face showing the mouth closed and open is required. This should be taken with due regard to perspective (see: Imaging in bite mark cases). Further images from both the front and the sides with the teeth in centric, lateral and protrusive positions are taken. Clear images of the occlusal and incisal surfaces of both arches are needed, as well as detailed images of any features including restorations, enamel chips, broken teeth or similar distinctive artefacts that may transfer to an injury.

Lighting of the images is important and this is often difficult to manage in the clinical situation, especially with an uncooperative patient. Use of two flash units to the sides of the camera on a bracket rather than an integrated flash above the lens is preferable, and diffusers help supply an even light source to reduce shadows and specular reflection. A ring flash will not significantly reduce specular reflection.

Dental impressions of the suspect

Dental impressions of each dental arch suitable for casting are required. It is important to obtain excellent, accurate impressions of the teeth and associated structures, so the impression must remain in the mouth undisturbed until it is thoroughly set. If this is difficult, then at minimum we need to have confidence in the accurate recording of the premolar and incisor teeth. The occlusal and incisal surfaces alone are not considered to be sufficient. With very young children, the best that might be achieved is to have them bite into some softened wax that is immediately soaked in chilled water.

Because multiple pours of impressions will be required, select an impression material that is suited to this. Polyether, polyvinyl siloxane or hybrids of these are a good choice. With an uncooperative suspect, a hydrophilic material such as a polyether may help avoid the need to dry the teeth prior to taking the impression. Disposable trays are good for this procedure because the impressions may be needed as exhibits in court.

It is good practice to have material specification sheets for any material used because this can forestall questions about their accuracy in court.

We recommend making at least three pours of each impression. The pouring technician or forensic odontologist should clearly label each dental cast on a surface visible in the occlusal view with a number indicating from which pour it was made. We recommend pouring all impressions in die stone, preferably under vacuum. If circumstances forbid, then at least the first pour should be in die stone to ensure the resulting casts are sufficiently robust to withstand the necessary handling, and subsequent pours can be made in dental stone. Plaster is insufficiently robust for use in any circumstance.

The first cast is the one used for the comparison process, as it will be the most accurate of the three and the most robust if it is the only one cast in die stone. The second cast forms a backup in case of an accident to the first. We recommend keeping the third cast pristine for use as a potential exhibit.

If the dental impressions are given to a dental laboratory to pour, they need to maintain a chain of custody as part of the process. Receipts should be exchanged for the impressions and models, and both parties should record and keep them for possible court purposes.

Before the return of dental casts and wax bites from the dental laboratory, the laboratory should be asked to code items for each suspect with a non-identifying number or label where there is more than one suspect. This should contain no information to identify the person from whom each set of items originates, and helps defend against any allegation of confirmation bias. We recommend that the laboratory provides the key linking the codes to suspects only to the police investigator. The forensic odontologist will therefore compare codes rather than named suspects with injuries and return a finding like 'cases 2A and 3C were eliminated on comparison, but case 1E could not be eliminated'. The police investigators can subsequently make the identity of the individual linked to the code available to a court. This strategy is even more effective if the forensic odontologist who performs the comparison is not the person who performed the examination of the suspects, in which case the laboratory or police investigators should supply no name to the odontologist even if only a single suspect is involved.

This is in contrast to the AuSFO Guidelines for the Conduct of Bitemark Analysis in Australia [3] which recommend using either identification numbers or names of the individuals from which the cast is taken.

Three-dimensional scanning

An alternative to taking dental impressions is three-dimensional scanning of a dentition and building a virtual model. This eliminates the need to select impression and casting materials and the use of a dental laboratory, but it has the potential disadvantage that if the scan is not perfect, the data will not be accurate. Modern intraoral scanners can achieve resolutions of approximately 20 μm.

A further disadvantage of not having cast impressions is the need to print a physical copy of the dentition using a three-dimensional printer if we are to make simulations of an injury later (see: Undertaking the case – bite mark analysis).

A stone cast is useful as both an aid and an exhibit in court. A three-dimensional printed model may not have the same level of familiarity to a jury as a stone cast, which requires little technology and is easily understood.

Bite registration of the suspect

We recommend recording the centric occlusion of the suspect by asking them to bite into a sheet of dental wax or bite-recording material in their normal closing position. Polyvinyl siloxane materials are better than wax because they are stable over time. It may be required as an exhibit for court. We use it to locate the relationship between the upper and lower dental casts. We find little advantage in recording lateral or protrusive excursions of the mandible. These provide little if any advantage in the comparison process unless there is an anomaly in the bite that permits them to demonstrate its significance.

We recommend that the forensic odontologist marks the bite record to indicate which arch is the upper and which is the lower for court purposes. It is also important to indicate the right and left sides on the record (we use the letters R and L). This avoids confusion during later imaging and presentation in court.

DNA sample

Taking a DNA sample of a suspect is a police responsibility in many jurisdictions, and the forensic odontologist should ask the police if they have already obtained one for comparison with DNA swabs of the victim's injuries. If they have not, then this is the time to request that they secure one if someone previously swabbed the victim's injuries for DNA in a timely fashion or if that opportunity is still available. However, in the case of an injury on a child, remember that mother may 'kiss it better' so due caution should be exercised in interpreting the result.

Bite mark analysis

The analysis phase of bite mark examination is separate from the comparison phase. We proceed to the comparison phase only if we are satisfied after the analysis phase that there are sufficient grounds to determine that the injury is a bite mark and there is enough information in the injury to make comparison with a dentition worthwhile.

Injury analysis in this context is about assessing the evidence provided by the injury and its recordings. It is possible that one may be able to view and assess the fresh injury at first hand, but experience suggests it is more likely that the police will ask that the images of the injury be examined, possibly long after they were taken.

In the analysis phase, we assess the class characteristics and individual characteristics of an injury or image(s) of an injury to determine the extent to which the injury satisfies the class characteristics, and if there is a sufficient level of individual characteristics to proceed. If only images are available, the quality of the images needs to be assessed to determine if they are truly representative of the injury without introducing further, possibly uncontrolled, distortions (see: Imaging in bite mark cases). If we view the injury clinically, then it needs to be evaluated to determine if it contains sufficient information to let us move forward to comparison.

Any of the following outcomes is possible:

- When we receive images without the opportunity to examine the injury directly, we conclude that any images we receive are of satisfactory quality or not. If they are not, we stop the examination at this point.
- We consider that the injury does or does not satisfy the class characteristics of a bite mark (see: Describing bite marks – conclusions based on the description of the injury). If it does not, we stop the examination at this point.
- If the above are positive, we may feel that there is sufficient information in the injuries to proceed to the comparison phase or not. If there is not, we stop the

examination. If there is and we elect to proceed, we should not guarantee the outcome of any comparison at this point.

The process is summarised in Fig. 8.18.

If it is felt that the injury does satisfy the class characteristics of a bite mark but does not feature sufficient individual characteristics to allow comparison, this should still be reported. The fact of the existence of a bite mark injury may still be important to a case, even if a comparison with specific suspects cannot be performed.

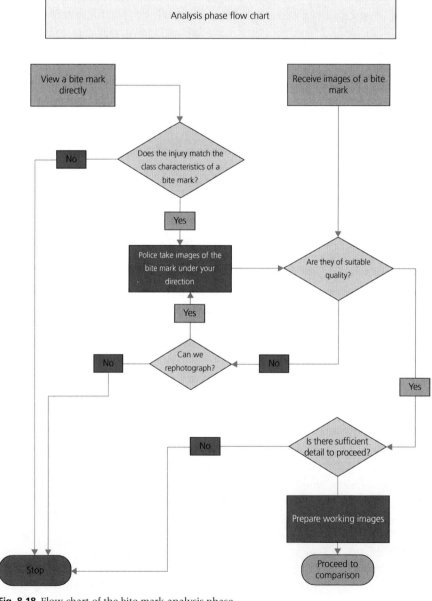

Fig. 8.18 Flow chart of the bite mark analysis phase.

For the purposes of this chapter, we used a simulated injury that we created by coating the surfaces of the teeth of a dental cast with lipstick and applying them to a skin surface with a small amount of drag. We removed the majority of the lipstick with a wet cloth before we photographed it. While we recognise that this does not replicate the features of a real bite mark injury, it permits us to demonstrate the principles of examination without using any actual criminal case materials.

1.   Selection and preparation of working images

A rough perusal will allow us to discard images (either received or taken by a police photographer under our direction) that are obviously unsuitable for further use. The criteria we use to select the images we wish to keep include:

- correct lighting;
- absence of specular reflection;
- appropriate distance between the camera lens and the surface with the injury; and
- correct use of a forensic scale, typically an ABFO No 2.

We will probably select only a small number of useable images, and we need to choose the best for the comparison phase. We require at least one image showing the overall locations of the injuries and their positions on the victim (the context image) (Fig. 8.19) and detailed images showing each of the injuries (Fig. 8.20).

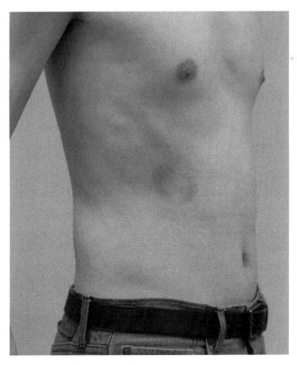

Fig. 8.19 A 'context shot' showing the location of the injury.

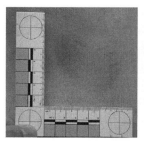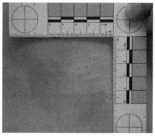

Fig. 8.20 Selected images showing the injury with the ABFO No 2 bite mark scale lower-left, upper-right and with no scale to demonstrate that the scale has not obscured any element of the injury. Note the absence of specular reflection. Images were taken from a distance of 1.5 m with a 150 mm lens.

We select images to show each injury with the forensic scale towards the lower right and again towards the upper left, and finally without the scale to demonstrate that no feature of the injury has been obscured by the scale (Fig. 8.20). The text and numbers on the ABFO No 2 bite mark scale are readable and not reversed, so we can be certain that the image is correct and we know which side is the right side and which is the left.

Each image is inspected to determine if the injury shown satisfies the class characteristics of a bite mark and, if it does, if there is sufficient detail showing individual characteristics to proceed. If there is not, the analysis is stopped here. If there is, the analysis proceeds to the next step.

If bruise colour is an issue in the matter, we may wish to colour-correct the injury images at this point. Because the 'neutral grey' patches on the ABFO No 2 scale are not reliable, it may be necessary to determine their colour and use them to correct unless a known grey card has been included in the field of view. Colour correction only makes sense if using a calibrated workflow and this must extend to any projector in the courtroom if we intend to project the images for later viewing.

Next, we select images of the dental casts of a suspect (Fig. 8.21).

Now we test the selected images containing forensic scales to ensure that the photographer has imaged them correctly and has not introduced errors or distortions (Fig. 8.22).

At this point, we wish to produce 'simulated injuries' by biting the casts into a substrate (in this case, Play-Doh® dusted with talcum powder for contrast). We produce simulations of the scraping pattern we expect with each cast as well. All of these are scaled and photographed exactly as the dental casts in Fig. 8.21 were imaged, ensuring the ABFO No 2 bite mark scale is in the plane of the surface we are imaging (Figs. 8.23 and 8.24). We also test these images to ensure we have not introduced any new distortions, just as we did with the dental cast images (Fig. 8.21).

With all the working images selected, we proceed to the comparison phase.

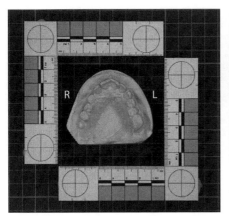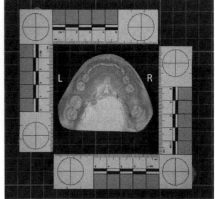

Fig. 8.21 Selected images showing the dental casts we photographed from a distance of 1.5 m using a 150 mm lens. The ABFO No 2 bite mark scale is level with the occlusal plane at the anterior teeth to ensure we have scaled these correctly. The right and left sides are clearly marked.

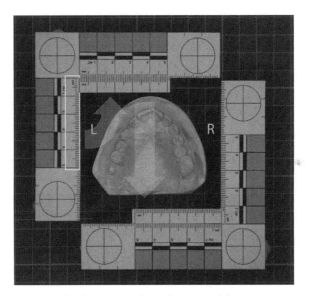

Fig. 8.22 Testing the images for distortions. This is the image of the upper suspect cast shown in Fig. 8.21 above. We have copied the left-hand vertical limb of the ABFO No 2 bite mark scale (white outline), and rotated and moved it to lie against the horizontal scale (curved arrow shows direction of rotation). We have then copied it again to compare with the horizontal limb of the right-hand horizontal scale (straight arrow). The scale limbs are the same length in both cases indicating that we have introduced no distortions in the imaging process.

2. Preparation of bite mark templates, or exemplars

Bite mark templates or overlays (also known as 'exemplars', mainly in the US) are traditionally considered to comprise outlines of incisal or occlusal edges of teeth used in the comparison process. In the view of the authors, using only

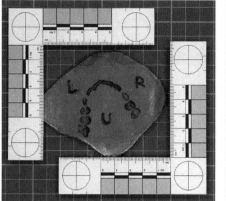
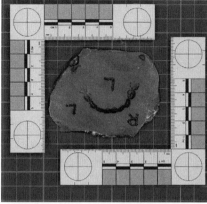

Fig. 8.23 Simulated injuries. We gently bite the dental casts into the surface of powdered Play-Doh® to record the pattern produced. We clearly mark the right (R) and left (L) sides of the dental arch to avoid confusion later, and label the simulations U (upper) and L (lower).

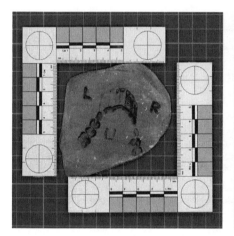
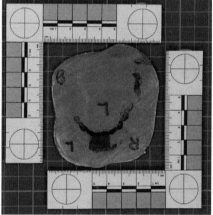

Fig. 8.24 Simulated scrape injuries. We lightly drag the dental casts across the surface of powdered Play-Doh® to record the pattern produced. We clearly mark the right (R) and left (L) sides of the dental arch to avoid confusion later, and label the scrapes U (upper) and L (lower).

the incisal edge outlines ignores the mechanics of the wide biting process and fails to document the palatal anatomy of the upper incisors, losing valuable information.

Bite mark templates have a long history. In 1943, Morgen [39] illustrated how all of the teeth on a dental model could be painted black except the incisal and occlusal surfaces. He photographed them and superimposed the resulting negative on a scaled negative of the bite. Gustavson [40, p. 151] illustrated the opposite technique, in which the edges of the teeth are inked or painted, although he does not explain if this is done with a transparent overlay or if the ink is placed directly on the teeth of the model. Ström [41] coated incisal surfaces and edges with lipstick, which rubbed off to leave a mark indicating contact with the teeth.

Some practitioners have advocated physically comparing the dental cast directly with an injury. However, it can create iatrogenic artefacts mimicking skin injuries which can be confused with actual injury patterns [42]. It is also difficult to present as evidence. It has now been discredited. Page et al. [43] reported that it was used in Australia for a small number of cases between 2002 and 2012.

The need for objectivity and reproducibility

Consistent outcomes from bite mark examinations by different experts require techniques for making objective and reproducible bite mark templates. A template is nothing more than an attempt to capture the characteristics of the relevant teeth in a dental arch for comparison with the details of an alleged bite mark injury. The perfect bite mark template would not only capture all of the relevant detail, but would be exactly reproducible by any independent expert consulted on the case. The technique for making it would therefore produce an objective result rather than a subjective one. The majority of techniques currently used do not meet this criterion, and many are selective and subjective in the characteristics that they record.

Transparent film has been a popular method of recording a template. The odontologist places it over a dental model and either indicates the incisal surface of each tooth with an indelible pen, or attempts to produce what is called a 'hollow-volume' overlay by drawing around the incisal edge of each tooth with a fine pen capable of marking the surface of the film, as explained by explained by Luntz and Luntz [44, p. 154]. Sweet and Bowers [45] determined that such templates fail to capture dental characteristics of interest and do not capture tooth rotation well. We have observed that they are subjective and do not produce consistent results, even when the same individual makes sequential attempts. We therefore do not recommend use of this technique.

The use of photocopiers in comparison of bite marks and teeth was illustrated by McCullough in 1983 [5], and using them to scan a dental model and then draw around the incisal edges on the resulting xerographic print was described by Dailey in 1991 [46]. Sweet and Bowers [45] found this technique poor, but more recently Khatri et al. [47] have suggested it is accurate. Apart from the potential for distortion introduced by the photocopier scanner and imaging anomalies introduced by the xerographic process (where there is no control over the moving light source), there is then the subjective step of manually tracing the tooth outlines from the printed sheet. We absolutely do not recommend this method.

Various computerised methods of creating templates or overlays have been proposed [30, p. 48]. Some depend on the use of a digital image selection tool, for example the 'magic wand' tool in Adobe Photoshop®, while others rely on edge-selection techniques in an image of the dental model [48]. Variations on these two techniques were evaluated by McNamee et al. [49] who found them generally reliable. If the images of the dental casts contain distortions caused by the imaging process, these will also be present in the bite mark template, and the templates themselves may vary depending on how the dental cast is lit to produce areas of light and shadow. Different lighting may produce different templates, even if the user feels that the process is 'objective'. The use of tools such as the Adobe Photoshop 'magic wand' are subjective, since obtaining exactly similar results on different occasions depends on selecting precisely the same shade of pixel in the image each time the task is undertaken. This subjectivity was recognised by Metcalf in 2008 [50] who advocated a more *objective* approach using ultraviolet light. He combined Morgen's painting technique [39] with the use of the Adobe Photoshop 'magic wand' tool to create a hollow-volume tracing. However, subjectivity still lies in the 'painting' element of this technique, which he performed with a special marker.

A variation on the creation of bite mark templates by impressing dental casts into soft wax was described by Luntz and Luntz [44, p. 154], in which the wax is placed on a sheet of paper and points of contact result in the white paper showing through when the cast is pressed down into it. A further variation is to transilluminate the wax bite, photograph it, and trace the outline of the bite on the scaled photograph with a digital imaging program [50]. Yet another variation is to place a sheet of transparent material over the bitten wax sheet and to trace the outlines of the individual marks by hand. A fourth variation occurs when the depressions in the wax produced by the teeth are filled with a radiopaque substance and then x-rayed to produce an 'objective' result [45, 51]. There is no specification about the amount of filling applied.

We believe that all of these techniques run the risk of subjectivity. In other words, different attempts would not necessarily arrive at identical results from the same starting point.

Digital contours as an objective bite mark template

Metcalf [50, p. 426] notes that: 'Dr Curtis Daley has presented a novel method where a dental stone cast of the suspect's dentition was embedded in stone of a contrasting colour, and then what are essentially serial horizontal sections are made through the occlusal plane with a dental model trimmer and these are sequentially photographed.' This appears to be the only mention in the literature of an attempt to create sections through a dental model. One of the authors (AF) and John Garner developed a similar process in Queensland in 1998.

Dental casts can be laser-scanned in three dimensions at very high resolutions (typically 20 µm), and the resulting digital models can be sectioned to produce contours representing sections at different depths from the occlusal plane as shown in Fig. 8.25. We can use these contours as a bite mark template because each can be viewed separately, and by drawing a line around the base of each

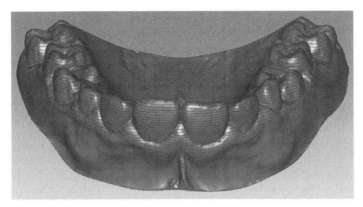

Fig. 8.25 A 3D laser-scanned dental model. We scanned this model at a resolution of 20 μm and then sectioned it at 0.5 mm intervals to produce digital contours, visible as thin lines in the region of the teeth. We can make the section interval as narrow or as broad as we wish. (Image courtesy of C Little.)

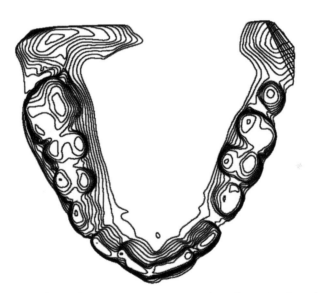

Fig. 8.26 A series of hollow-volume sections comprising a three-dimensional overlay. We can view the sections separately or in any combination, permitting us to examine the way in which the teeth engage with the tissue during biting and how this corresponds with bruising and scrape marks on the tissue. (Image courtesy of C Little.)

contour section, corresponding hollow-volume overlays are produced that represent the three-dimensional characteristics of the teeth in the cast (Fig. 8.26). The technique is objective, because if we specify the plane of section and the contour interval, anyone with access to the digital model and appropriate software can reproduce the results. We refer to this as a 'dynamic template' because we can turn the various contour layers on and off to examine the dynamics of the bite.

Because the model is dimensionally accurate to the specified resolution of the 3D scanner, there is no ambiguity whatsoever about the probity of the measurement and all of the potential distortions than can be introduced by imaging errors are eliminated.

Access to more of the tooth than just the incisal edge permits the comparison of tooth anatomy with contusions resulting from the contact between the palatal surfaces of the upper teeth and the tissue. We also gain a greater appreciation of the relationship between the features of the teeth and scrape marks caused by their dragging across the bitten surface.

A generic problem with the use of any bite mark overlay is that the odontologist was not present when the injury occurred, so we have to estimate the angle of the occlusal plane of each arch to the bitten surface. This becomes even more complex when the bite is on a curved surface. The preferred approach has been to estimate the greatest angle of the occlusal plane at the time of biting and then create contours at this angle. We repeat the process with the occlusal plane horizontal. Both sets of contours are now used in the comparison, recognising that these two planes represent the extremes and that reality lies somewhere between them. This allows us to demonstrate the extremes without misrepresenting the actual angle because of a poor guess.

Bite mark comparison

We make it completely clear that bite mark comparison is a pattern-matching exercise. Many factors can affect the transfer of information from teeth in a dental arch to a bitten victim and human tissue is a very poor impression medium.

The dimensions of the arch and its components that we see in a bite mark can be quite different to those in the causative dental arch. The elements that make up the pattern do not vary in relation to each other as much, although variations in overall dimensions can occur due to variables beyond our control (see: Sources of potential distortion and error in bite mark injuries). This renders bite mark comparison a difficult matter, and we need to demonstrate the basis for our conclusions clearly, taking all the features of injuries into account to maximise the amount of information we can use.

Our obsession with accurate measurement and elimination of introduced distortions in the images we use is therefore a matter of ensuring that the images we work with represent reality as closely as possible and do not introduce new errors into the process. We cannot account for factors we cannot control and may not even recognise, such as changes in the position of the portion of the body on which the injury is located since the victim received the injury.

There are probably as many different protocols for undertaking bite mark comparison as there are groups who undertake the task. We illustrate our method, developed by Mr John Garner (originally digital imaging expert and Senior Sergeant in the Queensland Police Service) and one of the authors (AF) over many years.

We recommend that a digital imaging expert carry out the actual digital image processing, and that they present that part of the process in court. This frees the forensic odontologist to concentrate on the interpretation of the comparison rather than on the technical processes leading up to it.

For our comparison, we use Adobe Photoshop®, but one can use any competent digital imaging program. The Gimp is an excellent free alternative, available on a GNU General Public License.

Protocol – testing hypotheses

A basic principle of bite mark comparison is not to make assumptions about anything. Even though we have previously discussed the wide bite and the different features of marks made by upper and lower dental arches (see: The process of biting and how it relates to bite marks), we still test the hypothesis that either arc of an injury can relate to the upper or the lower arch of teeth.

We will refer to each of the hemispherical groups of marks comprising one-half of the injury as an 'arc' in the following discussion.

We construct our protocol as a series of hypotheses that we test for each injury:

1 That there is no position in which the features of either the upper and lower simulated injuries match either arc of the real injury.

To test this hypothesis, we select one arc and digitally compare simulated injuries (see: Undertaking the case – bite mark analysis) from both dental arches, upper and lower, against it to exclude the possibility of a match. If we find a position where the comparison appears to match, we refute the hypothesis and we proceed to the second injury arc. Again, we compare simulated injuries from both dental arches with the second arc to try to exclude a possible match. If we find a position that appears to match with the simulated injury from the opposite dental arch, we test a second hypothesis.

2 That the centre lines of both dental arches, when projected along any apparent scrape lines (which indicate the direction of biting), will not meet at an appropriate location inside the area comprising the injury.

If we refute both of these hypotheses, then we have a potential match and we move on to a more detailed comparison of the minutiae of each dentition and the underlying injury.

Determine the size and resolution of the smallest image among the comparison images and scale the other images accordingly

A flow chart of the basic protocol appears in Fig. 8.27.

We cannot legitimately add information to an image by digitally increasing resolution or size. This causes the imaging program to 'create' new information (potential evidence) by interpolation. Therefore, the amount of information in the smallest image determines the parameters for all of the other images. Careful preparation of the images prior to the comparison process is important to ensure that the process runs smoothly. If the images of the dental casts, simulated injury

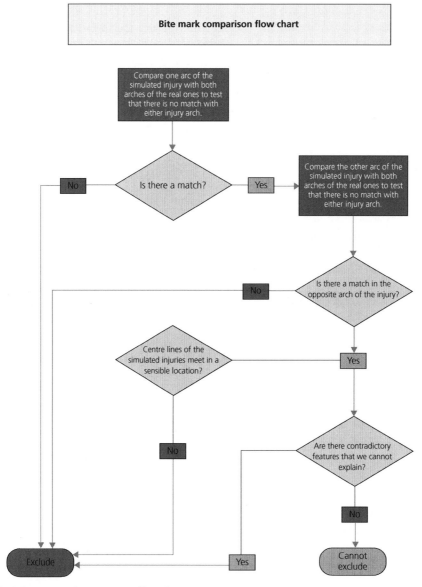

Fig. 8.27 Bite mark comparison flow chart.

and simulated scrape are all acquired using the same camera on the same tripod with the same lens at the same distance, they should all be scaled very similarly (minor variations may occur because we may move the forensic scale fractionally to lie in the plane of interest for a particular object). The images should therefore be scaled down to the size of the original injury image if it is smaller than they are, or vice-versa. The resolution of all the images must be identical before this step is undertaken (300 dpi is a good choice with today's technology).

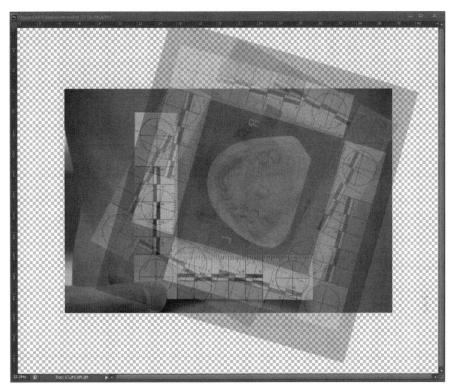

Fig. 8.28 The 'injury image' layer with overlying layers superimposed to demonstrate the value of a large canvas with a transparent background. The large canvas enables one to move and rotate layers with ease.

Base (injury) image

The first step is to open a blank transparent canvas and place the image of the injury we selected in the analysis phase on it as a layer named 'injury image'. The canvas should be larger than the actual image to permit us to move it freely (Fig. 8.28). Resolution for the canvas matches that of the source images. We verify that the vertical and horizontal limbs of the included forensic scale match.

Simulated injury

We believe that it is important to compare similar things. In this context, this means we wish to compare an injury with an injury, rather than an injury with a dental arch. We therefore open the 'simulated injury' images from both upper and lower dental casts (see: Undertaking the case – bite mark analysis – selection and preparation of working images). We ensure that the dimensions of their forensic scales match those in the original injury layer exactly.

We then proceed to move and rotate them for comparison of each with both arcs of the injury (Fig. 8.29). This tests the hypothesis that we can find no position in which the features of the simulated injuries and those of the 'injury

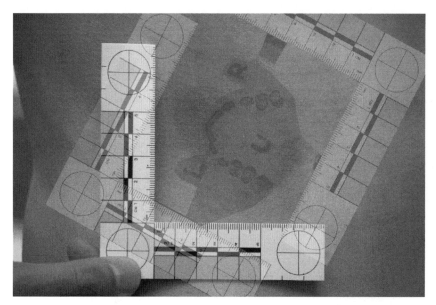

Fig. 8.29 Comparison between the 'simulated injury' of the upper dental arch and the injury image. The opacity of the simulated injury can be changed to visualise the injury image beneath it.

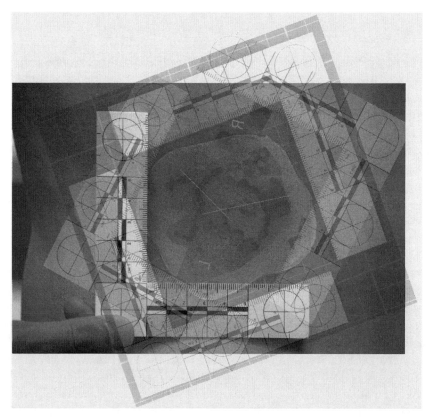

Fig. 8.30 Projection of the centre lines of both simulated images as compared with the injury image. Recall that this 'injury' was made by using a dental cast coated with lipstick against the skin, therefore this figure shows the principle only.

image' match. We only proceed to the next step if both the upper and lower simulated injuries clearly match with the features of opposite arcs of the original injury. If the match is clear, we identify the midlines of both dental arches and project them along the direction of movement during biting (Fig. 8.30) as determined by any scrape marks left during the biting process. We expect the projected centre lines to meet inside the circle of the injury at a sensible location, which is often nearer the marks caused by the lower teeth because these tend to move less during wide biting.

If there is any ambiguity about the match, then we look more closely at minutiae (see the following sections), and if this does not resolve the issue, we state that there is insufficient information to reach a conclusion.

If a non-match is obvious, this substantiates the hypothesis and we exclude the dentition.

If we have determined matching positions between simulations and the injury image, we provide the individual images to a second forensic odontologist to determine whether they reach a similar conclusion independently. They should reach the same result in order for us to move forward.

Scrape simulation

When two or more forensic odontologists agree that there is a unique matching position between the simulated injuries and the injury image, we use the simulated injuries to place the 'simulated scrape' into position (see: Undertaking the case – bite mark analysis – selection and preparation of working images). Once again, these layers are precisely scaled against the injury image layer, and the features of the scrape can then be compared with the scrape marks left in the actual injury (Fig. 8.31). It may take several attempts to produce a scrape simulation whose direction aligns with one in the actual injury.

In many respects, the scrape is like a bar code and seems to be quite specific for each dentition. Unlike the example shown, where we have coated a dental cast with lipstick and dragged it across a tissue surface, in real injuries the bruising occurs in regions of reduced pressure. Scrape marks therefore commonly represent embrasures between teeth, small divots in incisal surfaces, irregularities in the margins of restorations, and areas adjacent to high spots on the incisal or occlusal surface. This adds individual characteristics to the scrape. There are no studies on the degree to which these patterns are specific to any particular dental arch, but it seems a question worth examining.

Because of the mechanics of wide biting, upper teeth tend to drag further across the bitten surface than lower teeth. Scrape marks associated with the teeth of the lower arch therefore tend to be shorter and more distinct than those from the upper arch. This makes comparison between the simulation and the actual scrape easier and tends to produce a good result, especially when clear lower-arch scrape marks are present.

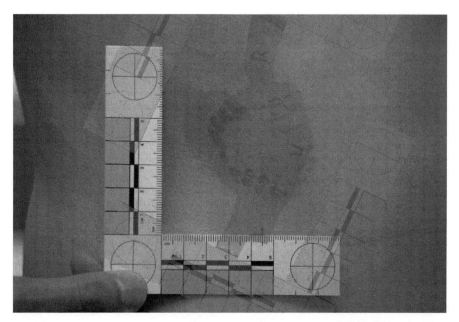

Fig. 8.31 Comparison between the simulated scrape from the upper dental cast and the scrape pattern on the injury layer. It can be challenging to simulate the direction of the actual scrape on the injury exactly. The opacity of the simulated scrape can be changed at will to make the visual comparison easier.

Dental cast

The position of the simulated injury is now used to correctly locate the dental cast image (Fig. 8.32).

Because of the geometry of the bite, the cast images need to be flipped horizontally to act as a 'rubber stamp', as shown in Fig. 8.33. The right side of each cast needs to match the right side of each simulated injury, scrape and the real injury. This step is potentially confusing, and is one reason why we mark the right and left sides of the casts, the simulated injuries and scrape simulations so we can ensure they match on the comparison images. If we fail to flip the casts, their images will not match the simulated injury and scrapes correctly.

Bite mark template (exemplar) and contour analysis

The bite mark template can now be added directly to the image (Fig. 8.34).

Comparison

With all the components for the comparison now in place, we can assess the degree to which a possible match may be present. Each template contour, the dental cast, the simulated injury and the simulated scrape are in separate layers on the canvas. Each can be managed individually, and we can turn them on or

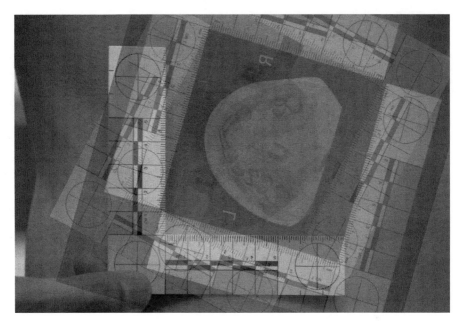

Fig. 8.32 The position of dental cast is determined by locating it with the impressions in the simulated injury.

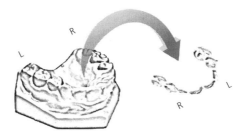

Fig. 8.33 The mages of upper dental casts must be flipped horizontally because the cast acts as a rubber stamp, leaving an inverted impression on the bitten surface. Flipped images of the lower teeth are not needed in this manner because they are oriented in the opposite direction during biting.

off at will or adjust their opacity as we desire. By using these tools to examine the match, it becomes relatively simple to determine if there are contradictions or unexplained aspects to the match. If no contradictory features are found, we can use the layers to explain the features seen in the injury.

Presenting bite mark evidence in court

Presenting bite mark evidence can be difficult because it is a technique replete with jargon and it can be very difficult for jurors to visualise. We use the tools we have described above to demonstrate the evidence visually.

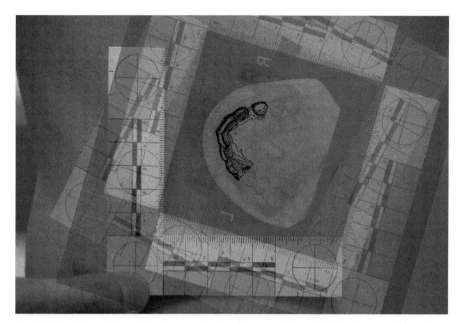

Fig. 8.34 The bite mark template contours for the relevant teeth are added to the composite image.

As previously stated, we have found it useful to have the photography and imaging performed by experts so they can present the processes in evidence, leaving the forensic odontologist free to concentrate on the interpretation of the bite marks. We have developed a template for this type of evidence presentation, which we use to build a suite of multi-layered images for court presentation (Fig. 8.35).

We place a panel on one side of the image window and colour it to help us recall what our finding was. We vary the colours we use from case to case so that barristers cannot anticipate what a colour means, but we always use colours that do not imply innocence or guilt (red or green). Yellow, blue and violet are useful. We use one colour to indicate we cannot exclude and another to indicate what we can exclude on the evidence we have. In complex cases with multiple suspects and possibly multiple injuries, it can be very difficult to remember exactly what the outcome of each comparison was and the colours provide a prompt. We do not volunteer to either prosecution or defence what the colours mean in any particular case.

Page [52] has suggested that visual presentation of evidence can lead to 'the contrast effect'. This happens when the images are shown repeatedly (if unintentionally) with a dental model or some other layer present. He states, 'the danger with the contrast effect is that forensic analysts, witnesses, and juries become susceptible to seeing associations that simply are not there, particularly on repeated exposure to evidence where associations may be borderline similar, but not necessarily representative of "matches"' [52, p. 71]. It may therefore be useful to ensure that the default state of the image on the template is with only the injury layer showing. This avoids inadvertently providing cues that could trigger the contrast effect.

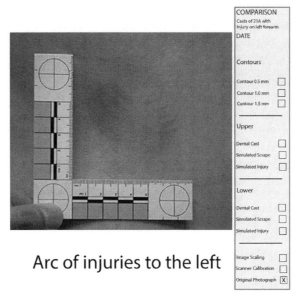

Arc of injuries to the left

Fig. 8.35 We use the template above for presenting the analysis and comparison in court. The labels in the Comparison box on the right represent the various layers we will demonstrate, and an 'x' appears in the check-box corresponding to the layer when it is shown, so observers always know what is occurring. In this case, the Comparison box is filled with one colour to connote 'can exclude' and a different colour to connote 'cannot exclude' as an aide memoire for complex cases where multiple injuries or suspects are involved. The numbers and text of the labels in the Comparison box vary according to the needs of the case. (Image courtesy of A Forrest and J Garner.)

Sources of potential distortion and error in bite mark cases

Distortions due to tissue properties and movement of a bitten body part

The human body is designed to move. When movement occurs, it may cause stretching or compression, changing the shape of a body part. For example, lifting an arm causes tissues over the breast, upper back and shoulder move and stretch. Bending or straightening a limb causes the tissues overlying muscles on either side of the moving joint to change their shape and length. Skin tension changes accordingly, and itself varies from one body part to another.

In 1971, DeVore [53] recognised that postural distortions were potentially a grave issue, citing a change in magnitude of a circular mark on the anterior thorax of up to 60% when the arm was flexed and raised.

Bush et al. [27] considered the issue of movement of body parts using cadavers. They showed that bite mark injuries generally stretched along the direction of movement, with extension usually leading to more distortion than flexion. Within the limits of their study, they noted that body movement tended to affect the entire injury or a part of it, but not single individual tooth marks alone. They also noted that every injury they made in their research looked different from every other one, and from the original dentition from which they created the bite marks.

Their results make for sobering reading, and emphasise to the thoughtful reader that perhaps we should think of bite mark comparisons as pattern-matching exercises rather than strictly metric ones.

Living victims might not recall specific details about their body position when they received an injury (or their memory may be incorrect). In deceased victims, we may have no way of knowing body positions at the time a bite mark injury occurred. It is therefore possible, even likely, that distortions that may not even be recognised might be present before we image the injuries. This is an example of an uncontrollable variable, and its extent can be considerable.

In summary, when we examine a bite mark, we need to consider both its location and the nature of the bitten tissue. In this context, we also need to recall our earlier discussion about distortion in injuries in relation to skin tension and Langer lines, and the mechanism of the biting action, which together will help us understand the factors in play. Performing an analysis of the dentition with the 3D contour overlays during the comparison phase is useful in helping to reconcile features of the injury with the distortions we observe.

While we need to undertake much further research on living subjects, it is clear that, based on cadaver studies, the potential effects of distortions due to tissue characteristics and the movements of body parts are one of the root causes of the caution needed when interpreting the outcomes of a bite mark comparison. They therefore place limitations on the strength of the conclusions that can be reached.

Distortions due to evidence collection

If we take impressions of a three-dimensional injury, some compression of the injury and surrounding tissues may occur during the application of the impression materials. If the final impression is not rigid, further uncontrolled distortions may occur, both as we lift the impression from the tissue surface and during casting.

Distortions due to poor imaging

In the authors' experience, this is one of the most common issues in bite mark analysis; we receive images of the alleged injuries, taken by a police officer without consulting the forensic odontologist, long after the date of photography. Consequently, photographic errors including parallax, perspective, lighting and low resolution may be inherent in the image. All too frequently, there is a lack of scale in the image, or it is in the wrong position and/or angle to the camera lens. Because the comparison between different items depends on accuracy of measurement, such images may be problematic at best, and often unsuitable for use in bite mark comparison.

Potentially controllable variables

- Distortions introduced by poor photography. Solution: correct the photographic technique (see: Imaging in bite mark cases).
- Distortions introduced by using a flatbed scanner to digitise a printed photograph. Solution: use a camera or measure and correct the distortion introduced by the calibration of the stepper motor.
- Distortions introduced by using a flatbed scanner to digitise a 3D dental cast. Solution: photograph the casts from a distance of 1.0–1.5 m with a lens of at least 100 mm focal length.
- Distortions introduced while taking impressions of an injury. Solution: use a 3D scanner with no tissue contact.
- Distortions introduced while taking impressions of teeth. Solution: allow the material to set thoroughly before removing it.
- Distortions to the injury caused by the forensic odontologist avulsing it. Solution: do not undertake avulsion of the injured tissue.

Potentially uncontrollable variables

- Distortions due to movement of a body part after injury: potentially significant and may not be obvious.
- Distortions due to the nature of the skin or tissue and the direction of bite: potentially significant but we can recognise the potential for this if we understand the tissue factors and tension lines involved.
- Distortions in bruising due to the travel of the bruise under the influence of gravity and repeated movement.
- Changes to the teeth of the assailant from dental treatment prior to the examination.
- Distortions caused by the victim pulling away from the assailant during the assault. This may result in multiple superimposed bite marks at the same site.
- Distortions due to the dynamics of the biting action and the tissue type involved.
- Other factors unique to the case (for example, biting through clothing).

Limitations of bite mark analysis and reporting the outcomes of bite mark comparisons

From the foregoing discussions, we know there are questions about the degree to which individual dentitions can be clearly distinguished at a level relevant to bite mark injuries and the accuracy with which the features of the dentition are transferred to bitten tissue.

Furthermore, it is apparent that many factors can affect the appearance of a bite mark injury. Some of these may be beyond our control, including those due to tissue properties, skin tension and body movements.

Others may already be present due to errors in photography when we receive images of injuries. We may create further such distortions ourselves during the process of imaging the various elements needed for analysis and comparison if care is not taken.

Some of these sources of distortion can be controlled, but much of the uncertainty (for example, the ability to differentiate among dentitions at the level relevant to bite marks) is inherent in human structure.

We must acknowledge these issues and reach conclusions that take account of them. This means that there are scientific limitations to the strength of the conclusions we can reach in any particular case.

On this basis, we reiterate that bite mark comparison is primarily a pattern-matching exercise. Metric analysis is important, but strict metric concordance between the injury and the comparison images does not always occur. This does not invalidate the possibility that we cannot exclude a suspect, but we do expect to see systematic distortions that can be explained in such cases.

We know that different individuals may have teeth that are difficult to distinguish at the bite mark level, so we cannot scientifically claim that only a particular suspect could have caused a bite mark except in extraordinary circumstances, where a specific and unique feature is present. However, we need to remember that we are examining from the pool of available suspects and conduct comparisons from this closed group, rather than with everyone in the world.

Because of these limitations, we recommend expressing the outcome of a bite mark comparison as one of only three options:

1 Can exclude the suspect.
2 Cannot exclude the suspect.
3 Cannot reach a conclusion because of insufficient detail to perform a valid comparison.

This differs from the recommendations of the American Board of Forensic Odontology [1, p. 117], which recommends five possible 'descriptions and terms' that relate a suspected bite to a bite mark:

1 The Biter.
2 The Probable Biter.
3 Not Excluded as the Biter.
4 Excluded as the Biter.
5 Inconclusive.

We believe that the nature of the evidence does not support conclusion 1, and we question the strength of conclusion 2 on the basis that we cannot quantify the chances of a match between a randomly selected dentition and a randomly selected bite mark injury.

The British Association for Forensic Odontology 'Guidelines for Good Practice in Bitemark Investigation and Analysis' (Updated August 2010) [54] include a category of 'Beyond reasonable doubt'. It is the authors' belief that this category is statistically unjustified and may be inappropriate in a legal setting as the use of that specific terminology may go to the ultimate issue at court.

The AuSFO Guidelines for the Conduct of Bitemark Analysis in Australia [3] suggest using the terms 'strong association', 'weak association', 'minimal association' and 'significant disparity' to describe the relationship between a bite mark and a dentition (p. 19).

Can we determine the age of the biter from the injury arch dimensions?

The 'ideal' bite mark results from contact with all six incisor and canine teeth of each arch, and sometimes features contact with additional teeth as well. In practice, this is not always the case, and we sometimes observe marks from partial arch contact. This may be due to the shape of the tissue bitten, to the bite being inflicted with the head turned to one side, or when anterior teeth are absent in the arch of the assailant. We are reluctant to consider comparison of 'partial' bite marks except in exceptional circumstances when the features of the injury and suspect teeth provide a compelling case.

The following discussion applies to all six incisor and canine teeth in an arch.

Arch widths in bite marks generally fall in a specific size range. The relevant work most commonly referred to in the forensic odontology literature is Barsley et al. [55], who found that the mean intercanine arch width of the adult (14–87 years) maxillary dental arch was 35.9 mm and the mandibular arch was 28.1 mm from a population of combined whites and blacks attending a dental school. They noted that blacks had a larger mean intercanine width in both arches than whites. The corresponding intercanine width measurements for white males were maxillary: 36.0 mm, mandibular: 27.8 mm, and for white females, maxillary: 34.4 mm and 26.8 mm. There were problems with this study, however. The intercanine width was measured from the labio-distal aspect of worn canines instead of from the centre of the worn area and, when canines were missing, the measurements were taken from the next most distal tooth unless no posterior tooth was present, in which case it was taken from the next most anterior tooth in the arch. The mean widths are therefore likely to have been over-estimated.

The more recent study by Thilander [56] examined a large sample of Swedish caucasoids with normal occlusion and tabulated intercanine widths of males and females aged 5, 7, 10, 13, 16 and 31 years [56, table 5 p. 114]. A question of interest is whether an adult or a child caused a particular bite mark injury. At first sight, this seems as though it should be an easy question to answer; after all, it seems to be intuitively obvious a child's mouth is smaller than an adult's is. In reality, the question is not so simple. Bernstein [20] maintains that bite marks arising from children are typically smaller than those of adults and feature smaller, rounded, bowlike arches. He holds that the mean maxillary intercanine width measures 28–29 mm from ages 3–6 years and the mean mandibular intercanine distance is approximately 22.6 mm. These mean measurements are broadly concordant with Thilander's results.

However, according to Thilander's data, a 5-year-old white female has a possible range of maxillary intercanine width from 25.6 mm to 32.3 mm, and a 31-year-old white female has a corresponding range of 29.1 mm to 34.5 mm. Clearly, there is a substantial overlap. The corresponding figures for a 5-year-old white male are 26.8 mm to 32.8 mm, and for a 31-year-old white male 30.1 mm to 37.5 mm. This illustrates the danger of relying on mean measurements when using arch width as a determinant of age.

While measurements of the arch widths in injuries are a good way of determining if a patterned injury is likely to be a bite mark when both canine teeth in an arch register in the pattern, we should be cautious about using this apparent intercanine width to estimate the age of an assailant. Other uncontrolled factors may affect the physical dimensions of the injury. If an injury features arch widths that fall substantially outside the ranges given by Thilander [56] without an adequate explanation, this would suggest that the injury is not a bite mark, and further investigation of the injury as a bite mark should cease at this point.

Can we visually age bite marks?

Visual aging of bite marks has been attempted in the past [57]. The current view is that attempts to age bruises (including bruised bite marks) on the basis of their appearance and colour is not sustainable and should not be undertaken [58, 59]. The best that we can offer might be an opinion as to whether the bruise is old or recent [59, 60]. This is supported by recommendation 2.4 of the AuSFO Guidelines for the Conduct of Bitemark Analysis in Australia [3, p. 8].

Swabbing for DNA

In some states in Australia, swabbing for DNA evidence is a police responsibility. In such jurisdictions, scientific police officers undertake it. As rules constantly change, you should verify if you are entitled to take swabs of injuries, or if you need a police officer to perform the task. In New Zealand, it is also a police responsibility and it is performed by Environmental Science and Research (ESR) scientists. We suggest always asking a police officer to take swabs on your behalf for probity. Police will take responsibility for any DNA samples from suspects.

Police should be advised to swab recent suspected bite mark injuries for potential assailant DNA as well. Forensic biology evidence is currently likely to be far stronger than evidence from any bite mark analysis. Concordance between the outcome of a DNA profile comparison with a suspect and the results of a bite mark comparison independently confirms the result of the comparison and provides valuable data about bite mark evidence. However, the forensic biologist needs to recognise that trace DNA from a third party can contaminate any surface or item, and appropriate caution is needed in cases involving trace samples. Mother may 'kiss it better' if the victim is a child.

The currently recommended swabbing technique is Sweet's Double Swabbing Technique [61], which is also recommended by the Australian Society of Forensic Odontology [3, pp. 2–3]. The protocol is simple:

Materials required
- Two sterile cotton swabs (no preservatives).
- 3 ml of sterile distilled water.
- Fitzpak swab box or similar (holds two swabs) (Cat No F06129; Invitro Sciences Inc., Welland, Ontario, Canada (invitro.sciences@sympatico.ca).

Method
DNA sample from the bite mark site
Dip the head of one sterile cotton swab in sterile, distilled water to moisten the tip thoroughly (~10 seconds). Roll the swab head over the saliva stain using circular motions and medium pressure to wash the stain from the surface. Place this swab in the evidence box to air-dry thoroughly (≥30 minutes).

Within 10 seconds of completing the first swab procedure, roll the tip of the other sterile cotton swab over the area of skin that is now wet from the first swab. Use circular motions with light pressure to absorb the moisture from the skin onto the swab head. Place this swab in the evidence box and let it air dry thoroughly (≥30 minutes).

Since both swabs come from the same site, we consider them to form a single exhibit. We therefore place them both in the same swab box, marking it with evidence continuity details and submitting it to the laboratory. We do not require control swabs from an adjacent site.

DNA reference sample from victim
A DNA reference sample is required from the recipient of the bite mark to allow interpretation of possible mixtures.

If the time to submission is longer than several hours, frozen storage (−20°C) and cold transportation (dry ice or frozen packs) are recommended.

Conclusion

Pretty and Sweet [62] report that increased caution is being exercised in the United States with regard to the use of bite mark evidence in the courts and this level of caution seems to be gaining general support. The report of the National Research Council in the US [63] noted that bite mark evidence is introduced into criminal trials without any meaningful scientific validation. Further, it is true that DNA evidence has exonerated a number of individuals convicted largely on evidence given by a bite mark 'expert' [64], and this fact alone should mandate great caution in the way in which bite mark evidence is examined and in the strength of the conclusions reached. However, this level of caution does not yet seem to extend to the categories that the American Board of Forensic Odontology suggests should be used to report the conclusions of bite mark comparison [1]. The question has arisen, is bite mark comparison junk science? Mary Bush [65] discusses this issue in a US context and it makes for thoughtful reading.

The authors believe that bite mark evidence does have a place in the courtroom provided we perform the analysis and comparison carefully, using defensible techniques. We maintain that every step we perform in the comparison should be reproducible by an independent forensic odontologist and that this level of review is mandatory before we submit a conclusion. We cannot sanction the use of any arbitrary process that can introduce error, so it is vital to carefully conceive and meticulously execute our techniques.

The existence of uncontrolled (and uncontrollable) variables places scientific limits on the level of certainty that can be reached, and these variables and consequent sources of uncertainty should be reported with our conclusions.

Finally, we believe that the most conservative opinion is almost always the correct choice, as this helps to avoid the weight assigned to the opinion in evidence being greater than is scientifically justified.

In summary:

- Bite mark evidence is usually circumstantial evidence in a case, unless the charge is one of biting.
- Case selection is a most important step in any case; examination of the injury is required to determine if it matches the class characteristics of bite marks, and if there is sufficient detail of individual features to support a comparison.
- Imaging procedures that correctly represent the injury and the other comparison materials such as dental casts without introducing new distortions are a requirement so that a valid comparison process can be undertaken.
- A clear and transparent comparison process that makes use of all the available information is also useful as a means of presenting the evidence in court in a way that the legal personnel and a jury can understand.
- Our conclusions should be in accordance with the scientific limitations of the technique and should not overstate the strength of the evidence.
- In our experience, whenever we need to express an opinion, the most conservative possible opinion is almost always the correct one.

Future directions

Further research on almost all aspects of bite mark analysis and comparison is needed, particularly in terms of determining the degree to which different dentitions can be distinguished, understanding the processes that lead to distortions of the injuries, determining error rates, and reaching an agreed methodology for conducting the process. The process must undergo proper scientific validation and, until then, we need to exercise due caution in our casework.

Until a standard methodology is developed, there can be no comparison between the results of different experts undertaking bite mark comparison, and therefore no determination of the strengths, weaknesses or error rates of the process. We should select this methodology to be defensible and not to introduce any avoidable further error.

Independent peer review of all comparison cases before we report them is a key factor in being able to ensure that opinions are actually valid and fairly represent analysis and comparison of the case material. The processes used in the bite mark analysis and comparison must be sufficiently transparent and well documented that independent peer review is possible. In our view, this should become a standard part of the examination.

These measures will address many of the current deficiencies in bite mark evidence, and will go a long way to ensuring a firm foundation for its future.

References

1 American Board of Forensic Odontology (2013) ABFO Diplomates Reference Manual Available from http://www.abfo.org/resources/abfo–manual/. Accessed July 2014.
2 Senn DR. (2011) History of bitemark evidence. In: Dorion RB (ed.) *Bitemark Evidence – A Color Atlas and Text*, 2nd edn, CRC Press, Boca Raton, London, pp. 4–22.
3 AuSFO (2013) Australian Society of Forensic Odontology: Guidelines for the conduct of bitemark analysis in Australia in (AuSFO, ed.) Australia.
4 Pretty IA, Sweet D. (2000) Anatomical location of bitemarks and associated findings in 101 cases from the United States. *Journal of Forensic Sciences* **45**, 812–814.
5 McCullough DC. (1983) Rapid comparison of bite marks by xerography. *American Journal of Forensic Medicine and Pathology* **4**, 355–358.
6 Bernitz H, Kloppers BA. (2002) Comparison microscope identification of a cheese bitemark: a case report. *Journal of Forensic Odontostomatology* **20**, 13–16.
7 Sweet D, Hildebrand D. (1999) Saliva from cheese bite yields DNA profile of burglar: a case report. *International Journal of Legal Medicine* **112**, 201–203.
8 McKenna CJ, Haron MI, Brown KA et al. (2000) Bitemarks in chocolate: a case report. *Journal of Forensic Odontostomatology* **18**, 10–14.
9 Kerr N. (1977) Apple bite mark identification of a suspect. *International Journal of Forensic Dentistry* **4**, 20–23.
10 Simon A, Jordan H, Pforte K. (1974) Successful indentification of a bite mark in a sandwich. *International Journal of Forensic Dentistry* **2**, 17–21.
11 Nambiar P, Carson G, Taylor JA et al. (2001) Identification from a bitemark in a wad of chewing gum. *Journal of Forensic Odontostomatology* **19**, 5–8.
12 Pretty IA. (2007) Development and validation of a human bitemark severity and significance scale. *Journal of Forensic Sciences* **52**, 687–691.
13 Souviron RR. (2012) A bitemark classification that makes sense. Paper presented at the American Academy of Forensic Sciences, Atlanta, GA, USA.
14 Dorion R. (2014) A proposed human bitemark classification. Paper presented at the meeting of the American Academy of Forensic Sciences, Seattle, WA, USA.

15 Gold MH, Roenigk HH, Smith ES et al. (1989) Human bite marks. Differential diagnosis. *Clinical Pediatrics* **28** 329–331.

16 Grey TC. (1989) Defibrillator injury suggesting bite mark. *American Journal of Forensic Medicine and Pathology* **10**, 144–145.

17 Goodbody RA, Turner CH, Turner JL. (1976) The differentiation of toothed marks: report of a case of special forensic interest. *Medicine, Science, and The Law* **16**, 44–48.

18 Kasper KA. (2011) A new trend for familiar patterned Injury? ASFO Case of the Month. Available from http://www.asfo.org/case–of–the–month–archives/. Accessed April 2014.

19 Sperber ND. (1990) Lingual markings of anterior teeth as seen in human bite marks. *Journal of Forensic Sciences* **35**, 838–844.

20 Bernstein ML. (2011) The nature of bitemarks. In: Dorion RB (ed.) *Bitemark Evidence – A Color Atlas and Text*, 2nd edn, CRC Press, Boca Raton, London, pp. 53–65.

21 Hermsen KP. (2014) A follow–up study of bitemark characteristics in live human subjects. Paper presented at the meeting of the American Academy of Forensic Sciences, Seattle, WA, USA.

22 Rawson RD, Ommen RK, Kinard G et al. (1984) Statistical evidence for the individuality of the human dentition. *Journal of Forensic Sciences.* **29**, 245–253.

23 Kieser JA, Bernal V, Waddell JN et al. (2007) The uniqueness of the human anterior dentition: a geometric morphometric analysis. *Journal of Forensic Sciences* **52**, 671–677.

24 Bush MA, Bush PJ, Sheets HD. (2011) Statistical evidence for the similarity of the human dentition. *Journal of Forensic Sciences* **56**, 118–123.

25 Thompson IO, Phillips VM. (1994) A bitemark case with a twist. *Journal of Forensic Odontostomatology* **12**, 37–40.

26 Miller RG, Bush PJ, Dorion RB et al. (2009) Uniqueness of the dentition as impressed in human skin: a cadaver model. *Journal of Forensic Sciences* **54**, 909–914.

27 Bush MA, Miller RG, Bush PJ et al. (2009) Biomechanical factors in human dermal bitemarks in a cadaver model. *Journal of Forensic Sciences* **54**, 167–176.

28 Langer K. (1978) On the anatomy and physiology of the skin. I. The cleavability of the cutis. *British Journal of Plastic Surgery* **31**, 3–8.

29 Langer K. (1978) On the anatomy and physiology of the skin: II. Skin tension by Professor K Langer. *British Journal of Plastic Surgery* **31**, 8–13.

30 Bowers CM, Johansen RJ. (2003) *Digital Analysis of Bite Mark Evidence using Adobe Photoshop.* Forensic Imaging Services, Santa Barbara.

31 David TJ, Sobel MN. (1994) Recapturing a five-month-old bite mark by means of reflective ultraviolet photography. *Journal of Forensic Sciences* **39**, 1560–1567.

32 Wright FD. (1998) Photography in bite mark and patterned injury documentation—Part 2: A case study. *Journal of Forensic Sciences* **43**, 881–887.

33 West M, Barsley RE, Frair J et al. (1992) Ultraviolet radiation and its role in wound pattern documentation. *Journal of Forensic Sciences* **37**, 1466–1479.

34 Golden GS. (1994) Use of alternative light source illumination in bite mark photography. *Journal of Forensic Sciences* **39**, 815–823.

35 Golden GS, Wright F. (2011) Photography. In: Dorion RBJE (ed.) *Bitemark Evidence – A Color Atlas and Text*, 2nd edn, CRC Press, Boca Raton, London, pp. 74–102.

36 Page M, Taylor J, Blenkin M. (2012) Context effects and observer bias–implications for forensic odontology *Journal of Forensic Sciences* **57**, 108–112.

37 McNamee AH, Sweet D. (2003) Adherence of forensic odontologists to the ABFO guidelines for victim evidence collection. *Journal of Forensic Sciences* **48**, 382–385.

38 Dorion R. (2011) Tissue specimens. In: Dorion RBJE (ed.) *Bitemark Evidence – A Color Atlas and Text*, 2nd edn, CRC Press, Boca Raton, London, pp. 167–194.

39 Morgen H. (1943) Zur Frage der Sicherung und Auswertung krimineller Bisspuren. *Zahnärztl Rdsch* **52**, 791–796.

40 Gustavson G. (1966) *Forensic Odontology*, Staples Press, London.

41 Ström F. (1963) Investigations of bite–marks. *Journal of Dental Research* **42**, 312–316.

42 Senn DR, Souviron R. (2010) Bitemarks. In: Senn DR & Stimson PG (eds) *Forensic Dentistry*, 2nd edn, CRC Press, Boca Raton, pp. 306–368.

43 Page M, Taylor J, Blenkin M. (2012) Reality bites – a ten-year retrospective analysis of bitemark casework in Australia. *Forensic Science International* **216**, 82–87.

44 Luntz L, Luntz P. (1973) *Handbook for Dental Identification*. JB Lippincott, Philadelphia and Toronto.

45 Sweet D, Bowers CM. (1998) Accuracy of bite mark overlays: a comparison of five common methods to produce exemplars from a suspect's dentition. *Journal of Forensic Sciences* **43**, 362–367.

46 Dailey JC. (1991) A practical technique for the fabrication of transparent bite mark overlays. *Journal of Forensic Sciences* **36**, 565–570.

47 Khatri M, Daniel MJ, Srinivasan SV. (2013) A comparative study of overlay generation methods in bite mark analysis. *Journal of Forensic Dental Sciences* **5**, 16–21.

48 Naru AS, Dykes E. (1996) The use of a digital imaging technique to aid bite mark analysis. *Science and Justice* **36**, 47–50.

49 McNamee AH, Sweet D, Pretty I. (2005) A comparative reliability analysis of computer–generated bitemark overlays. *Journal of Forensic Sciences* **50**, 400–405.

50 Metcalf RD. (2008) Yet another method for marking incisal edges of teeth for bitemark analysis *Journal of Forensic Sciences* **53**, 426–429.

51 Wood RE, Miller PA, Blenkinsop BR. (1994) Image editing and computer assisted bitemark analysis: a case report. *Journal of Forensic Odontostomatology* **12**, 30–36.

52 Page M. (2013) *Professional Forensic Evidence Practice*. In: Bowers CM (ed.) *Forensic Testimony: Science, Law and Expert Evidence*, 1st edn, Academic Press, San Diego, CA. pp. 57–77.

53 DeVore DT. (1971) Bite marks for identification? A preliminary report. *Medicine, Science, and The Law* **11**, 144–145.

54 British Association for Forensic Odontology (2010) Guidelines for Good Practice in Bite Mark Investigation and Analysis.

55 Barsley RE, Lancaster DM. (1987) Measurement of arch widths in a human population: relation of anticipated bite marks. *Journal of Forensic Sciences* **32**, 975–982.

56 Thilander B. (2009) Dentoalveolar development in subjects with normal occlusion. A longitudinal study between the ages of 5 and 31 years. *European Journal of Orthodontics* **31**, 109–120.

57 Dailey JC, Bowers CM. (1997) Aging of bitemarks: a literature review. *Journal of Forensic Sciences* **42**, 792–795.

58 Maguire S, Mann MK, Sibert J et al. (2005) Can you age bruises accurately in children? A systematic review *Archives of Disease in Childhood* **90**, 187–189.

59 Nash KR, Sheridan DJ. (2009) Can one accurately date a bruise? State of the science *Journal of Forensic Nursing* **5**, 31–37.

60 Langlois NE, Gresham GA. (1991) The ageing of bruises: a review and study of the colour changes with time. *Forensic Science International* **50**, 227–238.

61 Sweet D, Lorente M, Lorente JA et al. (1997) An improved method to recover saliva from human skin: the double swab technique. *Journal of Forensic Sciences* **42**, 320–322.

62 Pretty IA, Sweet D. (2010) A paradigm shift in the analysis of bitemarks. *Forensic Science International* **201**, 38–44.

63 National Research Council (2009) *Strengthening Forensic Science in the United States: A Path Forward*. National Academies Press, Washington.

64 Innocence Project. Wrongful Convictions Involving Unvalidated or Improper Forensic Science that Were Later Overturned through DNA Testing. http://www.innocenceproject.org/docs/DNA_Exonerations_Forensic_Science.pdf. Accessed August 2014.

65 Bush MA. (2011) Forensic dentistry and bitemark analysis: sound science or junk science? *Journal of the American Dental Association* **142**, 997–999.

CHAPTER 9

Forensic odontology in disaster victim identification

Hugh G. Trengrove

New Zealand Society of Forensic Odontology, New Zealand

Disasters and disaster planning

A disaster can be defined as an unexpected natural or manmade event that may result in personal injury, mass fatalities, property and infrastructural damage. These events can be a result of natural events such as earthquakes and typhoons, accidents (aircraft, rail, maritime, industrial), terrorist activities and conflicts. Disasters that include multiple fatalities can be classified as being 'closed', 'open', or a combination of both. A 'closed' disaster is a disaster where a list of probable victims is readily available, for example an aircraft crash where a flight manifest exists. An open disaster is a disaster where there is no readily available list of possible victims. An example of an open disaster is a shopping complex building collapse where the number and the identity of shoppers is unknown. Some disasters may be both open and closed, for example, an aircraft crash into a suburban area of a city where the resultant fatalities include those on the aircraft and people on the ground.

Given the very significant impact such disaster events have on society there is increasing awareness of the need for authorities and communities to make plans for responding to a disaster. The disaster response plan, the details of which may vary from scenario to scenario and from nation to nation, forms the basis of the emergency or disaster response framework. Disaster planning typically includes consideration of four principal phases: mitigation, preparedness, response and recovery.

The mitigation and preparedness phases focus on actions and activities aimed at reducing the adverse effects of an anticipated disaster and on optimising the effectiveness of the planned response to the disaster. The strengthening of buildings to resist earthquake damage and the prepositioning of disaster response equipment are examples of mitigation and preparedness undertakings.

Forensic Odontology: Principles and Practice, First Edition. Edited by Jane A. Taylor and Jules A. Kieser.
© 2016 John Wiley & Sons, Ltd. Published 2016 by John Wiley & Sons, Ltd.

The response phase to a disaster is centred on the actions taken as an immediate consequence of the disaster with a specific focus on rescue (saving and preventing further injury to the survivors of the incident) and evacuation, on protecting critical infrastructure, and on the retrieval of deceased individuals.

The recovery phase deals with the restoration of infrastructure and normalisation of operations and services. An important element of the recovery phase is taking the lessons-learned during the operational response to the disaster and incorporating these as amendments or additions in the disaster response plans.

Most nations have local or regional disaster plans and dedicated specialist resources to manage small to medium sized disasters and multiple fatality events. As the scale of the disaster increases and casualty numbers rise, more resources are needed, often requiring wider national and international support. The International Criminal Police Organization (INTERPOL, through the DVI Unit, part of the Operational Police Support Directorate), has a coordination and support role in multiple fatality disasters that have international ramifications, noting that the national authority where the disaster occurred retains jurisdiction over the actual disaster site [1]. The usual cultural and legal processes following death cannot be completed until formal identification of the deceased has been established. The timely and accurate identification of the deceased is essential for family, legal and societal reasons. Delays in the identification process results in emotional hardship for relatives and for communities. Therefore, the early recovery and identification of deceased individuals is a fundamental element in any disaster response.

Disaster victim identification

Disaster Victim Identification (DVI) refers to a respectful, systematic and orderly process undertaken in response to a multiple fatality incident with the aim of scientifically identifying the deceased casualties of the incident so that they can be returned to their relatives. The process involves matching post-mortem information from a deceased individual with ante-mortem information of a missing person and through this identifying the deceased individual. A DVI operation is typically part of the 'response phase' to a multiple fatality event and usually becomes fully operational at the conclusion of the rescue and evacuation part of the operation. DVI activities are initiated when it is clear that the disaster has resulted in multiple casualties, and commences with body recovery and concludes – following the return of the identified deceased individuals to their relatives – with a formal review (debrief) of the DVI operation. The threshold for activation of a DVI operation varies from jurisdiction to jurisdiction and is influenced by the nature and complexity of the disaster. A DVI response may be initiated when there are large numbers of deceased individuals or in situations with smaller numbers of deceased, but where the nature of the incident results in a complicated identification process, such as when there has been marked fragmentation or commingling of human remains. A DVI response may also be initiated when the number of deceased exceeds the resource capacity of the authority dealing with the incident. The prompt, definitive identification of the deceased individuals is the primary aim of a DVI operation.

DVI is a multi-disciplinary activity that relies on a range of comparative scientific and non-scientific methods to identify human remains. The DVI disciplines include those referred to as primary identifiers; forensic odontology, skin friction ridge analysis (typically finger, palm and sole-prints), and deoxyribonucleic acid (DNA) [2]. Secondary identifiers such as visual identification, descriptions of personal property, evidence of medical procedures, anthropological information, and circumstantial evidence also contribute to the identification process.

The usual requirement for corroborative evidence regarding identity requires the use of multiple methods of identification (information from multiple disciplines) when at all possible. The relative contribution to the identification process from each discipline in a DVI operation is dependent on the nature of the disaster, the state of the human remains and the requirements of the investigative authority (coroner). Irrespective of the methods of identification utilised, the authority ascribing the identity must be convinced that the data supporting the identification meets the required burden of proof.

DVI planning and organisation

It is essential that a DVI plan is developed as part of the larger overall disaster response plan and this preparation must be completed well in advance of a multiple fatality incident. The DVI plan provides an organisational framework around which a DVI response can be launched. The plan should be based on international best practice standards and outline the resources (personnel specialist/technical expertise, equipment, consumables, infrastructure) and procedures to be utilised following a disaster so that delays in responding to a multiple fatality incident are minimised. Early planning improves the likelihood that optimal outcomes are achieved from the DVI operation. A number of DVI planning tools and guides exist to assist with DVI preparation including those relating to: the US Department of Health and Human Services (Disaster Mortuary Operational Response Team DMORT), Pan American Health Organisation/World Health Organisation and INTERPOL. The INTERPOL DVI guide that was first published in 1984 and which has subsequently been revised in 1997 and 2009 is commonly used as the basis for DVI planning in Australasia [2]. This guide, for use by INTERPOL member states, provides information and recommendations on international standards and consistency when facilitating or participating in multinational DVI operations and is available on the INTERPOL website. The INTERPOL DVI Guide provides the key information from which a detailed DVI plan can be developed and contextualised for the local environment and disaster risks.

Multiple fatality disasters have many similarities, however no two are the same so a DVI plan must be sufficiently flexible to allow adaptation to the circumstances of a particular disaster (Figs. 9.1–9.3).

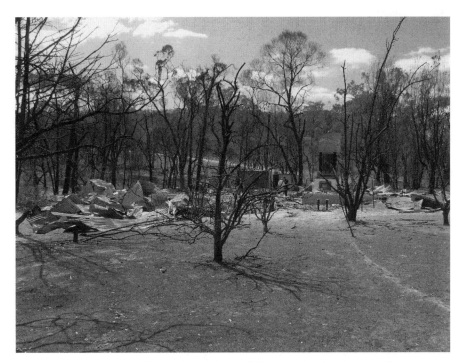

Fig. 9.1 House destroyed in the Black Saturday bushfires (2009), Victoria, Australia.

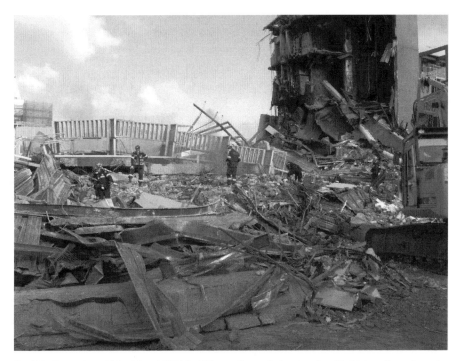

Fig. 9.2 Canterbury Television (CTV) building collapse following the Christchurch earthquake (2011). (*See insert for colour representation of the figure.*)

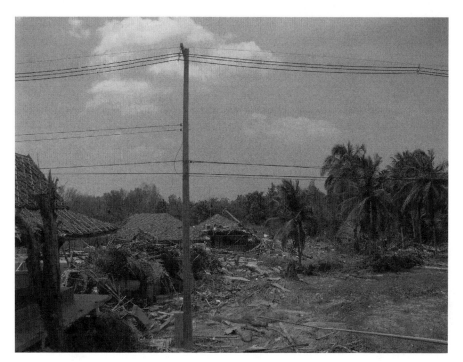

Fig. 9.3 Damage following the Boxing Day, Asian tsunami (2004).

Consideration needs to be given to the type and scale of the event, the resources available and the societal and cultural expectations of those affected by the disaster. In some situations severe constraints on DVI operations may exist because of the scale of the event or because of cultural and religious beliefs and customs of the affected communities. To ensure DVI plans are robust, disaster scenario planning (e.g. scenarios based on different disasters – earthquake, aircraft crash etc.) and 'on-the-ground' and 'desktop' exercises are useful. All DVI plans should be regularly reviewed and should be practised.

A DVI response involves a range of organisations and agencies working together in an integrated and coordinated way, so it is important that planning includes consideration of the functional responsibilities of those involved, the command and control relationships between the various groups and how communication and coordination will be managed between these groups.

DVI and forensic odontology

Forensic odontology has been utilised in the identification of deceased individuals in multiple fatality events for over 100 years, with the first reported use in Paris following a fire in the Bazaar de la Charité in 1897 [3]. Since then, forensic odontology has made a contribution in many major disasters with the role and relative contribution increasing significantly over the past 40 years. Forensic odontology has contributed to the identification of the deceased in many of the major international DVI operations involving Westernised countries with published accounts relating to many of these.

- *Airline disasters:* Air New Zealand Flight TE901 – Erebus disaster (1979), America Airlines Flight 191 (1979), Pan American Flight 759 (1982), Arrow Airways Flight 950 – Gander disaster (1985), Air India Flight AL182 (1985), British Airtours Flight 28M (1985), South African Airways Flight SA 295 – Helderberg disasater (1987), Air Inter Flight 5148 (1992), Korean Airlines Flight 801 (1997), Comair Flight 5191 (2006), Air France Flight 447 (2009), Colgan Air flight 3407 (2009).
- *Maritime disasters*: Townsend Thoresen sea ferry – Herald of Free Enterprise (1987), USS Iowa disaster (1989), Scandinavian Star ferry disaster (1990).
- *Fires*: Bradford City football ground fire (1985), North Sea Occidental petroleum oil rig disaster – Piper Alpha oil rig (1988), Bailen (Spain) bus accident – Aquitaine train crash (1997).
- *Terrorist activities*: Beirut Marine Headquarters bombing (1983), Pan American Flight 103 – Lockerbie bombing (1988), Oklahoma Federal Building bombing (1995), World Trade Centre – 9/11 attack (2001), Bali bombings (2005), London bombings (2005).
- *Natural disasters*: South Australia 'Ash Wednesday' bushfires (1983), Boxing Day Asian tsunami (2004), Black Saturday bushfires (2009), Christchurch earthquake (2011).

Forensic odontology has assumed an increased importance in DVI over this time for a number of reasons. Improvements in dental health and advances in dental restorative techniques in Westernised countries means that teeth are being retained for longer due to often having received more restorative interventions. This means that deceased individuals are more likely to have teeth and a history of dental intervention. Secondarily to this, forensic odontology DVI protocols and procedures have been refined and formalised, national and international forensic networks have been established and information and lessons learned shared. Forensic odontology continues to deliver a significant contribution to the identification of the deceased from multiple fatality events, and as a result of this forensic odontology is accepted as a key element of any DVI response.

Forensic odontology DVI planning

A forensic odontology DVI response plan should be developed as part of the overall DVI plan with its principal focus on the personnel and equipment requirements, and standardisation of processes and procedures. Typically a forensic odontology DVI response plan is organised around geographic regions and usually relies on volunteer dentists who have training and experience in forensic odontology. The forensic odontology response plan forms the basis for the actual operational planning that is required when an incident occurs. The response plan must be flexible and scaleable to allow adjustment and amendment when the specifics of the disaster are known. The plan should be regularly reviewed and exercised.

Personnel

The personnel component of the forensic odontology DVI plan underpins the entire plan and impacts directly on the capacity to respond to an incident. The development of a forensic odontology personnel deployment plan should be completed as an early response to a DVI incident. The nature and scale of the DVI incident informs the personnel deployment plan, particularly with regard to the role of forensic odontology (e.g. what forensic odontology involvement is required in each DVI phase) and the anticipated duration of the operation.

Personnel planning must consider the workload and work schedule to ensure that the operation is sustainable and the health and welfare of deployed personnel are not unnecessarily compromised. There is a common tendency for personnel to wish to work extended hours in a desire to get the casualties of the disaster identified and repatriated to their families. Working hours must be carefully balanced to ensure that the welfare of the personnel is guarded, that the operation remains sustainable over the required duration and that the outcomes are not compromised. Personnel planning should include consideration of managing working hours noting that working extended hours and shift-work may increase the risk of mistakes and accidents occurring. Working hours and deployment rotation length have a direct bearing on critical incident stress so it is essential that rest and stand-down periods are factored into work rosters and personnel rotation plans.

Personnel selection

DVI operations are potentially dangerous and are typically more technically challenging and 'environmentally' difficult than single identifications, and accordingly can be extremely physically and emotionally demanding. To optimise the likelihood of good outcomes and to mitigate potential long-term adverse effects on the individuals deployed, care must be taken when selecting personnel for deployment. Personnel should be selected based on their individual and collective training and experience (particularly in the 'odontology team' environment), and with regard to the specific requirements of the particular DVI operation. In addition to training in forensic odontology, personnel require training to facilitate their safe and effective work in the environment in which they are operating. The deployment of untrained and inexperienced personnel early in a DVI operation creates additional supervisory and support workload in what is typically an already resource-constrained environment, and so this should be avoided. Notwithstanding this, once the DVI infrastructure and processes are established, and provided there are sufficient experienced forensic odontologists available to provide support and mentoring, the deployment of less-experienced odontologists to learn and gain experience is a valid consideration.

To ensure a timely response to a DVI incident, a detailed and accurate list of forensic odontology personnel (contacts list) who have the training and experience, and who are able and interested in contributing to a DVI operation, is required in advance of an incident occurring. The contacts list information should include:

- Information on how to contact the forensic odontologists and auxiliary personnel, noting that a disaster may disrupt communication networks so it is important that all methods of contact are known. A key element of this is the agreed procedures regarding communication between the individual(s) planning the DVI operation (usually the forensic odontology coordinator) and those on the list: that is, who should contact who, when and how.

  Information regarding the availability of personnel to assist with a DVI operation is essential in ensuring an organised, efficient and timely forensic odontology contribution to a DVI operation. The required information includes: the individual's availability for a short-notice deployment and for the time they are prepared to be deployed, their availability for deployment out of their region, and for multiple rotations to the operation.

  Given that an individual's availability is subject to change, it is often helpful for those able to assist with a DVI incident to proactively contact the 'forensic odontology coordinator' with information regarding changes in their availability.

- Details regarding each individual's forensic and DVI training and experience, including specific information regarding experience in each DVI phase, is useful, as well as information regarding any leadership role the practitioner may have taken. This information is essential for personnel planning and also as part of the credentialing and quality assurance process.

- Information regarding the fitness and health of each individual is useful as these aspects may impact on the deployment, location, duration and tasking.

- Personal readiness. Having an understanding of the individual's family and employment situation is important as both have an influence on the psychosocial welfare of the individual whilst deployed. Good family support networks combined with backing from employers for the deployment assist in mitigating the social, emotional and psychological impacts of such deployments.

Collectively, this information allows for the optimal coordination of personnel resources to each phase of the DVI operation – the right person, deployed in the right role, at the right time for the right duration.

Other personnel considerations

Local personnel resources

It is usual for the forensic odontology personnel living in the area in which the incident occurred to form the basis of the initial or immediate local DVI response plan. They can usually be deployed with minimal delay and have the best understanding of the local DVI plan, resources and issues. However, it must be remembered that, unlike personnel who have deployed to a disaster scene from an unaffected area, local people, in addition to the DVI activities, have normal daily routines to manage. They may also have been personally affected by the disaster through loss or damage of property, injury or death of relatives, friends or colleagues, and may have experienced disruption in normal work and home routines. As such they are under increased risk of work overload and the development of acute and chronic critical incident stress. Managing the desire of local forensic odontologists and associated staff to assist with a DVI whilst protecting their emotional and welfare interests can be a challenging balance. Depending on the size and nature of the incident, to reduce the workload burden on the local personnel, consideration should always be given to deployment of personnel from out of the area to supplement local resources.

Regional and national personnel resources

When the scale of an incident exceeds the personnel resources available locally, additional assistance may be sourced through regional, national and international networks and arrangements. DVI planning must include consideration of how these additional staff will be integrated into the DVI response, particularly those personnel who come from other nations.

International personnel

Given the accessibility of international travel it is highly likely that a DVI incident will include deceased from other countries. The country in which the disaster has occurred has jurisdiction over the incident and is principally responsible for dealing with the victims of the incident; however, it is common practice for nations who have lost citizens in a disaster to be represented during the DVI. The representation will frequently include specialities such as forensic odontology. Some of the international DVI teams will arrive as a result of intergovernmental discussion and agreement and others will arrive unannounced. INTERPOL, at the request of the host country, will often facilitate DVI support through member states [2].

DVI response plans should consider the potential role of practitioners coming from other nations and how these individuals or teams can be usefully employed within the DVI response. Many countries have governmental bodies that regulate dentistry and that authorise practice in that nation. If this is the situation, then it is useful that the host nation has a process for the prompt registration of international practitioners in place well in advance of a disaster event. As a general principle, personnel from nations that have lost citizens in the disaster who are deployed to assist with the DVI should, whenever possible, be integrated into the DVI response. Noting that it is essential that the practice of overseas personnel meets professional and ethical standards and there is an expectation that these personnel will conform with the processes and procedures of the host nation.

Ethics and professionalism

High professional and ethical standards are expected of personnel deployed in support of DVI operations. Work practices must be of the highest standard and be conducted in compliance with the processes and protocols of the operation. It is important that practitioners only work in areas in which they have competence and in which they have operational authorisation. Practitioners must be mindful of the requirement to act ethically and responsibly with regard to information management and in particular with regard to unauthorised removal of victim and operational information and photographs. Personnel must comply with the specific operational rules regarding personal photographs and the disclosure of privileged information to any party. There is an expectation that practitioners will recognise and respect the cultural beliefs and practices of all participants in a DVI including those of the deceased who must be treated with dignity and respect.

Equipment and consumables

The equipment and consumable component of the forensic odontology DVI plan is usually focused exclusively on the odontology specific requirements (e.g. specialist items) for each operational DVI phase and requires the development of detailed lists. Other more general items, for example gurneys, waste containers, computer equipment, tables and so on are usually the responsibility of the DVI logistic planners who should be made aware of the general forensic odontology equipment and support requirements for each DVI phase.

An odontology 'specific' list of equipment and consumables details the items that are required and a scenario-based estimate made of the quality required of each item. If the equipment and consumables are not to be assembled and stockpiled in preparation for an incident, the plan should clearly detail from where these items will be sourced and arrangements as to how they will be accessed and assembled. An outline of forensic odontology equipment requirements is included in the sections discussing each DVI phase.

Procedural guidance

It is essential that the forensic odontology DVI response plan includes detailed procedural guidance documentation. Robust, integrated processes and procedures are essential in DVI operations to ensure optimal results are achieved and errors and omissions minimised. To ensure consistency these processes must be known and adhered to by all involved. The use of 'Standardised Operating Procedures' (SOPs) is a common method for detailing process requirements. The SOPs should be reviewed and, when necessary, amended during the operation to reflect the specific contingencies of the operation and to reflect any lessons learned. They should also be reviewed and amended following the final operational debrief.

Training and rehearsal

Training and rehearsal in DVI operations are essential elements in pre-disaster DVI planning, and the effectiveness of the training and practice has a direct influence on what is achieved during the operation. Training must not be solely focused on technical skills, but must also involve integrated team practice within a disaster scenario activity. Training allows the development, trial and refinement

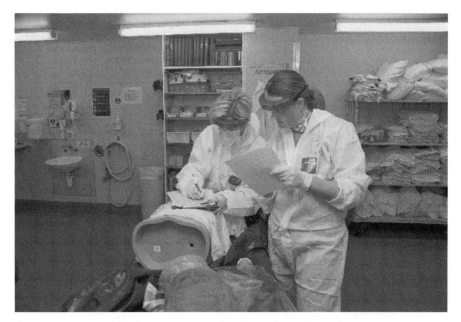

Fig. 9.4 Training provides the opportunity to familiarise themselves with DVI processes.

of processes and procedures in a controlled environment with participants taking an active role and therefore ownership of these. This ownership facilitates the implementation of, and compliance with, these processes in the operational setting. Training heightens the awareness of the physical and stress implications of DVI operations and may assist personnel in understanding and potentially managing the psychological and emotional effects of DVI work. In addition, when undertaken in a team environment, training facilitates the development of a team support network that can be useful for reducing the psychological and emotional impacts of the DVI work (Fig. 9.4).

DVI operations

The DVI process is centred on collecting ante-mortem and post-mortem data in a comprehensive and orderly manner that enables subsequent comparative and reconciliation processes. To facilitate this INTERPOL separates the DVI process into four operational phases (Phase 1: Scene, Phase 2: Ante-mortem, Phase 3: Post-mortem, Phase 4: Reconciliation) and one 'administrative' phase (Phase 5: Debrief). The DVI operation commences with the Scene phase and concludes with the Debrief phase. Each operational phase progresses independently of the other phases and, although the deceased's remains 'progress' through the phases sequentially, the operational phases frequently occur concurrently. A 'debrief' element is embedded into and is integral to each phase, with phase 5: Debrief being the final consolidating debrief. Forensic odontology has a role in all phases of a DVI operation.

DVI documentation

To ensure consistency in ante-mortem and post-mortem data collection, INTERPOL adopted a set of DVI forms that were developed in 1968, and these forms have subsequently been revised following practical application in DVI situations into what is now generally accepted as an international DVI form. These DVI forms provide a structured and detailed template against which data is collected. The INTERPOL DVI ante-mortem forms are yellow in colour and post-mortem forms are pink, with each set of forms being divided into various sections based on the specific information being sought. The INTERPOL DVI forms are available for download from the INTERPOL website.

Health and safety during DVI operations

Protecting the health and safety of personnel deployed in support of a DVI operation underpins the entire operation. Deployed personnel must be trained, equipped and resourced in a manner that mitigates the health and safety risks in the deployment area. There is usually complex interplay between multiple hazards in the environment and they need to be identified, removed, minimised or isolated.

Biological hazards

Infective agents can be transmitted from human remains to DVI workers by physical or airborne (aerosol) contact with the remains, by contact with contaminated instruments and equipment, and by penetrating injury from sharp contaminated items. DVI practitioners must take all practical steps to reduce transmission of infective agents by applying standard precautions. Standard precautions (previously referred to as universal precautions) are based on the concept that the body fluids and tissues of all persons are a potential source of infection, independent of diagnosis or perceived risk. Key elements of standard precautions in the DVI setting are personal protective equipment, protocols regarding the handling of remains and equipment (including sharps), and hand hygiene.

Physical hazards

The list of potential hazards in, and associated with, a disaster area is large and can include: radiological, infectious agents and pathogens, chemical and ongoing disaster events (e.g. earthquake aftershocks). Personnel must be provided with personal protective equipment (PPE) suitable for the task and must be trained and competent in using this equipment. Site safety plans and operating procedures must include details of what PPE is required to be worn and there should be processes in place to ensure compliance with these requirements. Incidents that involve chemical, biological, radiological or nuclear (CBRN) contamination will require specialised PPE and training. It is important that when using radiographic equipment radiation safety protocols are followed.

Psychological risks

Personnel working in a DVI environment, that by definition involves widespread and violent loss of life, will experience an array of emotional responses to the event and they are at risk of developing a range of physiological disorders. The stress responses maybe what would be expected as 'normal' stress reactions that subside within a short timeframe. Other reactions may be more pathological and may include acute stress disorder (ASD) and post-traumatic stress disorder (PTSD). The more 'extreme and intense' the event, the higher the psychological risk to personnel. A supportive 'team' environment is important in mitigating the psychological risks with team members 'looking-out' for and supporting one another. It is essential that there is organised and accessible psychological support during the post-operation period focused on identifying those demonstrating symptoms of ASD and PTSD, noting that both disorders are most amenable to treatment when the symptoms are identified early. Planned follow-up once the personnel return to their normal activities and good family support are key elements in managing post-traumatic stress reactions.

Personnel who have DVI experience may be at increased risk of PTSD when exposed to a new DVI event. Careful thought needs to be given to deploying personnel on multiple DVI rotations or on multiple DVI deployments over a short time period.

DVI phase 1: the Scene phase

The scene of a disaster requires specialist management and is attended by a variety of specialist groups, including personnel tasked with recovering human remains. Typically the disaster scene is first secured from unauthorised access and then is assessed as to how it is to be recovered taking into consideration the hazards in the scene, the resources available and the investigative priorities. Plans are then developed so that the scene is processed in a systematic and orderly manner to ensure that it is appropriately analysed, searched, human remains and other evidence recovered, and the control of the chain of evidence maintained.

Scene searching is conducted in an orderly and systematic manner following a search strategy developed with reference to the specific characteristics of that disaster. A variety of search patterns (grid, spiral, sector, expanding square) may be utilised depending on the topography, extent and nature of the debris field, the knowledge of 'high-interest' areas (areas where human remains are known or likely to be), and the personnel resources available. The scene management strategy must ensure that the entire scene is surveyed and mapped in a manner that facilitates the recording of the position of the human remains along with the contextual relationships with other relevant exhibits at the scene. The use of GPS technology is becoming increasingly important in this regard, particularly in large dispersed scenes.

The Scene phase of a DVI operation is focused on the orderly recovery of *all* human remains from the disaster scene and is generally controlled by police officers who are trained in victim recovery. The recovery of human remains usually commences after survivors of the disaster have been rescued and after the details of the scene have been carefully documented, commonly using mapping technology and photography (both still and video).

The role of the forensic odontologist at the scene

The forensic odontologist deployed as part of the recovery team to the scene of the disaster provides specialist expertise to assist with the orderly and complete recovery of human remains with the intention of enhancing the likelihood and timeliness of identifications. The nature and extent of the advice provided by the forensic odontologist depends on their individual training and experience relative to the personnel in the wider DVI scene team. A well-trained and experienced DVI recovery team may simply require specific specialist advice on the identification and management of orofacial remains. In other situations the forensic odontologist may assist with the development of search strategies, give advice on recovery and preservation techniques and provide leadership at the scene.

The nature and size of a disaster will influence decisions regarding the deployment of forensic odontologists. The decision to deploy a forensic odontologist to the scene is usually made by the DVI commander on the advice of the Scene phase commander and forensic odontology coordinator, taking into consideration the nature and safety at the scene, the utility and 'value' of the odontologist at the disaster scene and the forensic odontology personnel resources available (including timeliness, that is how long it will take to get the odontologist to the scene). It may not be practical, or good use of odontology resources, to deploy odontology personnel to disaster sites within scenes that extend over a wide geographic area, because of the large number of personnel, the equipment and other resources required to deal with the scene. Additionally, the decision to deploy a forensic odontologist to the scene will depend on the demand for odontology personnel for work in other phases of the DVI. The utility of the forensic odontologist at the scene is largely dependent on the nature of the remains. The odontologist's contribution may be relatively low in situations with intact bodies, but rises as the extent of skeletonisation, fragmentation, incineration and commingling increases (Fig. 9.5). The value in the deployment of forensic odontology personnel to disaster scenes such as these is well recognised [4–12].

Human remains at the scene

In disasters involving extreme traumatic forces and fire, the recovery may be complicated by the fragmentation and commingling of the human remains that may also be anisotropically distributed within disaster debris over the scene. When this occurs, a refined localised search is conducted around each set of human remains noting that in these situations it can be difficult to recognise

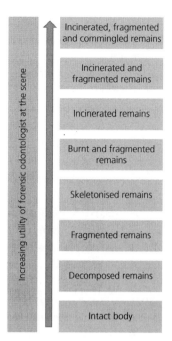

Fig. 9.5 The 'utility' of the forensic odontologist at the DVI scene increases as the extent of skeletonisation, fragmentation, incineration and commingling increases.

body parts and so there is an increased risk that remains will be overlooked. The likelihood that human remains will be missed increases when personnel unfamiliar with the recognition of body parts are tasked with body recovery.

The personnel searching the scene are often a different group from those recovering the remains, that is there are separate search and separate recovery teams. As human remains are encountered a DVI number is assigned and the remains are either clearly marked (often with a small flag or cone) for subsequent recovery or the recovery process is undertaken at the time the remains are located. Body parts are not matched to bodies at the scene but, rather, are treated as individual 'bodies' with the allocation of a separate DVI number.

Body labelling

All human remains should be assigned a unique DVI number following a defined protocol for the disaster. Unique numbering and adherence to a strict numbering protocol is essential to optimise efficiency and to reduce errors. A variety of numbering systems and materials are employed depending on the jurisdiction. DVI numbering typically includes a system for referencing the remains to the location where they were discovered, information about the personnel recovering them and a unique number for the specific remains. The materials used as DVI labels must be waterproof and durable, noting that they may need to withstand long periods in a moist environment and may be subjected to significant variations in temperature depending on body storage arrangements. Where possible, the labels should be attached to the body part and also be included on body-bags, containers and coffins.

Radio Frequency Identification

Radio Frequency Identification (RFID) tags are wireless communication devices that store information on a microchip that can be accessed by radio transmission to a reader connected to a computer. RFID tags can be passive where the power for obtaining data from the chip is sent from the reader, or 'active' RFID tags that have an inbuilt power source. RFID tags may also include a read/write function allowing additional information to be loaded and stored onto the microchip. Conceptually these devices have practical application in DVI settings as they can be inserted or attached to a body, storing information relating to that body. The opportunities for information storage are large, from simple identification numbers through to detailed records, for example regarding the recovery and examination of the remains. The use of RFID tags also potentially complicates the process compared with the existing inexpensive paper-based labelling systems. RFID technology requires additional equipment (tags and readers) and training and implicit in this are higher costs for maintaining satisfactory inventory levels and currency of training for those who will use the tags. RFID tags have been utilised in DVI situations [13, 14], but to date only limited practical development of RFID tracking of bodies has been completed.

Recovery of remains

All human remains should be recovered considering the respect and dignity of the deceased and in a manner that preserves the remaining tissues. The focus should be on prompt removal of remains to prevent further deterioration through environmental exposure and from decomposition. The need to remove the remains in an expeditious fashion must, however, be balanced with the requirement for careful and detailed recovery coordinated with any investigatory element at the scene. Early recovery from the scene means the post-mortem process is not delayed and the remains are removed from public view. Notwithstanding the need to complete tasks at the scene promptly, as is the need in all phases, quality in terms of following best practice processes and attention to detail must never be compromised because of haste.

Once the human remains have been located and labelled the recovery process is undertaken, noting that identifications should not be completed at the scene. The recovery process includes a written description of the remains in situ (including descriptions of the teeth if they are visible) and should be accompanied by high-resolution photographs showing, for orientation, the immediate wider scene and then photographs taken sequentially closer to the remains including close-up photographs of the face and mouth. Video footage is also useful, but should not be used in lieu of 'still' photographs.

Once the remains are photographed, the forensic odontologists' principal responsibilities relate to the orofacial elements. The remains should be inspected, in situ, to identify teeth, facial bones and the mandible. If the remains have been incinerated the teeth and supporting bone will be friable and teeth may have become loose in their bony sockets or lost from them. Prolonged burning, at high temperatures, frequently results in the enamel crowns of teeth being fractured or displaced intact from the underlying dentine. This tooth crown/tooth root separation is likely to be related to structural and compositional differences between dentine and enamel leading to differences in moisture content and coefficients of thermal expansion. Normal tooth anatomical shape and form is lost when the crown is displaced or fractured and additional burning and mechanical damage may further alter the shape. Burning can also produce a range of colour changes in bones and also in teeth. The changes in form and colour make recognition of tooth elements in the debris field even more difficult, and locating these is greatly assisted through the employment of forensic odontologists. An assessment of the level of destruction secondary to the incineration may be useful in determining the resources and personnel necessary for the recovery. Every effort must be made to recover all dental elements, as even the smallest tooth or restorative remnant may be useful in the identification process (Figs. 9.6 and 9.7).

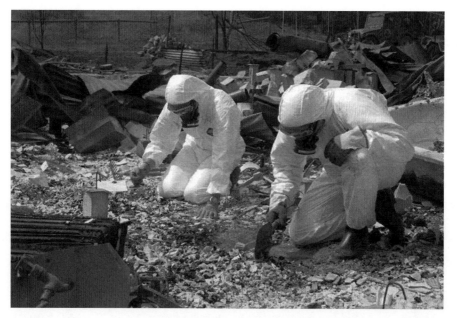

Fig. 9.6 Detailed searching is required to recover the human remains from a scene. (Courtesy of Karl Wilson.) (*See insert for colour representation of the figure.*)

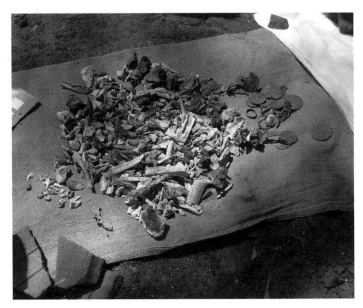

Fig. 9.7 Remains recovered following a detailed scene search.

During the recovery, forensic odontologists can also provide advice on human/ non-human remains and can assist in reducing the chance of iatrogenic commingling.

Protecting remains during recovery and movement

Fragile teeth that have fragmented or that may be susceptible to fragmentation must be protected during the recovery process and their subsequent transportation. The remains should be carefully supported and cushioned for recovery and movement noting the need to protect against mechanical damage due to crushing, vibration and jarring. Large elements, such as the face and head, should be carefully wrapped in a manner that avoids direct contact with, or pressure on, the fragile elements. Wrapping materials should be lightweight, flexible/adaptable and provide good cushioning. Plastic bubble wrap is commonly used, but other materials such as spun fibreglass, wool insulation and cotton wool contained in a plastic wrapping may also be suitable materials (Fig. 9.8). The packaging should provide a 'seal' around the remains, so that if fragile elements become dislodged during the recovery and subsequent transportation, they are contained within the wrapping material, reducing the need to search the entire contents of the body-bag for them during the post-mortem examination.

Smaller elements, such as bony fragments and individual teeth, should be placed into hard shell containers and packed securely, ensuring that they are not in contact with other fragments or with the container walls. Packing material should not compress these fragments, it should prevent them from moving around in the container. The container should be clearly labelled with the DVI number.

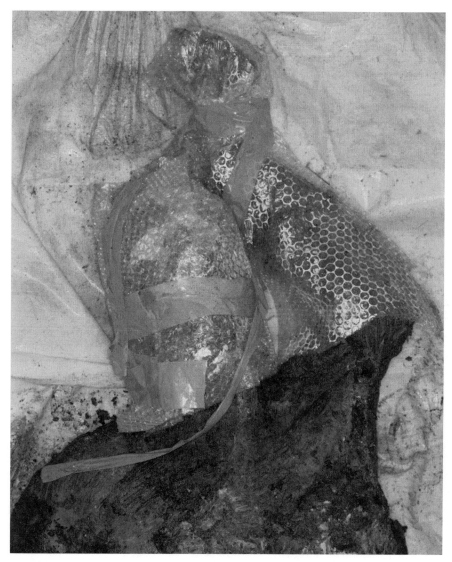

Fig. 9.8 Fragile elements should be carefully wrapped to reduce the chances of damage during recovery and transportation. Note that the hands have also been protected. (Courtesy of Karl Wilson.)

In situations of severe burning and calcination, cyano-acrylate is a reliable method of stabilising fragile teeth and bone. Cyano-acrylate should be used with some circumspection as once applied and dried, because of the complexity of various formulations and the porous nature of the incinerated tissues, it is impossible to remove (even with solvents) without damaging the remains. Care must also be taken to ensure the 'glued' specimen does not compromise or significantly complicate the subsequent post-mortem examination of the remains. For example, in situations where the teeth are in forceful occlusal contact due to heat-induced strictures of the facial tissues, the injudicious use of cyano-acrylate may bond together the maxillary and mandibular arches, complicating the subsequent post-mortem examination of the teeth. Caution should also be exercised when using cyano-acrylates in association with cotton wool as contact between the two may result in an exothermic reaction.

Once protected, the body and associated body parts are placed into a body-bag for further transportation. When the body or main body parts have been recovered, a careful review of the area must be undertaken to ensure all remains and associated property have been salvaged. This may require detailed sifting through the associated debris from the immediate and surrounding areas or, if this is not practical, the debris should be collected from areas under and around where the body lay for later examination. If debris is recovered it should be bagged, labelled and placed with the remains for transportation and subsequent examination. At the completion of the detailed search, the underlying earth or flooring should be free of debris (Fig. 9.9).

The human remains should be protected from damage during transportation, ideally by placing them in individual caskets, although this may not be practical in a large mass fatality event. As a minimum, measures should be taken to ensure that body-bags are not stacked on top of each other and their unrestrained movement around the vehicle floor should be minimised.

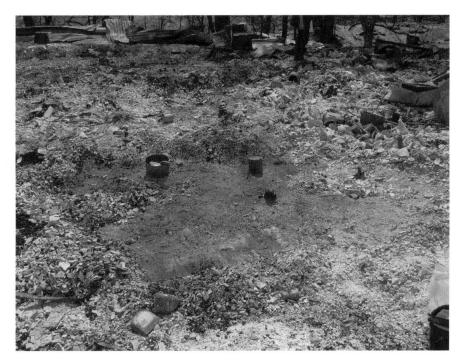

Fig. 9.9 Following a detailed recovery the underlying earth or flooring should be free of debris. (Courtesy of Karl Wilson.)

Scene training and experience

Forensic odontologists deployed to the scene must have appropriate training for their anticipated role, they should have extensive clinical and post-mortem experience and preferably be experienced in working in the disaster scene environment. The requirement that the forensic odontologists have forensic odontology and wide clinical experience should not be underestimated as the recognition of human orofacial elements that may be displaced, fragmented, discoloured and potentially commingled with non-human elements is challenging, even for experienced practitioners. Post-mortem experience is essential as the odontologist will be dealing with human remains. Working in an austere environment with the particular demands this brings requires the practitioner to be physically fit, resilient and sufficiently self-sufficient to cope with the physical, environmental and emotional demands of the scene so as not to be a burden to the wider recovery team. The ability to work as part of a team, commonly as the only forensic odontologist at the scene, is essential.

Personal protective equipment at the scene

In addition to the items suggested below, personnel deployed to the scene should dress appropriately for the environment they are entering and take necessary personal items such as sunglasses, a wide brim hat, sun-block, insect repellent and lip balm.

The odontologist at the scene requires PPE specific for the scene environment and usually requires a higher level of protection from mechanical or physical hazards than in other DVI phases. In determining the PPE requirements for a scene a detailed environmental hazard assessment is necessary and this should include consideration of the anticipated climatic conditions. Scenes that contain a CBRN element usually require enhanced and specialised PPE. Protective clothing and footwear must be fit for purpose and appropriate for the environment. For example, as a general rule for all scenes footwear should include robust sole and toe protection (steel cap and plate) and have good ankle support. The decision as to whether the footwear is rubber, leather or 'fabric', waterproof or 'breathable' will depend on the specific scene. In a hot, dry environment a leather boot may be more suitable than a gumboot. A combination of heavy duty gloves for handling debris and rubber gloves to protect against infectious risk are usually indicated. Respiratory protection is usually needed when working at a disaster scene. The level of respiratory protection required should be based on an assessment of the nature of the particulate and vapour hazards (aerosol, dust etc.) at the scene. This assessment will inform the type and design of respirator or mask that should be worn. In some situations a simple filter mask is all that is needed and in others, such as a chemically contaminated scene, self-contained breathing apparatus may be required. It is essential that masks and respirators fit and seal well on the face and are comfortable to wear. Masks and respirators must be maintained and replaced in accordance with the manufacturer's instructions, taking particular note of the service life of filters. Eye protection in the form of glasses, goggles or eye protection integrated with respiratory protection should shield against splashes, splatter and particulate matter. The lenses should offer UV protection and be scratch and impact resistant. Tinted lenses may be desirable depending on the environmental conditions. If the practitioner requires corrective lenses, the eye protection selected should include corrective lenses or allow spectacles to be worn beneath. Protective outer garments that prevent contaminants contacting clothing and skin are important. Outer garments are typically of a disposable, 'overall' type design and are impermeable. Depending on the nature of the scene and actual role of the forensic odontologist, auditory protection, a helmet, elbow and knee protection may be required. Typically PPE will be donned before entering the scene and removed following any decontamination protocols for the scene in dedicated areas at the periphery of the scene (Figs. 9.10 and 9.11).

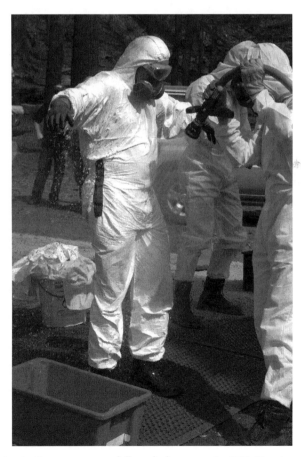

Fig. 9.10 Decontamination processes are followed when removing PPE. (Courtesy of Karl Wilson.)

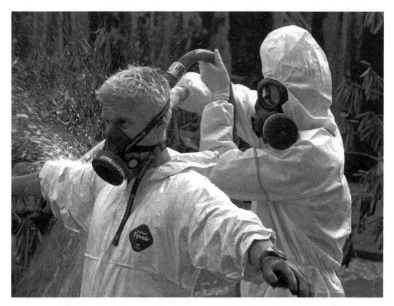

Fig. 9.11 Decontamination processes must be systematic with respiratory protection removed last. (Courtesy of Karl Wilson.)

Equipment

In addition to PPE appropriate to the scene environment, more specialised equipment may be required by the forensic odontologist. The type of equipment necessary will depend on the scene and the role of the forensic odontologist. For scenes involving severe incineration and fragmentation where the forensic odontologist expects to be sorting through ash and debris, a trowel, brushes and tweezers may be useful. Depending on the size of the scene and the amount of debris, sieves (various gauges) may have utility, noting that sieves separate material based on size and not shape so careful examination of the sieved material is required (Figs. 9.12 and 9.13). Sieving can also damage fragile elements and cause further dissociation of parts meaning they should be used judiciously.

Incinerated remains may have been reduced to component parts that are fragile and must be recovered and transported with great care. A range of stabilisation and packing materials (as discussed earlier) for these fragile elements is required. Depending on the nature of the remains and the way the remains will be recovered and transported, it may be useful if portable radiographic equipment is available for use at the scene. Fragile orofacial structures that may be damaged during recovery can be radiographed at the scene, mitigating the risk of loss or destruction during recovery and transportation. Radiography is best performed in the controlled mortuary environment and should only be employed at the scene after careful assessment of the relative risks and benefits.

Photographic equipment is essential as high-resolution images of the remains (and immediate surrounding area) before the recovery commences

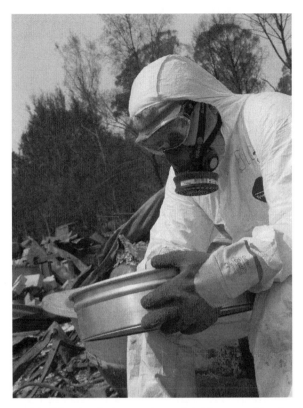

Fig. 9.12 When used judiciously, sieving can be useful when searching for dental remains. (Courtesy of Karl Wilson.)

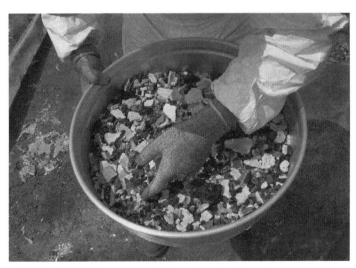

Fig. 9.13 Care must be taken when sieving to ensure fragile remains are not damaged. (Courtesy of Karl Wilson.)

(and as indicated during the recovery) are valuable for later comparative analysis and as part of the documentation of the 'chain of evidence'.

General considerations

Perimeter security or cordons and controlled access points are established at the scene boundaries to restrict access to the scene to only those personnel authorised to enter the area. Managing access is important to protect the integrity of the scene, to prevent the unauthorised removal of property, to exclude the curious, and to prevent unauthorised photography and reportage. Entry to the site is usually restricted to those individuals holding the correct identification and whose names are on the list of authorised personnel. The forensic odontologist must have the appropriate authorisations and identification to facilitate them accessing the scene.

Before entering the scene the forensic odontologists must be aware of the scene management guidelines that include: the scene safety plan including evacuation plan, scene boundaries, entry and exit points including decontamination areas, scene organisation (grid schema, rest and recovery areas, ablution arrangements, etc.) and protocols for reporting into and out of the scene.

DVI phase 2: the Post-mortem phase

In a DVI situation, the post-mortem process involves a detailed and systematic examination by teams of specialist personnel of not only the human remains recovered from the scene, but also the property and material associated with these remains. The primary aim of the post-mortem in these circumstances is to gain as much information as possible to facilitate the identification of all human remains (intact bodies and body parts). The post-mortem also has secondary purposes and, while not necessarily directly related to victim identification, these are nonetheless important. The post-mortem provides an opportunity to make an assessment as to the cause and timing of death and to retrieve possessions and property recovered with the human remains from the scene. While the role in facilitating the identification of the human remains is a key focus, the secondary roles are often important to the relatives and to the authorities reviewing what happened during the incident and the emergency response to the incident.

The relatives of the deceased commonly wish to know the detailed circumstances of their family member's death. The post-mortem may provide medical information regarding the mechanism of death and potentially the 'nature' of death; if the deceased died quickly or if their death was drawn-out. This information may also be useful in determining if the victim could have been saved (potential survivability) had the rescue actions been different or more timely. This knowledge is important in the 'acceptance' and grieving process for relatives.

The return of clothing and personal items that were recovered with the deceased, such as jewellery and wallets, can assist with closure for the relatives.

Authorities may be interested in post-mortem information from an investigative perspective in terms of the incident and the emergency response to the incident. The post-mortem information may be useful on a case-by-case basis as well as collectively and is usually considered in conjunction with information gained from the wider investigation of the incident. Such information can assist in determining the sequence of events that unfolded in response to the incident. This information is valuable when looking at the effectiveness (or otherwise) of systems designed to mitigate risks associated with an emergency event. In many situations the timeliness and nature of the rescue operation have a bearing on the survival of individuals who did not die at the time of the initial incident. The longer it takes to rescue trapped or injured casualties the more likely they will succumb to their injuries or to environmental causes. In the investigation into the emergency response to the collapse of the Canterbury Television (CTV) building following the Christchurch earthquake in February 2011, the cause and time of death of several victims was considered by the coroner in reviewing the effectiveness of the rescue operation [15]. The conduct of the rescue is also important in that the rescue itself may result in the death of individuals who survived the initial incident.

The post-mortem process is a carefully structured process centred on the examination and documentation of the human remains. A careful administrative process is followed to ensure the remains are registered into, and tracked through, the post-mortem process.

Mortuary

In a disaster situation, the mortuary (including body storage facilities) is a fundamental consideration when planning for, and responding to, a multiple fatality incident. It is usual, for logistic, administrative and welfare purposes, to conduct the post-mortem examinations in the same region as the disaster; however, consideration needs to be given to the viability and safety of this. Using local mortuaries is not always possible if there are inadequate mortuary resources (existing mortuary infrastructure or temporary mortuary arrangements) in the area, noting that in addition to the disaster-related work 'routine' mortuary cases continue or if there are ongoing safety risks secondary to the disaster event (e.g. earthquake aftershocks). In such situations it may be necessary to transport the remains to mortuaries in other regions (Figs. 9.14 and 9.15).

Post-mortem process

The DVI post-mortem examination involves a number of disciplines (specialist groups) each conducting a separate examination of the human remains. Typically the disciplines involved include: personal property and effects documentation, skin friction ridge analysis, forensic pathology, forensic biology, forensic odontology and

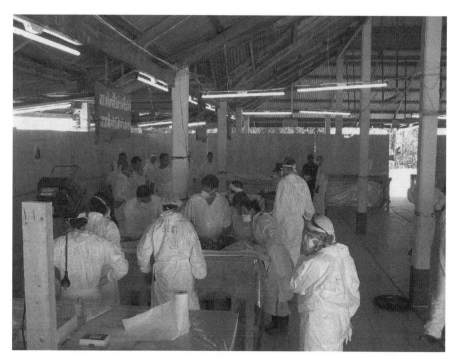

Fig. 9.14 Mortuary facilities at Wat Yan Yoa temple (Site 1), Khao Lak following the Boxing Day Asian tsunami (2004).

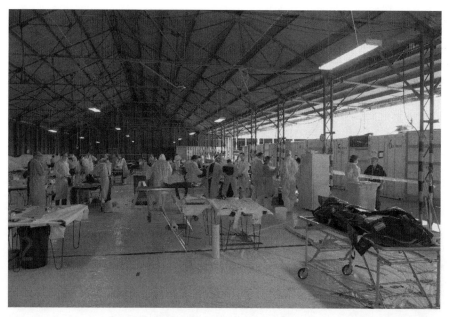

Fig. 9.15 Temporary mortuary established at Burnham Military camp after the Christchurch earthquake (2011). (Courtesy of Karl Wilson.)

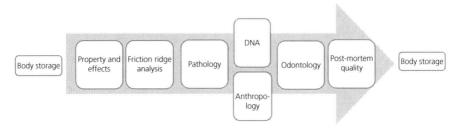

Fig. 9.16 During the post-mortem process remains pass through each examining discipline in a predetermined order.

quality control. Anthropology is also employed depending on the nature of the remains. All human remains are examined sequentially by each discipline and the examination findings recorded, images obtained and samples (as necessary) taken. To avoid errors and omissions each set of human remains is examined following the same sequence of disciplines. This means that if a discipline had not been able to complete the examination of a set of human remains at the end of a work-shift, those remains would be returned to that discipline at the commencement of the next work-shift. Typically the post-mortem examination follows the following sequence mirrored in the INTERPOL (Pink) Post-mortem Form (Fig. 9.16).

The order of examination by the disciplines can be adapted for a specific disaster dependent on the nature of the remains, the anticipated importance of the discipline in contributing useful post-mortem information and the risk that information will be lost due to deterioration of the remains if the post-mortem examination is delayed. For example, in the DVI operation that followed the 2004 Boxing Day Asian tsunami, in several mortuaries skin friction ridge analysis was the first examining discipline in the post-mortem process. The rationale for completing skin friction ridge analysis first was the anticipated importance of fingerprinting in the identification process and the likelihood that obtaining quality fingerprints would become more difficult over time. In this disaster many of the deceased had been immersed in water for some time. This, combined with advanced decomposition and the rigours of transportation of the remains in the disaster scene, resulted in the skin on the hands and feet sloughing off many of the bodies. In these circumstances there was a risk that fingerprint and sole print information would be lost, so to mitigate this, post-mortem skin friction ridge analysis was completed as the first discipline in the post-mortem process. In contrast to this, during the DVI operation following the 2011 Canterbury earthquake, skin friction ridge analysis was the last examining discipline in the post-mortem process. It should be noted that, while each discipline examines the human remains in a specific order, it is common to have dialogue and interaction between the disciplines as the remains progress through the post-mortem process. For example during the investigation (property) stage, the pathologist is frequently asked to give advice and guidance on a particular observation.

Personal property and effects documentation

Traditionally the first discipline to examine the remains is customarily the police or investigative section, often referred to as 'property and effects'. This is usually where the remains enter the post-mortem process, where initial photography is completed and clothing, personal property and associated material are separated from the remains. Detailed photographs are taken throughout the process commencing with the unopened body-bag. All personal items are removed from the body, cleaned, photographed and a detailed written description completed for each item. The contents of pockets, bags and wallets are carefully examined for papers and personal effects that may assist with the identification process. Examples of items of particular interest include: identity cards, driving licences, credit cards, 'SIM' cards from mobile phones and keys. These items are catalogued and packed into separate labelled bags that are usually stored with the remains. In some situations if the personal effects are valuable or where there is a risk of ongoing contamination, the effects may be stored securely separately from the remains. If removal of clothing, jewellery or property is likely to damage the remains it is usual for these items to be left in situ only to be removed during the pathological examination. Material, such as debris from the disaster, found associated with the remains, but that is clearly not important in the DVI process, is usually removed and discarded at this stage.

Skin friction ridge analysis

The traditional methods of obtaining skin friction ridge prints include ink/powders and scanning devices that can be used in the post-mortem setting. Though given the nature of the remains and the DVI environment using ink/powders and transposing the print onto fingerprint card is the technique most commonly employed. Whenever possible, prints are obtained from the fingers, palms and soles of the feet for each set of human remains. Specialised printing techniques may be required when the skin is decomposed, desiccated or macerated.

Forensic pathology examination

The nature and extent of the forensic pathology examination depends on the requirements of the coroner, the circumstances surrounding the disaster and the resources available. Typically the forensic pathology examination (autopsy) will include an external examination and physical description, and usually at least a limited internal post-mortem examination. The pathologist is also required to confirm that the person is in fact deceased (declaration of life extinct) and, occasionally, that the deceased does not have an infectious disease that would prevent airlines repatriating the deceased once released by the coroner. The external examination records the general state of the remains and, when possible, the sex and race, approximate age, measured height and weight, physical build, hair colour, scars, skin marks, tattoos, amputations, piercings and any other distinguishing physical characteristics. General photographs of the remains are taken as well as specific photographs of the unique physical features, such as scars and tattoos, and, if required, injuries. The photographs may be used later in the reconciliation process. The scope of the internal examination depends on a variety of factors including the number of deceased, the 'condition' of the deceased and the investigative requirements. The internal examination is used to obtain information useful in the identification process such as confirming sex (important given that some persons undergo sex reassignment surgery), looking for evidence of previous trauma (fractured bones) and surgery (e.g. hysterectomy), determining the presence of indwelling medical devices and prostheses and so on. Correlation of natural disease with medical records (e.g. known malignancies) may also aid the identification process.

If the decision has been made to determine the cause of death and potential survivability then the internal examination will be extremely important in documenting the full extent of the internal injuries, which can be extensive even with little evidence of external injuries. The usefulness of an internal examination is highlighted in deceased who are severely burnt. In these cases the question may be asked: was the person alive or deceased prior to the fire and did they succumb to the effects of the fire? The presence of soot in the major airways is conclusive evidence that the person inhaled smoke and was alive prior to the fire. Toxicology analysis then would confirm whether or not inhalation of products of combustion was the cause of death or at least a contributory factor. In some circumstances a more detailed pathological examination must be completed on specific individuals (if they can be recognised as such), for example, in an aircraft accident the captain and crew may be subject to a more detailed pathological examination. These would include investigations into the presence of drugs and/or alcohol and a more detailed investigation as to the cause of death, as well as the possibility of an incapacitating natural disease. These investigations may be useful in determining causality and culpability.

Post-mortem radiography

The use of conventional plane film medical radiography in forensic pathology is well established and provides information that assists with identifying fractures, foreign bodies and occult injuries as well as features useful in identification. In recent times, radiology, in the form of three-dimensional imaging, has assumed a greater importance during the forensic pathology examination. The development and refinements in three-dimensional imaging (multi-slice computed tomography (CT) and magnetic resonance imaging (MRI)) and improvements in the accuracy of these imaging techniques has provided the opportunity for a minimally invasive 'virtual autopsy' or 'virtopsy'.

These imaging techniques are useful for the triaging of remains prior to formal post-mortem examination; however, they are not a replacement for the autopsy itself. Such screening provides early information regarding the content of body-bags: determination of human versus animal, determination of sex, recognition of commingled remains, the identification of specific regions or sites of interest such as trace evidence (e.g. remnants of an explosive device that may have to be retrieved for further analysis). Importantly CT/MRI allows the pathologist to better plan and focus the autopsy and may assist in prioritising post-mortem work matched to the skills and resources available. The virtual autopsy does not displace the classic forensic autopsy in DVI situations; rather it is an adjuvant to such and is now accepted internationally as part of DVI best practice. Digital data storage of images also facilitates quality review and audit and if necessary re-examination long after the remains have been buried or cremated (aka 'digital exhumation').

Post-mortem DNA

To obtain a DNA profile it is necessary to collect suitable samples from the deceased body or body parts. It is common for the forensic biologist to obtain the necessary samples in conjunction with the forensic pathology examination. This is usually done at the conclusion of the pathology examination and in consultation with the pathologist. If teeth are identified as a useful source of tissue for DNA analysis, the forensic biologist will usually discuss this with the odontologists noting that the teeth are usually left in situ until the odontology examination has been completed. It is recommended that tissue samples for DNA analysis are obtained for each body or body part even if identification is likely to be confirmed using other methods.

Anthropology

An anthropological examination may also be completed at this time and may provide useful information regarding age, sex, stature, racial characteristics, medical conditions, congenital and developmental disease and trauma. The anthropologist can assist with distinguishing between human and non-human remains and with the separation of commingled remains.

Post-mortem odontology examination

The odontology post-mortem examination is typically undertaken following the pathological examination. The aim of the odontology post-mortem is to obtain as much dental and relevant orofacial information as possible to assist with the reconciliation phase. It is usual for the post-mortem information to be evaluated at later stages in the DVI process by odontologists who were not present at the odontology post-mortem. Therefore, the information gained at the post-mortem must be collected and recorded in a form and manner that ensures that the post-mortem findings are clear, complete and unambiguous so that further interpretation is not required. In some situations the post-mortem odontology group may be advised that there are no dental remains associated with a particular DVI number. Good practice requires that the odontology group confirm this by examining the remains and complete the odontology sections in the DVI forms.

As discussed in an earlier chapter, it is considered 'best practice' for two odontologists to conduct the post-mortem examination, often with support from auxiliaries. The two odontologists approach reduces the possibility of errors or omissions

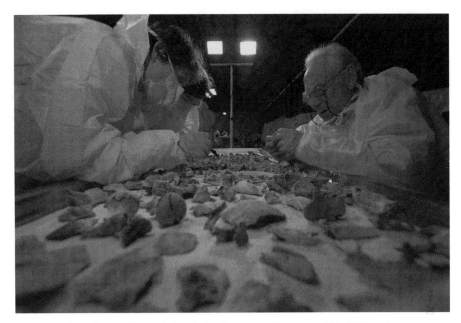

Fig. 9.17 Odontology staff examining skeletal remains. (Courtesy of Karl Wilson.)

occurring and provides an opportunity to confirm interpretations and examination observations. In some situations, depending on the complexity of the remains (e.g. severe burning, fragmentation and/or commingling), more than two odontologists may be involved with the examination (Fig. 9.17).

Before the examination commences it is essential that the DVI number linked to the human remains in question is checked against the number on the associated documentation. In a busy mortuary setting, with multiple examination lanes, it is possible that incorrect documentation can become associated with the incorrect remains and it is vital that any such error is identified and corrected promptly.

Traditionally one odontologist completes a systematic examination of the clinical status of each tooth and the surrounding orofacial structures with the other odontologist recording the dictated examination findings. At the conclusion of the examination the odontologists swap roles, with the recorder then examining the remains. This method of post-mortem examination provides a 'double-check' and increases the likelihood that accurate and complete records are obtained. In a DVI operation, swapping examiner and recorder roles may be impractical as it can be cumbersome and time consuming maintaining the 'clean/contaminated distinction', which usually requires the examining odontologist to decontaminate before they can assume the role of the recorder. To mitigate this, while maintaining a 'double-check' system, an alternative method is for the odontologist who recorded the examination findings to 'read back' what they have recorded while the examiner verifies this as they re-examine the remains (Fig. 9.18).

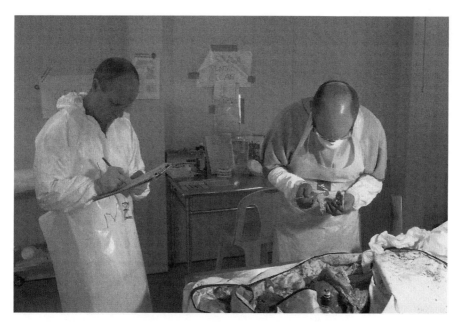

Fig. 9.18 Two odontologists examine each set of remains.

It is essential that adequate access to the dental elements is obtained for the post-mortem examination, and to achieve this it may be necessary to resect soft tissues or the jaws themselves. The purpose of resection or facial dissection is solely to gain access for the post-mortem procedures, thus resection should not be undertaken as a matter of course. The extent of the resection should be limited to what is essential to gain adequate access and resection techniques should be those that minimise tissue displacement and facilitate the return of the face to the pre-resection form. Resected tissues should not be stored separately from the remains from which they originate. If resection is deemed necessary, the approval of the coroner is typically required.

The odontology examination follows the format described in earlier chapters and the records taken include, at a minimum, written notes and descriptions usually made on the INTERPOL Post-mortem (pink) Forms (pages F1, F2 and G) or equivalent. The written records obtained must be clear, unambiguous and complete, using standardised charting conventions and abbreviations that are the same as those used in the other phases of the DVI operation. Where possible the electronic methods for recording the post-mortem findings in the mortuary should be utilised. Recording in this manner removes the need for later transcription and reduces the risk of transcription errors and thus has the potential to save time.

Radiology and photography

It is important that radiographs are obtained for all of the teeth, of any edentulous areas of the jaw and of structures that may be of forensic interest, for example bone screws and plates inserted following trauma or bony surgery. To optimise the chances of obtaining post-mortem radiographs that demonstrate a degree of equivalence with ante-mortem radiographs, a comprehensive range of post-mortem radiographs should be obtained. This is because the extent, type and orientation of ante-mortem radiographs available is unlikely to be known at this stage. Typically periapical radiographs are obtained for each tooth (including developing tooth germs) along with left and right posterior bite-wing radiographs. Radiographs should be taken using film positions and x-ray tube angulations that simulate those that would be used in clinical situations and ensuring that periapical views capture the complete root. Every effort needs to be made to avoid tooth or restoration overlap. The use of digital radiographic images is preferred over analogue or wet-film radiography as the radiographs can be quickly checked for adequacy at the time they are taken and can be repeated easily if necessary. If analogue radiography is used, the radiographic films should be developed and reviewed before the odontology post-mortem examination is concluded. Digital radiographic images should be labelled with the DVI number, saved in a predetermined digital format and form (disc, data stick) and included with the INTERPOL Post-mortem Forms. Analogue radiographs should be mounted and clearly labelled and included with the post-mortem documentation. CT imaging has been used in forensic odontology in age determination of human remains, but despite improvements in imaging technology and computer processing and analysis CT imagery does not, as yet, displace the requirement for conventional radiography in post-mortem odontology examinations. However, as technology develops there is an increasing likelihood that CT and other new imaging techniques will assume a greater importance.

Photographs should be obtained of all the dental elements and of any other orofacial features that may be useful in the identification process. Typical photographic views include right and left buccal views, anterior facial (teeth apart and with teeth together) and maxillary and mandibular occlusal views. Photographs of anterior teeth should be taken with lips retracted and the teeth together and also with the teeth apart. Removable appliances should be photographed in situ if possible and also out of the mouth. Digital photography is preferred as images can be checked for quality at the time they are taken and they provide greater utility over traditional film during the reconciliation process. The DVI number should be visible in all photographic images.

Teeth for DNA

In some situations the odontologist may be asked to remove a tooth (or teeth) for DNA analysis. This is best completed at the conclusion of the odontology post-mortem examination (that is after the odontology quality checking process). Teeth with the greatest amount of dental pulp, cementum and dentine should be selected as these tissues are the richest sources of DNA. Typically this implies an unrestored, pathology free molar tooth, which usually has the largest root surface area and more cellular cementum compared with single rooted teeth. The use of molar teeth for DNA sampling is recommended by INTERPOL [2] and the DNA Commission of the International Society of Forensic Genetics (ISFG) [16].

Notwithstanding these recommendations, the odontologist should be mindful that the important factor is the volume of DNA-rich tissue, such that a restored molar may be more suitable than an unrestored incisor tooth. If in doubt, advice should be sought from a forensic biologist. Given that robust evidence-based decontamination procedures for teeth harvested for DNA have not been established, bleaching and decontamination solutions should be avoided, with teeth being simply cleaned of gross debris by washing with 'DNA-free' water. Teeth taken for DNA analysis should be placed in a sterile container that can be sealed (e.g. a specimen container) and labelled with the DVI number. Details of what tooth has been removed must be included on the post-mortem forms.

Age assessment

Age assessment using tooth development and tooth eruption data can be of assistance in identifying children and young adults. Morphological changes such as wear, secondary dentine deposition and root dentine transparency may be of assistance for age estimation in adults. Age assessment can provide valuable information when dealing with situations where children of different ages have died, with and without issues of commingling, and in focusing on data sorting and searching efforts during the reconciliation phase of the DVI operation.

Odontology quality review

At the conclusion of the odontology post-mortem examination, and before the remains leave the odontology section, all of the odontology records and images obtained should be 'quality checked' for clarity, accuracy and completeness. The quality check is intended to reduce errors and omissions and to ensure the information obtained is sufficiently clear and comprehensive for an odontologist not involved with the post-mortem examination to have a clear understanding of the dental status of the remains (Fig. 9.19).

The quality check usually involves a review by an odontologist who was not directly involved with the post-mortem examination and who checks that the written records accurately reflect the radiographic and photographic details and that the documents are completed fully (annotations in all sections), are unambiguous and thorough and have been signed by those who performed the post-mortem examination. The photographic and radiographic images are also reviewed to ensure that all the necessary images have been taken and that they are of suitable quality. The remains should not be released from the odontology section until after the quality check, which effectively verifies that the odontology post-mortem examination has been completed and that all necessary records have been obtained.

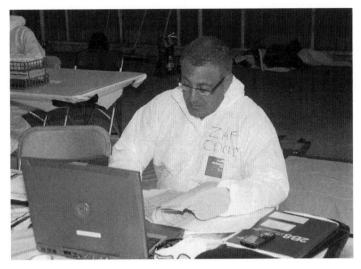

Fig. 9.19 The quality check ensures written records accurately reflect the radiographic and photographic details and that the post-mortem documents are completed fully. (Courtesy of Karl Wilson.)

Staffing in the mortuary

The DVI mortuary environment is complex and emotionally challenging and so it is desirable that personnel employed in the post-mortem phase of a DVI operation have mortuary training and experience. This is particularly the case in the early stages of a DVI operation where the processes and procedures specific to that mortuary are being established. Training and experience should, in addition to forensic odontology skills (including a working knowledge and understanding of the use of all the equipment and computer software being employed), include a robust understanding of mortuary processes and health and safety protocols.

The post-mortem process can be significantly enhanced through the use of 'dentally experienced' auxiliaries such as hygienists, dental therapists, technicians and chair-side assistants. The auxiliaries must have mortuary training and be experienced so that they can assist in a number of areas such as preparing the remains for examination, radiography, photography and record keeping.

Equipment and PPE in the mortuary

As discussed in an earlier chapter, personnel working in the mortuary must wear PPE appropriate for the task and with reference to the specific risks identified in the hazard assessment. The level of protection required from the PPE may vary from situation to situation; however, as a general rule skin (and underclothing), eye and respiratory protection is required. In some situations personnel will require specialised training with decontamination procedures and the use of PPE offering higher levels of protection. Incidents that involve CBRN contamination will require workers to take special precautions to protect their health and safety.

For example, the use of impermeable suits and respirators when dealing with remains that have been contaminated with chemicals. It is important that the PPE used fits well and is comfortable as in DVI situations this equipment must be worn for long uninterrupted periods.

Only minimal equipment is required for the preparation and examination of the remains. This equipment usually includes: toothbrushes and cleaning materials (gauze), dental mirrors, probes, tweezers, cheek retractors for photography, mouth props, scalpel blades and handles, and extraction forceps. The equipment needs to be replicated in each workstation. Equipment for resection may also be required (scalpels, a Stryker autopsy saw, tissue shears, bone mallet and chisels) (Fig. 9.20).

Radiology equipment including x-ray generators, radiographic film or digital sensors and processing equipment is required. The use of battery powered, hand-held x-ray generators is preferred to stand-mounted designs, as they provide greater portability and aligning the radiographic film to the x-ray generator is frequently easier. Radiographic film holders and materials to help position and support radiographic films/sensors and the remains such as 'Toley Bags' (bags full of sand in a variety of sizes) are helpful in attaining radiographic images

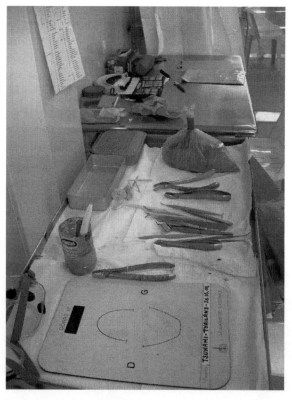

Fig. 9.20 Odontology post-mortem equipment.

replicating typical ante-mortem radiographic views. Soft wax is useful for holding individual teeth in position on radiographic films and sensors.

Photographic equipment is required and, as mentioned earlier, digital photography is preferred over standard film photography. High-resolution cameras with flexible focal length lenses that allow close-up photography are indicated, as are accessories such as lip and cheek retractors, front faced mirrors, external and ring-flash systems, photographic backdrop boards, and forensic scales (e.g. ABFO No 2 photomacrograhic scale). Depending on how the images are to be transferred and stored, multiple SD cards may be required.

Additional lighting, such as personal headlamps, is often necessary to supplement overhead lighting.

DVI phase 3: the Ante-mortem phase

The collection of ante-mortem data is an important early consideration in a DVI response and usually is a continuous process throughout the DVI operation. Ante-mortem data collection should commence as a priority as soon as possible after the incident, thereby taking advantage of what is usually high public interest in the incident. Delays in the ante-mortem data collection process may result in the holders of important ante-mortem records (e.g. dentists) not looking through their patient databases to see if any of the missing were patients of their practice. Once obtained, ante-mortem data must be kept secure and only authorised personnel should have access.

Missing persons database (list)
A missing person's database is developed for the disaster and ante-mortem data sought for those people on the database. Ante-mortem data is usually obtained more quickly in a closed disaster where the names of the missing are known (e.g. an aircraft crash with a passenger list) than with an open disaster where the list of missing people evolves over time.

Ante-mortem data collection
The ante-mortem data collection process typically involves a structured interview of relatives of the missing individuals in an attempt to obtain a wide range of ante-mortem material related to the missing individual. Ante-mortem information of importance includes: physical appearance, distinguishing features, descriptions of clothing and property, photographs, medical and dental records and fingerprints (if available). Recent photographs that show the teeth are helpful. Personal items may also be collected for fingerprinting and/or DNA sampling. Particular attention is paid to gathering information and descriptions of potentially unique physical characteristics such as scars, piercings and tattoos. A detailed and full ante-mortem record should be collected for each missing individual to provide a broad range of information

potentially useful in identifying the individual. Incomplete ante-mortem records where more data is available, or over-reliance on one aspect of the ante-mortem record, may cause unnecessary delays in the identification of deceased individuals.

Ante-mortem skin friction ridge records

Depending on the nature of the DVI incident, skin friction ridge analysis is usually a feature in the ante-mortem data collection process. In some countries, and in some specific situations, an ante-mortem fingerprint record may be on file (e.g. on identity documents or if the individual has a criminal record). Where a fingerprint record is not available, it may be necessary to obtain latent fingerprints from personal objects and surfaces that the missing person was known to have touched. If latent prints are to be collected, the sooner the collection commences the greater the likelihood of success. As time progresses the quality of latent fingerprints deteriorates and the likelihood of other individuals' fingerprints obscuring those of the missing increases. Both issues will complicate the fingerprint identification process. It is not uncommon, because of the protective effects of footwear, for the soles of the feet to remain intact long after fingerprint detail has been lost, such that at post-mortem sole prints can be obtained. It is important that as part of the latent print recovery attempts, consideration is made to recover sole prints from bathroom floors, bathroom scales and the like. Where latent prints are being obtained, reference prints from other household members may be required in order to eliminate these individuals from the latent print collections.

Ante-mortem DNA

It is relatively unusual for an individual to have an ante-mortem DNA record although increasingly such profiles (or stored samples suitable for profiling) are available. In situations where no such records are available, DNA profiles may be obtained from a variety of sources for direct matching (self-sourced sample), including stored blood and body tissue samples and from personal items. In New Zealand and some states in Australia a DNA profile may be obtained from the heel-prick blood samples (Guthrie cards) that are taken from most new born babies to screen for metabolic disorders (e.g. phenylketonuria). Improvement and refinement of DNA sampling and processing techniques means DNA can be obtained from an increasing number of personal items, such as hairbrushes, combs, razors, toothbrushes and the like. Care needs to be exercised when using DNA profiles obtained from such items, because these items may have been 'contaminated' by others sharing their use. Exfoliated primary teeth retained as a childhood memento can also be a useful source of DNA. As with fingerprinting, obtaining samples suitable for the isolation of a DNA profile is an important time-dependent ante-mortem data collection activity.

In situations where ante-mortem DNA information is not readily available or reliably obtained, reference samples suitable for DNA analysis can be obtained from direct relatives to determine if a kinship relationship exists between a set of remains and those individuals sampled.

Ante-mortem dental records

Ante-mortem dental records provide detail of dental and oral health procedures received by an individual prior to their death. The collection of ante-mortem dental data usually requires the relatives of the missing individual furnishing the details of the dental practitioners they may have seen. The relatives are also asked if the missing person had any dental records or dentally relevant material in their possesson. It is not unusual for an individual to retain extracted and exfoliated teeth, study models, old dental appliances, mouth guards, dental x-rays and the like, all of which may be useful. In situations where the dental practitioner(s) who has provided care to the missing individuals is unknown, then general requests to dental practitioners through registration authorities and professional associations can be useful in locating records (Fig. 9.21).

Ante-mortem records are usually requested from the relevant dental practitioner(s) by the police. It is important that a clinician from the dental practice providing the ante-mortem records is involved with reviewing and providing the records rather than this being a simple 'administrative action' delegated to an office staff member. This is important because clinical staff are best equipped to ensure that the records are clear and complete. Where necessary the clinician can

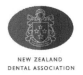

NEW ZEALAND
DENTAL ASSOCIATION

URGENT POLICE REQUEST

New Zealand police are seeking assistance in locating the dental records for the following person:

Last name:	**HUTCHINSON**
Given names:	Mary Rose
Date of Birth:	27 August 1987
NHI:	KBG1676
Last known address:	128 Waimea Road, Nelson

Ms HUTCHINSON is believed to have been a victim of the recent Rodenstock earthquake.

If you have the dental records or any information relating to Ms Mary Rose HUTCHINSON please contact:

Constable Kate Middlemass	Inquiry Officer, Operation RODENSTOCK
Telephone: + 64 4 565 4561	E-mail: kate.middlemass@rodenstock.pol.nz.
	Or
Dr David Keats	AM odontology coordinator - Op RODENSTOCK
Telephone: + 64 4 563 9981	E-mail: d.Keats@rodenstock.pol.nz.

Fig. 9.21 A request for ante-mortem dental records through professional associations can be made when the dental practitioner for an individual is unknown.

also provide clarification of the information contained in the records and other supporting information, such as details of other practitioners or agencies who may also have dental records of the missing person. This person also becomes a point of contact for the odontology ante-mortem phase leader.

It is essential that all available dental records are obtained including: written notes (electronic and handwritten), radiographs, plaster models (study and treatment), photographs, impressions, CAD/CAM and CAT scan data, clinical correspondence and dental and periodontal chartings. It is important that the original records are provided as the duplication process can introduce errors and may reduce the quality of the record. Some dental practitioners may be reluctant to provide the original records, citing 'medico-legal' concerns, in which case a 'clinician-to-clinician' (forensic odontologist to dentist) conversation, explaining why the originals are required and reassuring the clinician that the records will remain accessible to the treating clinician, can assist.

It is useful to have a forensic odontologist work with the police when collecting ante-mortem records. In addition to, as necessary, communicating with dental practitioners providing records, the odontologist conducts a preliminary review of the collected ante-mortem records and provides advice to the police as to the 'completeness' of these records and if the records suggest other dental practitioners may also have records. For example the presence of a referral letter, laboratory prescription, third-party claim and the like may prompt further record inquiries. The odontologist can also liaise directly with the dental practitioners providing the records, answering any questions and seeking additional information or clarification as necessary. Care must be taken to ensure that the chain of custody of ante-mortem records is documented and that the records are transferred and stored in a secure manner.

Once all the dental records have been obtained, these are reviewed and a consolidated summary (single master record) of the dental and oral status made, usually on the INTERPOL Ante-mortem (yellow) Forms (pages F1, F2 and G). An understanding of the dental nomenclature and charting systems used in the ante-mortem record is important to ensure that the records are understood and correctly transcribed and collated. As with the post-mortem findings, the consolidated ante-mortem record must be clear, unambiguous and annotations made in all sections should use standardised charting conventions that are the same as those used in the other phases of the DVI operation. It is usual that two odontologists are actively engaged with the interpretation and collation of each individual ante-mortem record. This approach minimises the likelihood that errors and omissions occur in the consolidated ante-mortem record. The consolidated record should then be reviewed as a part of the quality assurance process by an odontologist who was not part of the initial ante-mortem record analysis and transcription. The quality check focuses on ensuring the consolidated ante-mortem record details accurately, and without ambiguity, the information obtained from the various ante-mortem records.

The quality check also should confirm that the consolidated ante-mortem record is completed fully (an annotation in all sections) and is signed by the odontologists who performed the ante-mortem analysis.

Ante-mortem equipment

The principal items of equipment required in the ante-mortem odontology section are computers, printers, scanners, data storage devices and networks, general office equipment and consumables. Minimal specialist forensic odontology ante-mortem equipment is required and is usually restricted to radiographic viewers and access to specialised dental clinical record computer software.

DVI phase 4: the Reconciliation phase

Reconciliation is the process where the ante-mortem and post-mortem findings are compared and matched in an effort to establish a scientifically verifiable identification. The positive identification of a set of remains requires robust and substantive demonstration of individualism through the confirmation that a particular set of characteristics are unique to the deceased.

The reconciliation process involves two related activities, ante-mortem and post-mortem data matching and subsequently ante-mortem and post-mortem data comparison and validation. The matching process finds combinations of ante-mortem and post-mortem records that are similar and that merit more detailed evaluation. These record combinations are then studied in detail to determine if the records match sufficiently for an identification to be made. This process is undertaken for each DVI discipline. The data search and matching protocols are determined by each discipline with the search criteria based on characteristics determined for the specific DVI operation. Initially the matching searches are based on post-mortem key characteristics, as this data is most likely to be correct and can be verified by re-examining the remains. Data searches can be made with reference to the 'full' ante-mortem database or, in some situations, individual 'targeted' searching may be undertaken. Targeted searches are based on specific identifying information being available for a particular set of remains. For example, identification documents may have been found on an otherwise unrecognisable body. This information would then allow direct comparison of the post-mortem findings from those remains with the ante-mortem information for the individual described in the identification documents. A targeted search of this nature removes the need for a full ante-mortem/post-mortem database search for that set of human remains. Targeted searches speed up the identification process and may result in the early release of deceased individuals back to their relatives.

Skin friction ridge comparison (reconciliation)

The ridge characteristics of prints obtained during the post-mortem are compared with ante-mortem prints. Initial matches of ante-mortem and post-mortem prints may be made by fingerprint officers manually searching the databases, following possible matches that are identified using other information (e.g. circumstantial evidence), or from matches generated from specialised fingerprint data programs such as the automated fingerprint identification system (AFIS). The actual identification (or match) is carried out by a direct side-to-side comparison of the matched ante-mortem and post-mortem prints. The fingerprint officer will analyse the prints to determine if the skin ridge detail and characteristics of the ante-mortem and post-mortem prints match (or not) in terms of size, shape, sequence and spatial relationship to conclude if the prints are from the same source. The findings of this analysis are then verified by two other fingerprint officers. At the conclusion of this process a report is developed that includes a concise description of the findings and a statement regarding identification that may be; ante-mortem and post-mortem prints 'match' (identify), they do not 'match' (exclude) or the results are inconclusive.

DNA reconciliation

Reconciliation of DNA samples requires matching of ante-mortem DNA profiles from self-samples (e.g. blood cards), from relatives or from belongings with the DNA profiles obtained from the samples taken during the post-mortem. In a DVI situation, kinship searching or indirect matching may be complicated by the large volume of data. This makes specialist software capable of searching and matching data, completing kinship calculations and calculating the necessary statistics necessary. A report is compiled at the conclusion of this matching process, including a statement and statistical analysis, as to whether the ante-mortem and post-mortem DNA profiles correspond, don't correspond or if the analysis is inconclusive.

Odontology reconciliation
Data matching

The odontology reconciliation team take the consolidated post-mortem and ante-mortem data and review these to find key markers or characteristics that may subsequently be used as ante-mortem and post-mortem data-match search queries. Typically the key markers take one of two forms: first those that are general in nature (collective classification), such as sex and age (adult or child), that help reduce the number of records to be matched. The second group of key markers are noteworthy or uncommon dental features, such as missing teeth or complex restorations. From this a search algorithm is developed, for example a search algorithm may be post-mortem key characteristics – adult male, implant retained upper-left central incisor. Ante-mortem records with the same (or closely similar) key characteristics would be identified for subsequent detailed analysis.

There are several methods used for the initial comparative matching of odontology post-mortem and ante-mortem records. For disasters involving a relatively small number of sets of remains, simple visual comparisons (of DVI forms or using boards detailing key characteristics) or 'bingo hall' methods can be used. For visual matching of DVI forms, the consolidated ante-mortem forms are visually compared with each consolidated post-mortem form and likely matches identified and subsequently reviewed in detail. From a practical perspective, this usually involves placing the consolidated ante-mortem forms out on a table with the completed odontogram displayed (e.g. the INTERPOL F2 Form) and the odontologists comparing a single post-mortem odontogram sequentially with each ante-mortem form. Several odontologists can compare multiple records simultaneously. The 'bingo hall' method involves a number of odontologists each viewing the consolidated ante-mortem odontogram from several missing individuals. A consolidated post-mortem record is selected by the 'bingo master' who 'calls-out' the key characteristics from the post-mortem record. Each odontologist looks at their assigned ante-mortem records to see if any have the characteristics described. As more key characteristics are 'called out', possible matches are identified.

Computer-assisted data searching

As the number of deceased and/or degree of disassociation of remains rises, the amount of data increases, which further complicates the data-comparison process. Computer software programs that store, sort and compare ante-mortem and post-mortem data have been developed and are increasingly employed in DVI incidents. The use of DVI software greatly assists the reconciliation process as an initial matching and sorting tool. Once the ante-mortem and post-mortem data are entered, the reconciliation matching software searches the respective databases for key characteristic matches. The software and computer power allows prompt and almost limitless key characteristic matching combinations. These searches result in 'potential' ante-mortem/post-mortem matches that then require detailed comparative analysis (reconciliation) by forensic odontologists.

DVI software has the potential to enhance the speed and detail of ante-mortem/post-mortem data matching. The DVI computer programs have evolved and developed significantly since the first programs were developed in the early 1970s. The principles of data storage and matching are similar for all these systems; however, the systems vary in terms of the range of characteristics available in the database and the matching algorithms. DVI software systems in common use include: DVI System International (DVI Sys®), WinID3®, automated dental identification system (ADIS), Disaster and Victim IDentification (DAVID®), DMORT Victim Identification Profile (VIP), and the Unified Victim Identification System (UVIS) – dental identification module. INTERPOL currently uses DVI System International (Plass Data Software), which is a PC-Windows based Microsoft SQL database with functions based on the format of the INTERPOL DVI forms. World Dental Federation (FDI) tooth notations are used, and a comprehensive array of charting nomenclature and conventions combined with the use of the INTERPOL DVI form format enhances this system's utility in DVI operations involving multiple nationalities.

DVI software programs are currently unable to complete the formal detailed reconciliation required to meet evidentiary standards, thus final reconciliation must be completed manually by a forensic odontologist. This is an area of research interest and developments in image comparison technologies are showing promise.

Detailed reconciliation

Because data is frequently incomplete, data-match searches are likely to result in several potential ante-mortem/post-mortem matches that then require more thorough analysis. Each potential match is analysed in detail (individual comparison) and, based on comparative data, conclusions drawn regarding the likelihood that the ante-mortem record and post-mortem record relate to the same person. Any discrepancies that exist between the ante-mortem and post-mortem data must be explainable. If unexplainable differences exist, an identification cannot be made.

The reconciliation process usually involves two forensic odontologists who subsequently 'prove' any potential ante-mortem/post-mortem match to the reconciliation forensic odontology coordinator prior to a reconciliation report and statement being written (Fig. 9.22).

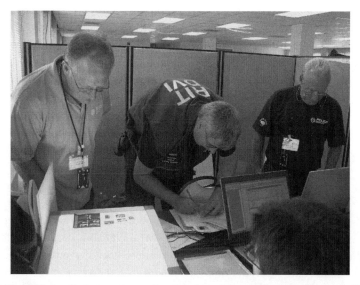

Fig. 9.22 Reconciliation findings are 'proved' to the odontology coordinator before being 'finalised'.

The reconciliation report details the findings of the ante-mortem/post-mortem comparative analysis and the reconciliation statement provides a concise description of the findings. INTERPOL suggest the following identification categories [2]:

- Identification (there is absolute certainty the post-mortem and ante-mortem records are from the same person).
- Identification probable (specific characteristics correspond between post-mortem and ante-mortem, but that either post-mortem or ante-mortem data, or both, are minimal).
- Identification possible (there is nothing that excludes the identity, but that either post-mortem or ante-mortem data or both are minimal).
- Identity excluded (post-mortem and ante-mortem records are from different persons).
- No comparison can be made.

Formalisation of identification

Reconciliation is completed by each discipline, usually independently of one another, and a reconciliation statement or report developed. The reconciliation results for each discipline are subsequently consolidated, along with consideration of any circumstantial evidence gathered at the scene and from the ante-mortem and post-mortem phases, to produce a definitive reconciliation report. This process requires that the various disciplines work cooperatively to ensure any inconsistencies are addressed and agreement reached.

The Identification Board is generally composed of the coroner, representation from the command and leadership elements of the DVI operation and experienced experts representing each discipline. The reconciliation information (ante-mortem/post-mortem match data) is provided to the Identification Board who consider the report, including the recommendations provided by each discipline, and reach a conclusion as to whether the proposed ante-mortem and post-mortem data match constitutes a scientifically verifiable identification. If the Identification Board is satisfied of this then the remains are released to the relatives. If the Identification Board finds that there is insufficient evidence to assign an identification then those remains are retained within the DVI process for further evaluation.

DVI phase 5: the Debrief

An essential element of a DVI operation is the 'debrief'. Debriefing should occur as an integral part of routine operational activity (daily meetings) so that issues can be identified promptly and remediation taken as necessary. At the conclusion of a DVI operation a final debrief is completed. This provides the opportunity to review the conduct and outcomes of the operation with the intent of identifying and documenting the lessons observed and applying this information to inform changes in operational processes and procedures in preparation for future events. The final debrief also provides the opportunity to bring those involved with the DVI back together for mutual reflection, sharing and psychological support. Participants in a DVI are exposed to traumatic events and are likely to suffer from fatigue and may experience high levels of stress; the debrief is an important opportunity to undertake critical stress debriefing both individually and collectively. The shift in emotive state from working in a DVI response to that of 'normal daily life' is significantly facilitated through group debriefing and good organisational support.

Administrative arrangements and information management

The administrative, logistic and information technology arrangements to support a DVI operation are extensive and complex. Careful planning and dedicated administrative and IT staff are usually required, noting that the portfolio of responsibilities is extensive – ranging from personnel management (including travel, accommodation, credentialing, security clearances, orientation) through to catering, supplies and IT infrastructure (e.g. computer cabling, hubs and networks). It is usual during a DVI operation for an 'Information Centre' to be established where the information and data gained from the scene, and from the post-mortem and ante-mortem process, is assembled and stored (Fig. 9.23).

A huge amount of information is generated during a DVI operation and it is essential that there are detailed and robust protocols for managing this information.

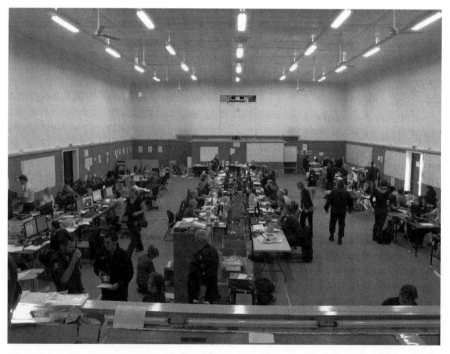

Fig. 9.23 Information Centre at Burnham Military Camp following the Christchurch earthquake (2011). (Courtesy of Karl Wilson.)

Standardisation of language, nomenclature and forms is essential. The detailed protocols governing the movement and tracking of files within and between each DVI phase is important. Bar-coding of documents to allow easy tracking and accountability can be useful. Data from the respective phases is usually digitalised and is consolidated centrally facilitating file management, data analysis and the sharing of information. Data must be protected from being lost (backed up) and from unauthorised access.

DVI and the people

The success of a DVI operation is fundamentally dependent on the people leading, managing and working within the operation. DVI situations are typically subject to significant local, national and international public and political interest and scrutiny. It is essential, therefore, that there is a clearly defined organisational structure that details command and control responsibilities. This ensures that operational activities are conducted in an orderly and coordinated way, it facilitates the passage of reliable and timely information, and creates and maintains an environment where the contributors can complete their tasks with minimal interference and distraction.

Forensic odontology team organisation

There are several forensic odontology DVI organisational structures that can be applied to a DVI operation, all of which are based around a coordinated team of practitioners with leadership in each phase (section).

The DVI odontology team is usually headed by the coordinating or lead forensic odontologist who takes overall responsibility for the odontology effort and who provides the interface with the various phase leaders and command elements in the wider DVI operation. The coordinating forensic odontologist is responsible for assigning or sub-delegating responsibilities to 'odontology phase leaders' who are tasked with leading and managing a specific phase with an emphasis on the maintenance of quality control and a focus on the task at hand.

Responsibilities

The key responsibilities of the forensic odontology leadership group are interrelated and require compliance with standardised operating procedures, effective communication and operational management as summarised below.

The forensic odontology coordinator is responsible for the overall coordination of odontology personnel and resources, and the provision of odontology identification reports to the Identification Board. The forensic odontology coordinator tasks include:
- Personnel selection and their respective phase deployment.
- Authorising operational protocols and procedures.
- The development and maintenance of an operational timetable.
- Maintaining communication and the flow of information to, and between, the forensic odontology staff in all phases.

- Providing specialist advice and technical support to the odontology team.
- Liaison and communication with the DVI command elements (at the appropriate level) and leadership, between the coordinators of the other disciplines, and with the coroner.
- The final review of reconciliation reports prior to submission to the Identification Board.
- The health and welfare of the odontology personnel, including oversight of matters relating to occupational safety and health.
- Reporting to operational authorities.
- As necessary, liaison with other relevant agencies and organisations.

The ante-mortem odontology phase leader is responsible for the completion of composite ante-mortem odontology records for the missing persons. They are also responsible for the operational management of odontology personnel deployed to the ante-mortem section, the application of standard operating procedures and protocols and the maintenance of best-practice standards. The ante-mortem odontology phase leader provides liaison within the ante-mortem section as a whole, liaison (as necessary) with other odontology phase leaders and with those practitioners providing ante-mortem records.

The post-mortem odontology phase leader is responsible for obtaining complete and accurate post-mortem odontology records for each set of remains. They are also responsible for the operational management of odontology personnel deployed to the post-mortem section, the application of standard operating procedures and protocols (including permissions regarding the resection of remains), the occupational safety and health of the odontology personnel and the maintenance of best-practice standards. The post-mortem odontology phase leader manages the timing and duration of work shifts, including breaks for meals and rest. They provide liaison with the other post-mortem disciplines, the mortuary management group and liaison (as necessary) with the other odontology phase leaders.

The odontology reconciliation phase leader is responsible for searching and comparison of the ante-mortem and post-mortem composite odontology charts to identify likely matches, and then the reconciliation analysis of matches including the development of 'identification reports and statements'. They are also responsible for the operational management of odontology personnel deployed to the reconciliation section, the application of standard operating procedures and protocols and the maintenance of best-practice standards. The odontology reconciliation phase leader liaises with the forensic odontology coordinator for the final review of reconciliation reports prior to submission to the Identification Board. The odontology reconciliation phase leader liaises with other disciplines in the reconciliation section to ensure any reconciliation inconsistencies are addressed and agreements are reached. They also actively communicate with the other odontology phase leaders to ensure that the odontology ante-mortem, post-mortem and site information is presented in a form and in a manner that facilitates the reconciliation process and to clarify any issues or ambiguities with this information.

References

1 INTERPOL Disaster Victim Identification [Internet]. [Place unknown]: INTERPOL (2014) Available from: http://www.interpol.int/INTERPOL–expertise/Forensics. Accessed August 2015.

2 INTERPOL Disaster Victim Identification Guide, [Internet]. [Place unknown]: INTERPOL (2009) Available from: http://www.interpol.int/INTERPOL–expertise/Forensics. Accessed August 2015.

3 Bruce-Chwatt RM. (2010) A brief history of forensic odontology since 1775. *Journal of Forensic and Legal Medicine* **17**, 127–130.

4 Solheim T, Lorentsen M, Sundnes PK et al. (1992) The 'Scandinavian Star' ferry disaster 1990– a challenge for forensic odontology. *International Journal of Legal Medicine* **104**, 339–345.

5 Botha CT. (1986) The dental identification of fire victims. *Journal of Forensic Odontostomatology* **4**, 67–75.

6 Griffiths CJ, Bellamy GD. (1993) Protection and radiography of heat affected teeth. *Forensic Science International* **60**, 57–60.

7 Hill AJ, Lain R, Hewson I. (2011) Preservation of dental evidence following exposure to high temperatures. *Forensic Science International* **205**, 40–43.

8 Hill AJ, Hewson I, Lain R. (2011) The role of the forensic odontologist in disaster victim identification: lessons for management. *Forensic Science International* **205**, 44–47.

9 Bassed RB, Leditschke J. (2011) Forensic medical lessons learned from the Victorian Bushfire Disaster: Recommendations from the Phase 5 debrief. *Forensic Science International* **205**, 73–76.

10 Pittayapat P, Jacobs R, De Valck E et al. (2012) Forensic odontology in the disaster victim identification process. *Journal of Forensic Odontostomatology* **30**, 1–12.

11 Berketa JW, James H, Lake AW. (2011) Forensic odontology involvement in disaster victim identification. *Forensic Science, Medicine and Pathology* **8**, 148–152.

12 Berketa JW. (2014) Maximizing postmortem oral–facial data to assist identification following severe incineration. *Forensic Science, Medicine and Pathology* **10**, 208–216.

13 Meyer HJ, Chansue N, Monticelli F. (2006) Implantation of radiofrequency identification device (RFID) microchip in disaster victim identification (DVI). *Forensic Science International* **157**, 168–171.

14 Hinchliffe J. (2011) Forensic odontology, part 2. Major disasters. *British Dental Journal* **210**, 269–274.

15 Coronial Services of New Zealand. (2014) Inquiry into the deaths of Dr Tamara Cvetanova and others. [Internet]. New Zealand: Coronial Services of New Zealand. Available from: http://www.justice.govt.nz/courts/coroners-court/christchurch/ctv. Accessed August 2015.

16 Prinz A, Carracedo WR, Mayr N et al. (2007) DNA Commission of the International Society for Forensic Genetics (ISFG): recommendations regarding the role of forensic genetics for disaster victim identification (DVI). *Forensic Science International: Genetics* **1**, 3–12.

CHAPTER 10

Forensic anthropology

Denise Donlon[1], Russell Lain[2] and Jane A. Taylor[3]

[1] *Discipline of Anatomy and Histology, University of Sydney, Australia*
[2] *Oral Surgery and Diagnostic Imaging Department, Sydney Dental Hospital, Australia*
[3] *Faculty of Health and Medicine, University of Newcastle, Australia*

The scope of forensic anthropology

This chapter is not intended to be an instruction manual for the practice of forensic anthropology, but rather an overview of the fundamentals of the discipline along with a discussion of the state of the art with a list of useful references. A chapter on forensic anthropology is included because of the cross-over between the disciplines of anthropology and odontology in a forensic setting. Both disciplines have an interest in the skull and dentition and both aim for the identification of remains from bones and/or teeth.

Forensic anthropology is the study of skeletal remains for medico-legal purposes and particularly for the identification of unknown individuals. Forensic anthropologists are trained in anatomy and/or anthropology and often in archaeological techniques for the recovery of remains. They work with skeletonised, decomposed, burnt and dismembered remains, rather than fleshed remains, which are the domain of the forensic pathologist. While their main function is in the production of a biological profile, they also assist with assessing post-mortem interval and trauma.

This chapter will give an overview of the assessment of features important in the production of a biological profile, such as the assessment of ancestry, sex and age of skeletal remains. In addition we discuss the problem of confusion of non-human with human bones and teeth and make suggestions on how to help resolve this confusion. It is not uncommon for bones of non-forensic interest to come our way, and so we will also discuss the identification of historic indigenous and non-indigenous remains and remains from historical military conflicts.

Assessment of ancestry

The term 'ancestry' will be used in this chapter rather than 'race'. The concept of race may be useful in some instances, but is not biologically valid, and is an outdated concept to geneticists and most anthropologists. The majority of alleles

---

Forensic Odontology: Principles and Practice, First Edition. Edited by Jane A. Taylor and Jules A. Kieser.
© 2016 John Wiley & Sons, Ltd. Published 2016 by John Wiley & Sons, Ltd.

have worldwide distribution and variation is clinal; that is, 'races' blend into each other, although there is some clustering of alleles according to geography. As physical variation develops as an adaptive response to wide-ranging and varied environments, people tend to view their own variation not as clinal, but as part of a discrete group. They identify as part of a group, and thus the idea of ancestry may be a useful concept to the forensic anthropologist and to police for investigative purposes.

As this book is principally directed at odontologists, the discussion of assessment of ancestry will be limited to the skull. This is appropriate, as most of the defining features of ancestry are in fact found in the skull.

Worldwide ancestral groups were traditionally known as Caucasoid, Australoid, Mongoloid, Polynesian, Melanesian and Negroid. Methods for identification of the major population groups in the region (indigenous and non-indigenous) are summarised and the difficulty of their application discussed by Littleton and Kinaston [1]. The terminology used to discuss ancestry varies and descriptions of so-called major racial groups have become outdated and replaced by descriptions of people as originating from particular geographic regions. This section will focus on Australia, Oceania and South East Asia, and in the Australian and New Zealand context European may be used instead of Caucasoid, Aboriginal used instead of Australoid and Asian instead of Mongoloid.

Importance of assessment of ancestry

In forensic casework the assessment of ancestry may be important in order to eliminate a large percentage of missing persons from an investigation. The assessment of ancestry is also important in order to allow appropriate management of remains, as it has implications for whoever takes responsibility for the body. An example may be when skeletal remains are Aboriginal and prehistoric or historical (Aboriginal or non-Aboriginal), in which case they are managed by the relevant heritage body, or alternatively they may be recent suspicious coronial cases. Historically, coroners have not been concerned about possible criminal involvement in a death if the post-mortem interval is greater than 70 years. Additionally, methods used to assess sex and age are often dependent on assessment of ancestry and the concept of ancestry is very important for timely separation of people in mass disasters. Individuals of mixed ancestry may identify with more than one group. They may display features of one ancestry more than another and this may not necessarily be the group with which they identify. This is sometimes the case with those who identify as indigenous. It is important, therefore, that features indicating different ancestries, however minor, are described.

Approaches

There are two main approaches to the assessment of ancestry from the skull: morphologic and metric. Morphologic methods involve observation of the shape and development of features of the skull. Areas of particular interest are the overall

European	Asian	Aboriginal

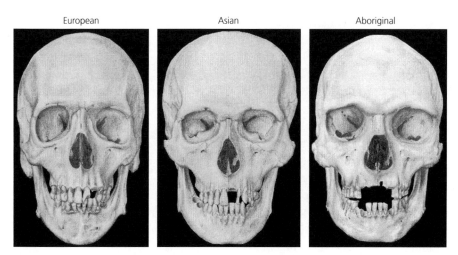

Fig. 10.1 Illustrations of European, Asian and Aboriginal skulls.

shape of the cranial vault, the flatness of the frontal bone, the shape of the eye sockets, the degree of development of the supra-orbital region, the prominence of the inter-orbital area, the breadth of the nasal aperture, the sharpness of the lower border of the nasal aperture, the degree of prognathism, prominence of zygomatic arches, robustness of mandible, development of the chin and dental arch shape [2]. There are also differences due to cultural activities, such as the presence of tooth avulsion and severe dental attrition in pre-contact Australian Aboriginals. Assessing ancestry this way is fast and accurate (85–90%) for those who are experienced in this method, but it is somewhat subjective. These features are illustrated in Fig. 10.1.

Metric methods usually use a combination of measurements of the cranium and involve discriminant functions [3–6]. Discriminant function analysis is a statistical method of classification that assigns individuals to a group. The multiple regression equations used in discriminant function analysis are derived from groups of known sex and ancestry. CRANID and FORDISC are two computer programs that give the probability of an unknown cranium belonging to a group in the database. CRANID (osteoware.si.edu) assesses a skull's probable biological ancestry. FORDISC 3.1 is an interactive computer program that runs under Windows for classifying adults by ancestry and sex using any combination of standard measurements (http://fac.utk.edu/fordisc.htm). The Forensic Anthropology Data Bank provides the database for FORDISC so that up-to-date ancestry, sex and stature estimation criteria are available from over 2000 skeletal cases.

Tooth size and non-metric traits

In Australian Aboriginals the length and breadth of the tooth crowns of deciduous and permanent teeth exceed those of European and Asian groups [7–9]. There are also differences between the size of teeth in Europeans and Asians from the Sydney region, as shown by discriminant function analysis [10].

Shovel-shaped incisors are probably the most useful dental morphological variant in assessment of ancestry, and their frequency may be as high as 100% in Asians and as low as 1% in Europeans [11, 12]. Winged incisors are also more common in Asians [13]. Carabelli's cusp, an additional cusp on the lingual surface of the first and sometimes second upper molar, has the highest frequency in populations of north-western European origin [14].

There is a need for further study of ancestry. Australia and neighbouring regions contain very diverse groups of people whose skeletons show regional variation in sex, age and stature and there are increasing percentages of mixed ancestry. A mass disaster, such as an aircraft accident, will most likely result in increased diversity of ancestry of the remains.

Assessment of sex

In biological and forensic anthropology the term 'sex' rather than 'gender' is used. Sex refers to the biological and physiological characteristics that define men and women, whereas gender refers to the socially constructed roles, behaviours, activities and attributes that a given society considers appropriate for men and women.

Sexual dimorphism is the systematic difference in form (including bone and dental morphology and size) between individuals of different sex in the same species. Bone growth is both genetically and hormonally controlled. The production of sex hormones increases around puberty, resulting in sexually dimorphic skeletal characteristics. When it comes to size, the degree of sexual dimorphism in humans is quite small – approximately 10% – which is less than that observed in most other primates. Morphologic features, especially those in the pelvis, are often the most reliable to use for assessment of sex.

There are a number of possible errors associated with the assessment of sex from a skeleton. There are effects of variation due to ancestry, thus methods should be population specific. Diet and lifestyle factors, such as activity levels, can affect sexual dimorphism as can random individual maturation. To be forensically valuable any method used should be at least 75% accurate. Depending on the types of bones present, identification should be possible in 80–90% of cases. When reporting conclusions, it is preferable to use a number of categories, such as definitely female, possible female, indeterminate, possible male and definitely male, rather than just male, female or undetermined.

Approaches

The pelvis is the most reliable part of the skeleton for assessing sex due to its obstetric function in females. There are a number of morphological differences related to this obstetric function. In the female pelvis the height is lower, the relative breadth greater and the subpubic angle is greater than in the male (Fig. 10.2).

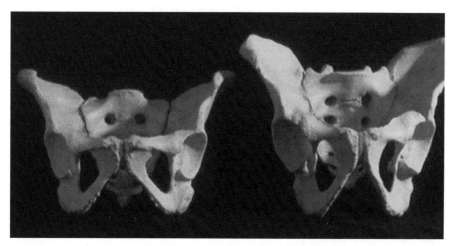

Fig. 10.2 Female (left) and male (right) pelves.

In the female a ventral arc is often present, as is a broader greater sciatic notch and a deep preauricular sulcus. The Phenice method uses a single hip bone (also called innominate bone or os coxa) to assess sex. It uses three features: ventral arc, sub-pubic concavity and medial aspect of the ischio-pubic ramus. If one of these criteria is ambiguous it is disregarded. The accuracy of this method is 96–100% in adults [15]. In females, parturition pits may be located on the dorsal surface of the pubis just lateral to the pubic symphysis. These pits are never present in males, but they may be present in females who have not been pregnant, and are thought to be due to the effect of hypertrophy of ligaments on the bone surface [16].

Metric methods include the ischio-pubic index and again the use of discriminant functions. The ischio-pubic index is useful if all that is available for analysis is a single hip bone. The index is an indication of the greater lateral growth of the pubis. The formula for ischio-pubic index is given here:

$$\text{ischio-pubic index} = \text{pubis length} \times 100 \,/\, \text{ischium length}$$

In Europeans, if the index is below 90 then it indicates male, if between 90 and 95 it indicates indeterminate sex and if over 95 it indicates a female. The index is usually 15% higher in females, regardless of the ancestry. This is because the overall size of the pelvis differs from one population to another. For example, Australian Aboriginals have narrow pelves regardless of sex.

Research has been carried out using other bones of the skeleton to assess sex and techniques may involve single measurements, indices or discriminant functions [17]. Generally, female bones are shorter and thinner with less marked bone surface features for muscle attachments, although there is a great deal of overlap in raw measurements. The proximal end of long bones is larger in males due to greater weight support, while the distal end is larger due to heavier muscle attachments. The diameter of the head of the femur is often used; as an example, for Europeans a measurement of less than 42.5 mm indicates female, between 42.5 and 43.5 mm indicates a possible female, and between 43.5 and 46.5 mm is indeterminate and sex cannot be assigned. A measurement of between 46.5 and 47.5 mm indicates possible male and over 47.5 mm indicates male [18].

For any measurable trait, the ranges of values for males and females overlap to a greater or lesser extent. The smaller the area of overlap the more often sex can be assigned with reasonable confidence. Use of multiple discriminant function analyses minimises overlap when using several traits at a time.

When using the skull to assess sex, again both morphologic and metric methods may be used. Differences may be seen in the development of the supra-orbital ridges, flatness of the frontal bone, prominence of the glabella and the development of muscle attachments on the temporal bones, nuchal region, ramus of the mandible, external occipital protruberance and mastoid process (Fig. 10.3). These features have been shown to be 80% accurate in assessing sex of unknown skulls [17, 18].

Discriminant function analyses have been devised for skulls by Giles [19], and Giles and Elliot [20] produced discriminant function analyses for sex estimation in American Whites and American Blacks (using old terminology). FORDISC and

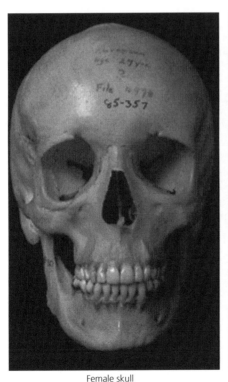 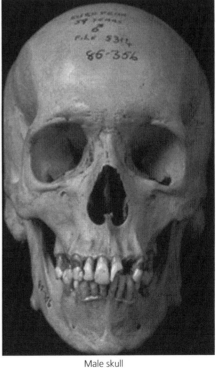

Female skull   Male skull

Fig. 10.3 Male and female skulls.

CRANID can be utilised for populations with greater variability. For Australian Aboriginal skulls, a method using a combination of morphology and measurements was produced by Larnach and Freedman [21].

Sexual dimorphism in the dentition

There is a small but significant degree of sexual dimorphism in the size of the permanent dentition. Multivariate analysis is the most useful tool to differentiate between male and female. The most commonly taken measurements are the bucco-lingual diameter and mesio-distal diameter. The absolute size differences are very small (0.4–0.5 mm) so measurement error is an important factor to consider. Children over the age of 6 years most commonly have a mixture of deciduous and permanent teeth. Measurements of a combination of permanent and deciduous dentition produced discriminant functions that were 76–90% accurate [22]. Few studies have been undertaken using deciduous teeth only. A study of cusp sizes in deciduous teeth of Australian children found significant sex differences in the metric crown traits of the deciduous canines and molars, and the accuracy of sex determination was between 70.2% and 74.8%, when using all parameters or mandibular parameters [23].

Sexual dimorphism in juveniles

Sex assessment in juvenile skeletons is extremely difficult. Few collections of juveniles of known sex exist. One is the Spitalfields collection of the London Natural History Museum. In this collection there are 37 males and 24 females of documented age and sex, which have been dated to the seventeenth century and range in age from birth to 5 years. Schutkowski [24] found three characteristics to be fairly reliable for assessing sex: the depth of the greater sciatic notch, the 'arch' criterion and the curvature of the iliac crest. The reliability of this work, however, has not been established, as the results have not been able to be repeated.

Fazekas and Kosa [25] used two measurements to assess sex in foetal skeletons, but their method correctly assigned only 70% of skeletons on a collection of known sex from Czechoslovakia. Weaver [26] found a non-metric feature, termed auricular surface elevation, to accurately assign 75% of female and 92% of male skeletons, although it was more useful for foetal rather than neonatal or infant skeletons.

Research into sexual dimorphism has been conducted on most bones in the skeleton. The product of such research may be especially useful in Disaster Victim Identification (DVI), where isolated body parts or bones may be all that is present to analyse; although many methods use North American population samples and thus may have limited application to other groups. As stated previously, reference samples should be from the same population group as the case study, which is difficult in many countries where skeletal collections of the population do not exist. The use of computed tomography (CT) scans may remedy this problem in the future. The use of nuclear deoxyribonucleic acid (DNA) is often the only method for sex assessment of juvenile skeletons.

Assessment of age

Age estimation of the skeleton is best achieved by examination of the complete skeleton, but this section will focus on the skull. Methods of ageing may be divided into those applied to juveniles and young adults (<30 years) and those applied to older adults (>30 years). Methods of ageing juveniles and young adults are based on development and growth, which is largely under genetic control, while methods for middle-aged and older adults are mainly based on degenerative changes.

Methods of ageing juvenile and young adults (<30 years)

Methodologies include age estimation from the dentition (not discussed in this section), studies of epiphyseal union and diaphyseal length measurements. Epiphyseal fusion is most useful in adolescents, especially between ten and 20 years of age, as many epiphyses fuse with the diaphysis at or around puberty. The timing of epiphyseal union does not differ significantly between people of different ancestries. On average, epiphyseal union in females tends to occur two years in advance of males. There is a range of four years between the completion of fusion in early maturers and completion in late maturers. The medial end of the clavicle is particularly useful in age estimation as it is the last epiphysis to fuse. Fusion begins around 16 to 21 years, and completion of fusion does not usually take place until 30 years of age. One cranial suture – the basilar suture or spheno-occipital synchrondrosis – is a particularly useful feature in adolescents as it closes at 14 to 16 years of age.

Diaphyseal length measurements are useful from before birth to mid-adolescence. Only the diaphysis is measured, not the epiphyses. In contrast to epiphyseal fusion, growth rates, as measured by diaphyseal length, vary between people of different ancestry and between sexes.

In foetal or neonatal skeletons, age is best estimated from the length of the long bones of the limbs and the appearance of specific bone ossification centres. The best reference source is Fazekas and Kosa [25].

In the juvenile post-cranial skeleton, the best age-estimation methods utilise the lengths of the long bones of the limbs and the stages of fusion of the bone epiphyses. Standard references include Kosa [27], Scheuer et al. [28] and Scheuer and Black [29].

Ageing of middle-aged to older adults (>30 years)

The primary methods of age estimation in the adult relate to morphologic changes in the pelvis, particularly the pubic symphysis. A number of methods have been proposed [30–33] and exemplar casts for the Suchey–Brooks method are widely used. Other methods include the sacroiliac articulations [34], the bone/cartilage interface (costochondral junction) of the ribs [35, 36] and in cranial sutures [37]. Osteoarthritis becomes apparent in older individuals, but it does not allow for the accurate ageing of a skeleton [38].

Apart from the basilar suture, the remainder of the sutures of the skull commence fusion anywhere between 25 and 40 years. Sutural closure is extremely variable; however, endocranial fusion is more reliable than ectocranial fusion. A recent method proposed by Meindl and Lovejoy [37] has been found to be of some value. This method scores the stage of closure of ten sites; lateral, anterior and ectocranial vault sites. Mann and colleagues [39] have offered the four maxillary sutures; incisive, interpalatine, intermaxillary and palatomaxillary, and their rates of closure as reliable age estimators.

A recent Australian study evaluated the Suchey–Brooks method of age estimation in a European Australian subpopulation of known age using CT of the pubic symphyseal surface [40]. The accuracy of age estimations was 63.9% of males and 69.7% of females correctly classified.

Chronological age – how old we are – rarely corresponds to our physiological age, which is how old our bodies appear due to wear and tear and diet. Thus some bones may age faster than others. No method is close to 100% accurate, and good forensic practice is to always provide a range (e.g. ±5 or ±10 or ±20 years of age). The older the skeleton, the wider the range will be, for instance for an adult age estimation sources of uncertainty will mean including an interval in the order of plus or minus five to 20 years. Providing a wide range for age estimation can be vital in any investigation so as not to erroneously exclude an individual from the investigation.

Comparative anatomy

The need to discriminate between human and non-human bones and teeth in a forensic situation is not a trivial one. The percentage of non-human bones mistaken for human bones reaching mortuaries averages 50% [41]. At the World Trade Centre in New York in 2001 over 2000 non-human bones were identified [42]. Thus significant time and resources of both police and anthropologists are spent on identifying and managing such bones. The bones most commonly confused with human bones in Australia are those of sheep and macropods (wallaby and kangaroo) (Fig. 10.4). Many of these animal bones not only are of comparable dimensions to human bones, but also are widespread throughout the country. Chicken bones, specifically the femur, can be mistaken for the bones of children by the untrained. The chicken, of course, is a mature animal when prepared for human consumption, so the femur exhibits epiphyseal fusion which would not be present in a child of comparable size.

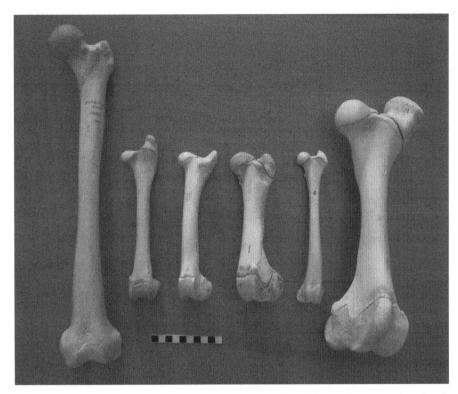

Fig. 10.4 Human, kangaroo, sheep, pig, dog, cow femora (from left to right). (Reproduced with permission from Dr S Croker.) (*See insert for colour representation of the figure.*)

Teeth and fragments of teeth may be recovered from disaster scenes or crime scenes, where it is important to differentiate human from animal teeth. Human teeth are basically a generalised design, reflecting the omnivorous diet of humans. Animal teeth have evolved into more specialised forms and arrangements, reflecting omnivory (as in the pig), carnivory (as in canids) or piscivory (as in seals). There are differences in the dental formula, with eutherian or placental mammals as well as metatherian or marsupial mammals having multiple incisor teeth and different numbers of molar teeth in upper and lower jaws. There are obvious differences in tooth form related to tooth function, and differentiation of most teeth as human or non-human is readily achievable. Some teeth are distinctive, such as the blade like arrangement of carnassial teeth in canids (dogs and dingoes) or the continuously erupting incisor of the macropods. The animals that graze on grasses, which contain abrasive silica, have high crowned or hypsodont teeth to allow for wear. Humans have low crowned or brachydont teeth.

Animal teeth likely to be found in the Australian context that could be confused with human teeth are cattle incisors, pig molars and burnt teeth where only the root or shattered crown remains [43]. The deciduous incisors of cattle are not unlike human teeth, but have a more flared crown tapering to a narrow root. Cattle permanent incisors are larger than human incisors and tend to exhibit significant wear. Both of these are mandibular incisors – animals with horns do not have maxillary incisors. The pig molar is longer mesiodistally than a human molar and has multiple low rounded cusps and an opaque colour.

There are differences in the microstructure of human teeth and the teeth of fauna likely to be found in association with human remains in South East Asia, Australia and Oceania. It should be noted that the anthropoid apes, such as the gibbon and orangutan found in Asia, have the same dental formula as humans, the same Dryopithecus pattern on mandibular first molars of three buccal cusps separated by a Y-shaped fissure and two lingual cusps, and even the same tendency, albeit much less frequent, of impacted third molars. There are of course significant size differences, although if presented with individual teeth there could be initial confusion.

Microstructural differences are also detectable under relatively low-power light microscopy; for example, marsupials (with the exception of the wombat) have tubular enamel rather than the prismatic enamel of humans. In the practicality of the DVI or casework identification process, however, teeth and bones are assessed at the macroscopic level. An additional consideration is that frequently anthropologists and odontologists do not deal with perfect exemplars. An extra difficulty can be added in cases of severe incineration, particularly where the remains have smouldered in embers for many days before recovery. Such a situation occurred in the Black Saturday bushfires in Victoria, Australia in 2009. Some victims of these fires perished in close proximity to family members and with their pets, leading to considerable commingling of remains. Differentiation between human and animal remains can be challenging, but is extremely important. The mandible of a medium-sized canid is not unlike that of a child. The canid mandible has a distinctive distally projecting angular process, but this was commonly found to be burnt away. The molar roots of canids resemble human deciduous molar roots, with a larger pulp chamber and different root form. This again was found to be altered by prolonged burning, and in combination with the loss of distinctive canid crown structure and the charring of the remains created difficulties in differentiating human and canid [43].

Apart from day-to-day casework, practitioners need to be prepared for quick elimination of non-human bones in a disaster situation. There are few large comparative anatomy collections in Australia and also few books or guides particularly for the Australian range of non-human taxa. There is a need to build comparative collections for use in mortuaries. Useful guides that include marsupials and some introduced animals include Wood-Jones [44], Merrilees and Porter [45], Triggs [46] and Oxenham and Barwick [47]. There are also books solely devoted to either European animals [48–50] or North American animals [51–53]. Additional research into testable methods for elimination of non-human bones from casework is also necessary.

Many of the differences between human and non-human bones have been summarised by Croker [54, 55]. If a bone is complete, or at least still has an epiphysis attached, then external morphological methods may be used with a high success rate. These are well described in the books and guides mentioned above. Difficulties may of course arise with juvenile human bones and non-human limb bones with unfused epiphyses. Some success in these cases has been made with more specialised methods, such as protein radioimmunoassay [56] and serology [57]. Some preliminary studies have used radiography in the hope that differences in trabecular bone may be used to distinguish between human and non-human limb bones [58, 59].

Another area in which more research is needed is in the examination of microscopic differences between human and non-human bone [60]. Some differences have been found in the Haversian canals between taxa [61]. Human bone is more likely to consist entirely of Haversian systems that are very densely packed, while non-human bone is more likely to show primary osteons that are more neatly arranged. Random areas of Haversian systems are possible and are also sometimes arranged in bands in non-human bone.

Mulhern and Ubelaker [62] have found microscopic differences between human, sheep and pig bone. Plexiform structure is often seen in the cortical bone of fast-growing non-human mammals. Cuijpers [63] also found differences between human, horse and cattle bone. Cattaneo and colleagues [64] looked for and found some differences between burnt human and non-human bone. Possible differences in cortical thickness between human and non-human bones have been examined recently by Croker and colleagues using radiography [65, 66]. There is a large amount of overlap, plus variation between non-human taxa and skeletal elements, although it may be a useful method for certain elements, such as the femur.

DNA analysis has great potential for differentiating between human and non-human bone, but is currently expensive, time consuming and destructive. The cytochrome b region has been identified as a region of the mitochondrial DNA (mtDNA) genome that is highly species specific, and resistant to post-mortem degradation.

Historical remains

Anthropologists occasionally are asked to examine human remains that may have no medico-legal significance. Examples include archaeological specimens of indigenous people, historical remains of no interest to the coroner, trophy skulls, teaching/reference specimens, cadaver specimens and religious material (e.g. from the Freemasons). The legal requirements that apply to the excavation of human remains, of historical, archaeological and medico-legal significance in various jurisdictions, have been outlined [67–70].

Archaeological remains may be identified as such by radiocarbon dating, bomb pulse dating and/or osteological analysis. Associated cultural items and artefacts may also assist in such identifications. The date of some remains will always be difficult to determine, especially if they fall into that period between 200 years and 60 years before present when radiocarbon dating is not very useful.

Australian anthropologists and odontologists have worked together in the recovery of military personnel missing in action (MIA), particularly in the areas such as Papua New Guinea, Indonesia, Vietnam, Malaysia, East and West Timor and France. Chapter 9 describes the elements of DVI from the civilian perspective. Anthropology plays a role in contemporary civilian DVI, but a much greater role in historical military identification. Recovery of MIAs can be regarded as a DVI operation spread over many scenes and an extended time scale. The same legal and operational principles apply and the same social drivers of restoring identity to deceased persons and returning remains to families hold.

However, there are some significant differences. Apart from the anthropological aspects, there is the issue of uncertainty over the actual location of the scene, due to the passage of time, loss of maps and inaccuracy of old maps due to the change in the earth's magnetic field in the 70 years since the end of the Second World War. There is a requirement for historians and researchers with an understanding of military processes to be part of the team, and also the sometimes confounding role of informants in the form of former soldiers of either side or local villagers, who are invariably very old and have faulty or embellished memories. There are issues of varying social status among informants, with more credence possibly given to the memory of those of higher status. The scene needs to be managed by an archaeologist to determine the extent of any grave(s) to ensure maximal recovery of remains and artefacts, and the DVI team needs to be aware of the possibility of unexploded ordnance associated with any remains. There is also a different importance given to property in these recoveries. Property is only a secondary identifier in civilian DVI and identification processes, but the presence of military equipment, uniforms, weapons, unit and rank insignia associated with remains carries more importance and identifying weight in a historical military recovery process.

In terms of the anthropology and odontology in these situations, the odontologist needs to be familiar with historical civilian and military restorative materials and techniques, both for the Australian soldiers for which the team has responsibility, and for the enemy soldiers or local civilians whose remains may be present. Some knowledge of local fauna and their dentition is required. The anthropologist will be dealing with bone fragments and/or poorly preserved and commingled remains. The assessment of ancestry between European, Asian and Melanesian in this situation is challenging and not always possible.

Following are two examples of recovery and identification of the war dead in order to illustrate the work of the forensic anthropologist.

In November 1941, just before the Japanese bombing of Pearl Harbour, the Australian cruiser HMAS Sydney was lost after a battle with the German raider

HSK Kormoran and there were no survivors of the crew of 645 men. Eleven weeks later a life raft containing one deceased person was recovered from waters off Christmas Island, 2500 kilometres from the site of the sinking. The body was examined, presumed to be a sailor from HMAS Sydney and buried. The location of the grave was lost.

In 2006 a team led by a Naval officer and consisting of an anthropologist, an archaeologist and two odontologists located the skeletal remains of a man suspected to be the unknown sailor from HMAS Sydney. The entire skeleton was present, although parts were fragmented as a result of post-mortem damage. A small piece of shrapnel was embedded in the left side of the frontal bone. All teeth were present with the exception of the maxillary right lateral incisor and the mandibular left first molar. Both teeth had been lost ante-mortem with the space closed. Numerous restorations in both amalgam and gold were present. The anterior teeth were somewhat misaligned with a midline shift and anterior open bite – a distinctive dentition. Slight shovelling (stage 2 in Turner's dental morphology classification [71]) was present on the maxillary central incisors. The cranial features of sharp inferior nasal sill, round/oval shaped eye sockets, moderately prominent glabella, narrow nasal aperture, narrow and prominent nasal bones, prominent nasal spine, long face, narrow rami of mandible, prominent mental eminence and obtuse inside angle of the mandible at the gonial region suggested the skeletal remains were European. Sex assessment was based primarily from the shape of the pelvis, which exhibited male characteristics of a very small pre-auricular sulcus, and a small subpubic angle, although the greater sciatic notch was broad. The vertical diameter of the head of the right femur was 49 mm, and the maximum diameter of the right humeral head was 50 mm, which both indicated a male. In addition, the skull showed male features of a deep palate, large mastoid processes, moderately prominent glabella, well-developed zygomatic tuberosities and a square chin.

Age was assessed using fusion of the epiphyses of the bones, the condition of the pubic symphyses, auricular region of the innominate and the sternal end of a rib. An age range of 22 to 31 years was indicated by the age-related changes in the skeleton. The distal end of the radius, proximal tibia, acromion of the scapula and the iliac crest were all fused, indicating an age of equal to or over 22 years. The medial end of the right clavicle displayed a well-defined fusing flake indicating an age of between 23 and 31 years. The condition of both left and right pubic symphyses was classified as Phase II (early stage) of the Suchey–Brooks method [34] indicating an age range of 24 to 30 years. This man had a long narrow face with a prominent chin and would have been missing his upper right lateral incisor when he enlisted in the Navy. A smiling photograph may show both these facial features as well as his distinctive dentition. Unfortunately the skeleton has yet to be identified despite attempts to match DNA with possible relatives.

Different challenges were presented in an operation to recover the skeletal remains of two Australian MIAs from the Vietnam War. The location was

Nui Gang Toi, Dong Nai Province in Vietnam. The site was actually located and partially excavated by Vietnam veterans, some of whom had fought in the area. As a result there was unfortunately some commingling of the bones and especially the teeth. The recovery team was led by the Australian Army and consisted of an anthropologist, archaeologist and two odontologists. Both skeletons, described as Nui Gang Toi North and Nui Gang Toi South, consisted of highly fragmented skulls, loose teeth, the shafts of the long bones of the upper and lower limbs and a small number of bones of the hands and feet and a partial clavicle. The bones were in very poor condition with roots growing through their medullary cavities and along the surfaces. These bones were heavily leached and there was extensive erosion of the bone surfaces, probably due to humic acids. In contrast, the bones of the feet were in reasonably good condition, almost certainly due to the protection given to them by the boots. There was no evidence of animal gnaw marks, cut marks or projectile marks. Ancestry assessment was difficult because of the incompleteness and poor condition of the bones, particularly the skulls. Incisor shovelling was not present in either individual, which supported the identification of these individuals as being of European Australian ancestry and not of Asian (Vietnamese) ancestry [72].

Sex assessment was made using measurements of the long bones as the pelves were not present and the skulls were very fragmented. The most useful measurement was the mid shaft circumference of the femora. Age estimation was difficult as all of the epiphyses of the long bones were missing, as were the pubic symphysis, the ribs, the auricular surface of the pelvis and the medial ends of the clavicles. The odontologists indicated that the teeth of Nui Gang Toi North suggested an age of over 16 years and Nui Gang Toi South an age of over 18 years. The size of the long bones and muscular development on the bones supported the view that they were both adult. An attempt was made to distinguish between the two individuals on the basis of the size of their bones and this was reasonably successful on the basis of femoral diameter and femoral cortical thickness. While the anthropological analysis assisted with the biological profile and the problem of commingling, the dental examination provided the identification, due to the location of Army dental records which included a bite-wing radiograph in the ante-mortem record of one MIA and a record of an acrylic partial denture that was recovered and found to be in excellent condition for the same MIA. This was supported by property in the form of the identity tags that had the names and service numbers of the missing men. Interestingly, the Vietcong fighters who had searched the bodies of the Australian soldiers in 1965 had reported that they had recovered these tags. The reconciliation of this inconsistency is an example of the skillset required for anthropologists and odontologists when dealing with historical recoveries.

The commingling of the teeth and their exfoliation from the jaws offered a similar challenge in this field case to the Black Saturday fires of 2009. The need for improved and current competency in dental anatomy was one lesson from this recovery [43].

Conclusion

The forensic odontologist is part of a team of investigators whose activities are often directed at identification of human remains. The United Nations has stated that identity is in fact a basic human right. There is a natural relationship between the forensic anthropologist and the forensic odontologist in many identification activities. It behoves aspiring odontologists to familiarise themselves with the postcranial skeleton and anthropological issues and debates in order to effectively extract the most benefit from this relationship and commonality of purpose.

References

1 Littleton J, Kinaston R. (2008) Ancestry, age, sex and stature: Identification in a diverse space. In: Oxenham M (ed.) *Forensic Approaches to Death, Disaster and Abuse*, Australian Academic Press, Brisbane, pp. 155–176.

2 Larnach SL, Macintosh NWG. (1967) The use in forensic medicine of an anthropological method for the determination of sex and race in skeletons. *Archaeology and Physical Anthropology in Oceania* **2**,156–161.

3 Giles E, Elliot O. (1962) Race identification from cranial measurements. *Journal of Forensic Sciences* **7**, 147–156.

4 Howells WW. (1973) Cranial variation in man: a study by multivariate analysis of patterns of difference among human populations. Papers of the Peabody Museum, Harvard University, **67**.

5 Wright RVS. (1992) Correlation between cranial form and geography in *Homo sapiens*: CRANID – a computer program for forensic and other applications. *Archaeology in Oceania* **27**, 128–134.

6 Jantz RL, Ousley SD. (2005) Fordisc, version 3.0: Personal Computer Forensic Discriminant Functions. University of Tennessee, Knoxville.

7 Barrett MJ, Brown T, Luke JI. (1963) Dental observations on Australian aborigines: mesio-distal crown diameters of deciduous teeth. *Australian Dental Journal* **8**, 299–302.

8 Barrett MJ, Brown T, Arato G et al. (1964) Dental observations on Australian aborigines: buccolingual crown diameters of deciduous and permanent teeth. *Australian Dental Journal* **9**, 280–285.

9 Brown T, Margetts B, Townsend GC. (1980) Comparison of mesiodistal crown diameters of the deciduous and permanent teeth in Australian Aboriginals. *Australian Dental Journal* **25**, 28–33.

10 Chui A, Donlon D. (2000) The value of dental metrics in the assessment of race and sex in Caucasoids and Mongoloids. *Dental Anthropology* **14**, 20–39.

11 Hrdlicka A. (1920) Shovel-shaped teeth. *American Journal of Physical Anthropology* **3**, 429–465.

12 Carbonell VM. (1963) Variations in the frequency of shovel-shaped incisors in different populations. In: Brothwell DR (ed.) *Dental Anthropology*, Pergamon Press, Oxford, pp. 211–234.

13 Turner CG, Swindler DR. (1978) The dentition of New Britain West Nakanai Melanesians. VIII. Peopling of the pacific. *American Journal of Physical Anthropology* **49**, 361–371.

14 Kieser J. (1984) An analysis of the Carabelli trait in the mixed deciduous and permanent human dentition. *Archives of Oral Biology* **29**, 403–406.

15 Phenice TW. (1969) A newly developed visual method for sexing the Os pubis. *American Journal of Physical Anthropology* **30**, 297–301.

16 Kelley MA. (1979) Parturition and pelvic changes. *American Journal of Physical Anthropology* **51**, 541–545.

17 Krogman WM, Iscan MY. (1986) *The Human Skeleton in Forensic Medicine*. Charles C. Thomas, Springfield.

18 Stewart TD. (1979) *Essentials of Forensic Anthropology*. Charles C. Thomas, Springfield.

19 Giles E. (1970) Discriminant function sexing of the human skeleton. In: Stewart TD (ed.) *Personal Identification in Mass Disasters*, National Museum of Natural History, Washington, pp. 99–107.

20 Giles E, Elliot O. (1963) Sex determination by discriminant function analysis of crania. *American Journal of Physical Anthropology* **21**, 53–68.

21 Larnach SL, Freedman L. (1964) Sex determination of Aboriginal crania from coastal New South Wales, Australia. *Records of the Australian Museum* **26**, 295–308.

22 De Vito C, Saunders SR. (1990) A discriminant function analysis of deciduous teeth to determine sex. *Journal of Forensic Sciences* **35**, 845–858.

23 Adler CJ, Donlon D. (2010.) Sexual dimorphism in deciduous crown traits of a European derived Australian sample. *Forensic Science International* **199**, 29–37.

24 Schutkowski H. (1993) Sex determination of infant and juvenile skeletons: 1. Morphognostic features. *American Journal of Physical Anthropology* **90**, 199–205.

25 Fazekas IG, Kosa F. (1978) *Forensic Fetal Osteology*. Akademiai Kiado, Budapest, pp. 1–287.

26 Weaver DS. (1980) Sex differences in the ilia of a known age and sex sample of fetal and infant skeletons. *American Journal of Physical Anthropology* **52**, 191–195.

27 Kosa F. (1989) Age estimation from the fetal skeleton. In: Iscan Y (ed.) *Age Markers in the Human Skeleton*, Charles C Thomas, Springfield, pp. 21–54.

28 Scheuer L, Musgrave JH, Evans SP. (1980) The estimation of late fetal and perinatal age from limb bone length by linear and logarithmic regression. *Annals of Human Biology* **7**, 257–265.

29 Scheuer L, Black S. (2000) *Developmental Juvenile Osteology*. Academic Press, New York.

30 Todd TW. (1920) Age changes in the pubic bone: I. The male white pubis. *American Journal of Physical Anthropology* **3**, 285–334.

31 McKern TW, Stewart TD. (1957) Skeletal age changes in young American males. Quartermaster Research and Development Centre, US Army Natick MA. Technical Report No EP–45.

32 Gilbert BM, McKern TW. (1973) A method for ageing the female os pubis. *American Journal of Physical Anthropology* **38**, 31–38.

33 Brooks S, Suchey JM. (1990) Skeletal age determination based on the os pubis: a comparison of the Acsadi–Nemeskeri and Suchey–Brooks methods. *Human Evolution* **5**, 227–238.

34 Lovejoy CO, Meindl RS, Pryzbeck TR et al. (1985) Chronological metamorphosis of the auricular surface of the ilium: a new method for the determination of age at death. *American Journal of Physical Anthropology* **68**, 47–56.

35 Iscan MY, Loth SR, Wright RK. (1984) Age estimation from the rib by phase analysis: white males. *Journal of Forensic Sciences* **29**, 1094–1194.

36 Iscan MY, Loth SR, Wright RK. (1985) Age estimation from the rib by phase analysis: white females. *Journal of Forensic Sciences* **30**, 853–863.

37 Meindl RS, Lovejoy CO. (1985) Ectocranial suture closure: a revised method for the determination of skeletal age at death and blind tests of its accuracy. *American Journal of Physical Anthropology* **68**, 57–66.

38 Stewart TD. (1958) Rate of development of osteoarthritis in American Whites and its significance in skeletal age identification. *Leech* **28**, 144–151.

39 Mann RW, Symes SA, Bass WM. (1987) Maxillary suture obliteration: Aging the human skeleton based on intact or fragmentary maxilla. *Journal of Forensic Sciences* **32**, 148–157.

40 Lottering N, MacGregor DM, Meredith M et al. (2013) Evaluation of the Suchey–Brooks method of age estimation in an Australian subpopulation using computed tomography of the pubic symphyseal surface. *American Journal of Physical Anthropology* **150**, 386–399.

41 Donlon D, Croker S. (2013) A 20 year review of anthropological casework involving non–human bones in an Australian forensic setting. Australasian Society of Human Biology Conference, Sydney.

42 Mundorff A. (2009) Human identification following the World Trade Center disaster: Assessing management practices for highly fragmented and commingled human remains. PhD thesis, Simon Fraser University.

43 Lain R, Taylor J, Croker S et al. (2011) Comparative dental anatomy in Disaster Victim Identification: Lessons from the 2009 Victorian Bushfires. *Forensic Science International* **205**, 36–39.

44 Wood-Jones F. (1923) *The Ancestry of Man: Man's Place Among the Primates*. Gillies, Brisbane.

45 Merrilees D, Porter JK. (1979) Guide to the identification of teeth and some bones of native land mammals occurring in the extreme south west of Western Australia. Western Australian Museum.

46 Triggs B. (1996) *Tracks, Scats and Other Traces: A Field Guide to Australian Mammals*. Oxford University Press, Melbourne.

47 Oxenham M, Barwick R. (2008) Human, sheep or kangaroo: a practical guide to identifying human skeletal remains in Australia. In: Oxenham M. (ed.) *Forensic Approaches to Death, Disaster and Abuse*, Australian Academic Press, Brisbane, pp. 63–94.

48 Cornwall IW. (1974) *Bones for the Archaeologist*. Littlehampton, London.

49 Schmid E. (1972) *Atlas of Animal Bones: for Prehistorians, Archaeologists and Quaternary Geologists*. Elsevier, Amsterdam.

50 Hillson S. (1992) *Mammal Bones and Teeth: An Introductory Guide to Methods of Identification*. Institute of Archaeology, University College London.

51 Ubelaker DH. (1989) *Human Skeletal Remains: Excavation, Analysis, Interpretation*. Taraxacum, Washington.

52 Bass WM. (2005) *Human Osteology: a Laboratory and Field Manual*. 5th edn, Missouri Archaeological Society, Columbia.

53 France DL. (2009) *Human and Nonhuman Bone Identification: A Concise Field Guide*. CRC Press, Boca Raton.

54 Croker SL. (1999) The distinction between human and non-human mammal bone: an Australian forensic perspective. Unpublished Honours thesis, University of Sydney.

55 Croker SL. (2011) Comparative cortical bone thickness in human and non–human mammal long bones: Biomechanical and forensic perspectives. PhD thesis, University of Sydney.

56 Ubelaker DH, Lowenstein JM, Hood DG. (2004) Use of a solid-phase double antibody radioimmunoassay to identify species from small skeletal fragments. *Journal of Forensic Sciences* **49**, 924–929.

57 Harsanyi L. (1993) Differential diagnosis of human and animal bone. In: Grupe G, Garland N (eds) *Histology of Ancient Human Bone: Methods and Diagnosis*, Springer, Berlin, pp. 79–94.

58 Chilvarquer I, Katz JO, Glassman DM et al. (1987) Comparative radiographic study of human and animal long–bone patterns. *Journal of Forensic Sciences* **32**, 1645–1654.

59 Robinson M. (2004) Mistaken identity: human foetal and neonate bones on forensic anthropology. Unpublished Honours thesis, University of Sydney.

60 Hillier ML, Bell LS. (2007) Differentiating human bone from animal bone: A review of histological methods. *Journal of Forensic Sciences* **52**, 294–263.

61 Owsley D, Mires AM, Keith MS. (1985) Case involving differentiation of deer and human bone fragments. *Journal of Forensic Sciences* **30**, 572–578.

62 Mulhern DM, Ubelaker DH. (2001) Differences in osteon banding between human and nonhuman bone *Journal of Forensic Sciences* **46**, 220–222.

63 Cuijpers A. (2006) Histological identification of bone fragments in archaeology: telling humans apart from horses and cattle. *International Journal of Osteoarchaeology* **16**, 465–480.

64 Cattaneo C, DiMartino S, Scali S et al. (1999) Determining the human origin of fragments of burnt bone: a comparative study of histological, immunological and DNA techniques. *Forensic Science International* **102**, 181–191.

65 Croker SL, Reed W, Donlon D. (2009) The feasibility of using radiogrammetry in comparing cortical bone thickness in human and non–human tibiae *The Radiographer* **56**, 25–31.

66 Croker SL, Clement JG, Donlon D. (2009) A comparison of cortical bone thickness in the femoral midshaft of humans and two non-human mammals. *HOMO – Journal of Comparative Human Biology* **60**, 551–565.

67 Donlon D, Littleton J. (2011) A brief history and current state of physical anthropology in Australia'. In: Marquez–Grant N, Fibiger L (eds) *The Routledge Handbook of Archaeological Human Remains and Legislation. An International Guide to Laws and Practice in the Excavation and Treatment of Archaeological Human Remains*, Routledge, Abingdon, pp. 633–646.

68 Tayles N, Halcrow S. (2011) A brief history and current state of physical anthropology in New Zealand. In: Marquez–Grant N, Fibiger L (eds) *The Routledge Handbook of Archaeological Human Remains and Legislation. An International Guide to Laws and Practice in the Excavation and Treatment of Archaeological Human Remains*, Routledge, Abingdon, pp. 647–656.

69 Halcrow S, Tayles N, Pureepatpong N et al. (2011) A brief history and current state of physical anthropology in Thailand. In: Marquez–Grant N, Fibiger L. (eds.) *The Routledge Handbook of Archaeological Human Remains and Legislation. An International Guide to Laws and Practice in the Excavation and Treatment of Archaeological Human Remains*, Routledge, Abingdon, pp. 623–632.

70 Bedford S, Regenvanu R, Spriggs, M et al. (2011) Introduction: A brief history and current state of physical anthropology in Vanuatu. In: Marquez–Grant N, Fibiger L (eds.) *The Routledge Handbook of Archaeological Human Remains and Legislation. An International Guide to Laws and Practice in the Excavation and Treatment of Archaeological Human Remains*, Routledge, Abingdon, pp. 657–670.

71 Turner CG, Nichol CR, Scott GR. (1991) Scoring Procedures for key morphological traits of the permanent dentition: The Arizona State University Dental Anthropology System. In: Kelley MA, Larsen CS (eds) *Advances in Dental Anthropology*, Wiley-Liss, New York, pp. 13–31.

72 Hillson S. (1996) *Dental Anthropology*. Cambridge University Press, Cambridge.

CHAPTER 11

Applied forensic sciences

David C. Kieser[1], Terry Lyn Eberhardt[2], Gemma Dickson[3] and J. Neil Waddell[4]

[1] Christchurch Hospital, New Zealand

[2] PestLab, AsureQuality Ltd, New Zealand

[3] Victorian Institute of Forensic Medicine, Australia

[4] Faculty of Dentistry, University of Otago, New Zealand

Introduction

The word 'forensic' comes from the Latin word *forensis*, meaning 'of or before the forum'. Forensic science is therefore the process of collecting and examining the information about past events to be used in a court of law.

The field of forensic science is a rapidly growing area, now supporting thousands of scientists worldwide. Historically, witness statements and torture were used to force confessions; however, nowadays forensic science has expanded into every facet from macroscopic crime scene analysis to microscopic genetic analysis.

The earliest known legal decision on a homicide was in 1850 BC and was written on a clay tablet. This was the case of a temple employee, who was murdered by three men who were later executed in front of the victim's house after nine witnesses testified against them. The wife of the victim also knew of the murder, but was spared from the death penalty because two witnesses told the court that her husband had abused her and that she did not take part in the murder. This case illustrates the historic reliance on witness statements that remained the keystone to legal verdicts for centuries. Nowadays, witness statements still remain integral, but not conclusive, in forensic analysis.

The use of deduction, as opposed to simple witness statements, to solve crimes can be traced back over 2000 years. For example, Archimedes (287–212 BC) used water displacement to discern that the goldsmith had diluted the density of the golden crown made for King Hiero II with elements of silver.

The first use of medicine in forensic science is recorded over 1000 years later in the book *Xi Luan Lu* (Translated 'Washing Away of Wrongs') written in 1248. Post-mortem analysis and an understanding of the effects of violence on internal organs began with Ambroise Pare (1510–1590), a French surgeon who studied the effects of violent death on internal organs. Although this advance allowed the clinician to diagnose a violent death, it failed to determine the criminal, and it

Forensic Odontology: Principles and Practice, First Edition. Edited by Jane A. Taylor and Jules A. Kieser.

was only in the 18th century that evidence-based forensic science began to evolve, with torture and forced confessions losing favour to scientific evidence in the eye of the law.

Fingerprint analysis was introduced into forensic science a century later by Sir Francis Dalton (1822–1911) in his book *Finger Prints*, where he described the rate of two individuals having the same fingerprint being 1 in 64 billion [1]. Fingerprinting has now become an integral part of forensic analysis.

More recently, forensic science has expanded, driven both by increasing demands and social interest, such as the novels about Sherlock Holmes and more recently TV series of forensic analysis. In 1984, Sir Alec Jefferys introduced DNA profiling into forensics and this has now become a mainstay of criminal and victim identification.

Forensic science now includes a multitude of avenues including computational forensics, criminalistics, archaeology, chemistry, botany, engineering, entomology, accounting, pathology, psychology, serology, toxicology, blood back-spatter analysis and of course odontology, to name a few.

Forensic odontology is an important niche of forensic science. It is important that the forensic odontology practitioner understands the scope of other forensic science disciplines and has an appreciation for the role of these disciplines should the need arise to work together during an investigation.

This chapter cannot hope to cover such a large field, but aims to introduce the topic via discussion of a few disciplines to encourage further reading in this fascinating area.

Crime scene protocols

With such high stakes not only for the suspect's future, but also closure for the victim's family and the future safety of the community, it is imperative that crime scenes are accurately reported and analysed, with minimal contamination by weather, environmental conditions, animals, civilians, medical personnel, law enforcement officers and the forensic team.

There is the chance that the crime scene may only be found after significant contamination has already occurred, which in turn may affect the accuracy of forensic analysis. An example is that of mass graves that are discovered and studied centuries after their creation. Similarly, in the acute setting with a surviving victim, medical personnel aiding the injured take priority over forensic analysis and, as such, their contamination will need to be accounted for by the forensic team.

However, once a scene is identified, it is imperative that only essential personnel enter the area and contamination is kept to a minimum.

Multiple crime scene protocols have been developed to aid investigators in the analysis of crime scenes, all of which aim to document, report and analyse the scene thoroughly and conclusively without the influence of inadvertent or deliberate contamination during the analysis.

The first step in this process is ensuring that the scene is safe, so as to ensure the safety of the investigative team. This is usually done simultaneously with securing the scene. A cordon will be placed around the scene, and ideally the larger the cordon the better, but this is limited by the location of the scene and the disruption to the community. For example, a crime in a farmhouse may allow the entire farm to be cordoned off, whereas a crime in a room of an apartment of a high-rise complex may only allow the relevant room to be cordoned off. These are decisions that need to be made early and may have dramatic implications on the outcome of the case.

Once the cordon has been established, all persons that had entered the area prior to the cordon need to be identified, so that their contamination may be traced. For example, a crime scene along a muddy path may retain the footprints of the criminal, but also those of the paramedics and police who entered the scene prior to the cordon. The police and paramedics' boots will need to be reviewed for their boot prints so that the criminal's footprints may be identified from the myriad of footprints retained in the mud.

If the scene is exposed to the environment, it needs to be protected, often with the erection of a forensic tent over the scene or suitable alternative. Again, the erection of such a structure must not contaminate the scene.

From this point forward, all personnel need to be dressed accordingly and suited to enter the scene. Not unsurprisingly there are protocols on what to wear, how to dress, how to don gloves, contain hair and apply a mask. A degree of common sense will aid the investigator in such matters provided they understand that all of these protocols are aimed at reducing contamination. It would be advisable to become familiar with the local protocols in the area of investigation.

It has been stated that a picture is worth a thousand words, and in crime scene analysis this could not be truer. Crime scene photography requires an experienced photographer, a measurement scale, a date and a time. Photographs should be taken in a systematic fashion starting from broad shots capturing the entire scene and then focusing closer and closer onto even the smallest of objects. All photographs require a perspective, which includes a measurement scale and at least two different angles of each frame. Videography is often used to aid in the three-dimensional review of the scene and should be considered standard practice. In contrast, photography adds more accurate resolution of the scene and important facets, such as blood spatter, the weapon, footprints and so on. The facets requiring specific photographic recordings should be performed in consultation with the lead crime scene analyst.

Once the scene has been photographed, it should be globally analysed by a crime scene expert. This is done in an unbiased fashion, with the expert attempting to reconstruct the event. However, this simply gives the expert a perspective, the ultimate reconstruction may take months to discern. The scene then needs to be recorded in print, paying particular attention to specifics, such as the distance from one object to the next.

Samples are then taken from the scene, starting with fluids and tissue samples, which are sent for pathological review and DNA profiling in sterile labelled containers. The body is then cloaked in an autopsy bag and transported to the morgue for a post-mortem to be performed. All samples are to be escorted, under the chain of command, to ensure that tampering of the evidence is prevented.

Fingerprinting is then performed on pertinent areas, including weapons, doors, tables and so forth. The scene is then deconstructed with non-biological samples being labelled and packaged for transport to the forensic laboratory for further testing. Photography and videography of the procedure should be considered to validate its sterility and accuracy.

Clearly, there are many facets to a crime scene investigation, and thus the American Society of Crime Laboratory Directors/Laboratory Accreditation Board (ASCLD/LAB) has attempted to develop a protocol for each one. It would be worth the interested reader and any crime scene investigator becoming familiar with these protocols.

Forensic entomology

The relationship between insects and humans is fraught with conflict as well as diverse in benefits. The focus of much of the study of entomology is based on the impact of certain insect species on the products and lifestyle of humans. Insects can have an enormous detrimental impact upon food production (e.g. crop infestation) as well as being known vectors of disease (e.g. malaria). Several benefits humans enjoy resulting from insect activity include the production of silk, beeswax and honey. The ecological role of pollination of plants and the role of food source to many species of animals are also beneficial and necessary to the continuation of life in an ecosystem. Often overlooked, however, is the vital role of insects in decomposition.

Decomposition is a naturally occurring phenomenon essential to the continued prosperity of an ecosystem. Essentially a recycling program, decomposition is responsible for the breakdown and redistribution of nutrients no longer in use by a living organism. Several species of organisms, such as bacteria, fungi, insects and vertebrate scavengers, have evolved into highly specialised facilitators of this process. Insects and their offspring have long been associated with decomposing plant and animal, including human, remains.

Carrion is an ephemeral habitat and the temporary nature of this resource results in the development of a unique, transitory invertebrate community. There are four ecological classifications pertaining to the relationship between insects and animal remains. The first is the necrophagous species, which are the insects that feed directly on the remains, predominantly the larvae of several fly species. The second classification includes both the predaceous and parasitic species. These species include insects such as ants, which feed directly on the eggs and larvae of flies on the remains, and parasitic wasps, which parasitise the same eggs and larvae. The third category is that of the omnivorous species, represented primarily by beetles, which feed on both the remains and other arthropods associated with the remains. The last category contains the adventive species, which are those insect species that use the remains simply as an extension of their natural habitat.

Insects make no distinction between human and other animal remains. The process of decomposition and the role of insects in this process have been well documented. Indeed, insects are now an integral part of death investigations and the science of forensic entomology, the application of the study of insects to legal issues, has become accepted and is considered defensible in the courts of law.

The primary use of insects as evidence is in estimating a post-mortem interval. This interval is defined as the time elapsed between the death and the discovery of the body. The time elapsed since death is one of the fundamental questions that require an answer during the investigation of a suspicious or unexplained death. Establishing this interval is crucial as it serves to focus the investigation on the correct period, and when decomposition is well advanced, insect evidence may be the only reliable method that can estimate when death occurred.

The predominant insects associated with remains are blow flies and their larvae, commonly referred to as maggots. Blow flies and other fly species frequently associated with remains have predictable life cycles and rates of development, and are capable of locating remains within minutes of death, which makes them ideal for use as indicators of when death may have occurred. The ecological niche of these species is that of a necrophagous insect responsible for the breakdown, or recycling, of remains.

The life cycle of the typical blow fly begins with a female finding a suitable substrate in which to deposit eggs or larvae (some blow flies lay live larvae instead of eggs). A suitable environment would be moist, provide protection from predators and harsh environmental conditions, and allow easy access to food. The most common areas where fly eggs or young larvae are initially found are the natural orifices of the body, which are concentrated in the head region. They may also be found in the genital region, if exposed, or near ante-mortem wounds.

Once emerging from the egg, the larvae pass through three stages called instars. For the fly species that lay live larvae, life begins as a first instar. Each larval stage is dominated by feeding behaviour. As the larvae grow and develop they almost continually feed upon the food source in which they were laid. Upon nearing the end of the third instar stage, the larvae enter into a post-feeding stage. During this time the larvae may be found migrating away from a now depleted food source in search of an appropriate site for pupariation. Once a suitable site is found, the cuticle of the larva hardens providing a protective shell, a puparium, in which the larva becomes a pupa. It is during pupariation that the morphological changes from larva to adult fly occur. The new adult fly then emerges from the puparium to search for food and a mate and the life cycle continues.

A post-mortem interval may be estimated by evaluating insect evidence in two ways. First, an estimate may be derived from the age of the fly larvae collected at the time of the discovery of the remains. Without complications such as adverse weather conditions or restriction of insect access through burial or tight wrapping of the remains, this estimate often coincides with the minimum amount of time that has elapsed since death.

In determining the minimum time elapsed based on larval age, data from several different sources must be obtained. Identification of first and second instars is often difficult, if not impossible, and a portion of these larvae needs to be reared to adulthood in the laboratory for confirmatory species identification. The remaining larvae are preserved as soon as possible and represent the age of the larvae found with the remains. Once identified to species, the appropriate species-specific development data is obtained. As the rate of development is temperature dependent, the temperatures to which the larvae and the remains were exposed must be determined. This requires the comparison of temperatures taken at the scene with those of the nearest weather station.

Through the combination of data on the identified species, weather and scene temperature data and species-specific developmental data, a retrospective calculation can now be made. This calculation provides an estimate of the time required for the larvae to develop to the age as found when they were collected from the remains. As blow flies may arrive at remains and begin laying eggs within minutes of death, determining the age of the fly larvae recovered from the remains will provide a minimum time elapsed since insect activity began, which often coincides with the elapsed time since death.

The second method of post-mortem interval estimation is based on the pattern of succession. As decomposition is a natural process, the attractiveness of the remains to different insect species changes over time. As the remains decompose and the suitability of the remains as a resource for a particular species changes over time, the dynamic interactions between insect species colonising the remains result in the development of a somewhat stable, if temporary, insect community. This results in insect species utilising the remains in a predictable order, and the post-mortem interval estimate is based on the diversity of insects recovered at the time of the body's discovery.

The collection of the variety of insects found with the remains can provide a snapshot in time of the community's development. Ample specimens must be collected to provide the consulting entomologist with a surplus of individuals to increase the chance of providing species that may be represented by only a few individuals.

Based on known successional patterns for a particular locality, an estimate of the time elapsed for a community to develop to the stage represented by the diversity of the collection, represents the estimated elapsed time since death. An increased number of species will strengthen the estimate of the post-mortem interval determined by insect succession.

This method is often used to complement post-mortem interval estimates based on the age of fly larvae. When larvae are no longer found with remains, such as during the later stages of decomposition, the pattern of succession may also be used independently.

Such an estimate, however, is only as accurate as the data upon which it is based. The natural variation found in the insect community is dependent upon climate, geographic location, season, habitat and even altitude. Although the process of decomposition is universal, the insect species associated with remains vary widely with changes in these parameters. The species that may be found also vary depending upon the deposition of the remains. For example, insect species found with buried remains or remains found indoors differ from those species found with exposed remains.

For these reasons, the use of forensic entomology as an investigative tool requires a foundation of knowledge on the life histories and habits of local insect species associated with remains. This includes developmental data for each forensically significant species as well as a succession database, based on experimental studies, that establishes the order in which insect species may be expected to colonise remains.

Insect evidence may also be valuable to an investigation in other ways. The knowledge of the biology and behaviour of these insect species may provide contextual information related to the circumstances of death. Interpreted correctly, insects may be valuable indicators of location or an association between places and persons.

Insect species may have both a temporal and spatial distribution. Some insect species are only found at a certain time of year. In temperate climates, there is an obvious increase in the number and variety of insects found during the summer months as opposed to the winter months. This can be of value during the investigation of older remains where only remnants of the insects' presence, such as pupal cases, are found. If, for example, the remnants are of those insects found only in summer, this indicates that death likely took place during the summer.

Some insect species have a worldwide distribution. These are primarily those insects associated with stored products that have been transported around the world through trade and commerce. Some fly species are synanthropic, meaning they are associated with humans and human activities, and also have a worldwide distribution. The distribution of most insect species, however, is limited by habitat. Habitat may refer to larger geographic areas, such as where host plants, in particular agricultural crops, and suitable temperatures and humidities are found. Most species will be found in different habitats based on their food source and other biological requirements. For example, some insect species require a source of water for egg laying or a particular prey species for feeding upon. The preferred habitat may also be quite localised, such as an area where several habitat features such as plants, water and food sources are found together. For example, a small clearing with a pond within a forest or even a particular height within a forest canopy may serve as the perfect habitat for some insects.

It is the distribution of the insect species found associated with remains that may provide an investigation with valuable evidence. For example, the fly species found colonising remains in a bush or forested habitat may be different from those present in an urban habitat (unpublished data). This means the species present on the remains can indicate whether or not the remains have been moved between these habitats.

Insects, or other arthropods such as mites, found with both the remains and a suspect are indicative of the suspect having been near the remains [2] or present in that habitat [3]. This may also be combined with the seasonal or even weekly temporal distribution of the insect. The identification of several insect species and their distribution has also been used to determine whether or not a vehicle has left a region. In this instance, the insects found on the radiator were used to support the theory that a vehicle driven by a suspect had crossed the country to the location of the crime scene [4].

An additional consideration for the use of insects as evidence is based upon their feeding habits. Fly larvae in particular, as they feed directly upon remains, ingest the materials within the tissues of the remains. They can, therefore, be considered as a possible source for DNA evidence and may also be useful for toxicological analyses. This may become especially important if the tissue itself has become too decomposed to be used for such analyses.

Insects as evidence is not restricted to cases of suspicious death, insects may be useful whenever a determination of time or place is required. The contamination of food products, fresh or stored, by insects is a common problem of worldwide concern. The identification of these insects may provide an indication as to the country of origin of the insects and become evidence useful to insurance claims.

There may also be a criminal element involved when it is illegal plant material that is transported from one location to another. In New Zealand, entomologists were asked to examine a seizure of cannabis plant material for insects to see if the country of origin could be determined [5]. The known distributions of the insects found were helpful in determining that, indeed, the plant material had originated from overseas.

Entomology is a well-established scientific discipline. The knowledge of insect biology, behaviour and distribution can all play a vital role in providing answers to questions, or support or contrast to theories that arise during many investigations. It is the logical interpretation of science-based information that makes forensic entomology one of the robust and reliable forms of scientific evidence.

Forensic microbial aquatic taphonomy

The accurate reconstruction of events surrounding the death of an individual and thereafter until the body is discovered (including the timing at which these events occurred and the duration of post-mortem submersion) are essential components of any aquatic death investigation. However, as the post-mortem submersion interval (PMSI) increases, its reliable estimation becomes increasingly difficult. Gaining a clear understanding of the post-mortem degradation and modification of human remains in their depositional context as they transition from the biosphere into the hydrosphere – central goals of forensic aquatic taphonomy – is therefore of vital importance for accurate reconstruction of post-mortem events and PMSI estimation. In order to achieve these goals, consideration of the interactions taking place between the body and its surrounding environment is fundamentally important. Surprisingly, aquatic decomposition researchers have paid little attention to this important taphonomic concept and have largely ignored the potential contribution that could be made by aquatic microorganisms to bring about post-mortem change of bodies immersed in aquatic environments. Novel research suggests such organisms play key roles in the aquatic decomposition process and may enable forensic practitioners to more accurately estimate PMSI.

Decomposition of bodies in water begins almost immediately upon immersion and, as on land, initially follows two parallel processes: autolysis, the enzymatic self-destruction of cells; and putrefaction, the post-mortem degradation of soft tissues through the actions of microbes [6]. Destruction of the soft tissues into smaller constituent elements may also come about through physical factors specific to the surrounding environment, such as current or tidal action or predation by scavengers, eventually leaving the skeletal elements susceptible to disarticulation and further degradation through a process known as diagenesis [6]. Although an important source of such putrefactive bacteria is the gastro-intestinal tract, saprophytic bacteria from the environment immediately surrounding the cadaver may also exert a significant influence on the decomposition of a body – a concept that had, until recently, been largely overlooked for cadavers in aquatic environments.

For the first time, a series of recent studies [7, 8] explored the interactions between decomposing mammalian remains and marine microorganisms, the most prolific degraders of organic matter in the ocean, and their potential role as agents of taphonomic change. The use of partial remains, rather than whole carcasses, meant that the post-mortem changes resulting from exogenous bacterial action could be separated from those brought about by endogenous, particularly gastro-intestinal, bacteria. Submerged remains underwent clear and repeatable patterns of decompositional change over time, progressing through a number of distinct stages (Fig. 11.1, a–e). Visible features of these stages were attributable to exogenous putrefactive bacterial action, such as the early appearance of coloured

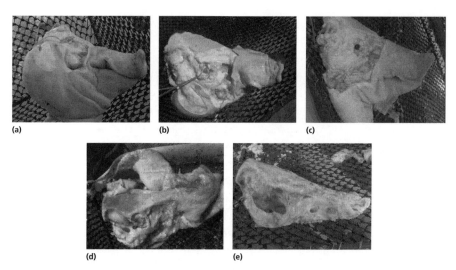

Fig. 11.1 Stages of decomposition for partial pig remains. (a) Fresh; (b) early putrefaction; (c) advanced putrefaction; (d) advanced decay; (e) skeletonised. (Dickson et al. 2011. Reproduced with permission from Elsevier.)

bacterial growths on the skin surface (Fig. 11.1, b), the rapid formation of an extensive slimy biofilm over the entire carcass (Fig. 11.1, c), and disintegration of soft tissues beneath the biofilm (Fig. 11.1, d). Such unique taphonomic changes indicate the significance of marine bacterial involvement in the decomposition of mammalian remains submerged in a natural aquatic environment and hint at important ecological processes taking place.

Mammalian remains in water form a localised, ephemeral habitat that may realistically be considered an 'aquatic cadaver decomposition island' (ACDI) in much the same way as previously proposed for cadaver decomposition in terrestrial environments [9]. Importantly, such remains act as a 'decomposition hub' for a number of opportunistic microbial species intimately involved in the cycling of carbon and other nutrients within marine and freshwater environments. Some bacterial groups are considered nutritional 'generalists', while others prefer, or are capable of, utilising only certain molecules. Thus it is proposed that the sequential breakdown of cadaver tissues and release of different combinations of organic compounds over time render the remains agreeable to successive groups of microorganisms over the course of the post-mortem period [8]. Especially for cases in which endogenous microbes of the body are absent or their actions suppressed, saprophytic bacteria within the surrounding environment will play an even greater role in the continued decay of human tissues into their constituent elements than was previously thought [7, 8].

A variety of methods have been suggested for PMSI estimation of bodies recovered from aqueous environments, and these can be divided into three broad approaches: analysis of post-mortem biochemical changes within the body [10];

consideration of the physical condition of the body [11, 12]; and identification of the colonisation and/or succession patterns of mobile aquatic organisms associated with the body [13]. However, each of these approaches has shown limited applicability for bodies recovered from marine environments and/or those with long submersion periods; as such, no reliable method of PMSI estimation currently exists.

Environmental saprophytic bacterial colonisation of submerged remains and subsequent changes in community composition over time has significant potential to provide information on submersion interval, but has so far received little attention. Such bacteria are attractive as potential PMSI indicators for several reasons: they are numerous and ubiquitous components of both marine and freshwater environments; they are prolific degraders of organic matter; and molecular methods to aid in their identification are now routine and relatively inexpensive.

Dickson [8] and colleagues [7] employed a molecular approach in their studies of microbial marine decomposition, which are, to date, the only experimental studies to examine specifically the patterns of exogenous bacteria that colonise mammalian cadavers in a natural aquatic environment. Marine bacteria were shown to rapidly colonise partial pig remains submerged in coastal marine locations. Discernible shifts in the dominant groups of bacteria took place over the course of the post-mortem submersion period, thus indicating a sequential pattern to saprophytic marine bacterial colonisation associated with the progressive decomposition of submerged cadavers. Several groups of bacteria were also found to be uniquely present during certain submersion intervals. Dickson and colleagues [7] proposed that dynamic changes in bacterial community composition over the course of the submersion period and the identification of bacteria unique to a particular post-mortem decomposition stage or submersion interval would function as 'biomarkers' or 'indicators' useful for predicting PMSI of recovered remains. Indeed, the microbial succession concept has since shown potential for its application to PMSI estimation in human death investigations involving cadavers recovered from water [8].

Many factors pertaining to the surrounding environment and to the body itself – similar to those that affect the progression of cadaver decomposition in aquatic environments – are also likely to influence the presence and colonisation patterns of certain aquatic bacteria on cadavers in water (Table 11.1). The qualitative effects of several important variables, such as water temperature and season, on marine bacterial colonisation patterns have recently been explored [7, 8], but many others, such as the impact that clothing has on such colonisation patterns, are yet to be investigated.

Water temperature is the most important environmental factor governing microbial aquatic taphonomic processes and bacterial community structure, and closely related to this is the season of submergence [7, 8]. These factors have direct effects on bacterial growth and metabolic function; warmer water temperatures

Table 11.1 Factors likely to affect the presence and type of aquatic bacteria colonising cadavers in aquatic environments.

Exogenous	Endogenous
Water temperature	Clothing
Season	Partial or complete remains
Geographic location	Submerged or floating
Scavenging/predation	Residual skin microflora
Salinity	Type of body surface tissue
Water quality/pollution	Antibiotics
Water depth	
Currents or water flow rate	
Dissolved oxygen concentration	
Water pH	
Commensal and inhibitory relationships between bacteria	

have a positive effect on the actions of bacteria, thus accelerating biofilm formation and the rate of decay, while colder temperatures slow down enzymatic processes and may preclude the presence or activity of certain bacterial species in the environment altogether during colder seasons. Certain bacterial groups may be better able to adapt physiologically to changing ambient conditions, outcompeting other groups for resources [14], which may partly explain the presence of several season-specific bacterial groups on remains submerged during different seasons [7, 8].

Dickson [8] discovered that bacterial communities recovered from the skin of pig remains submerged in two geographically distinct marine locations during summer displayed a degree of geographical specificity. These communities comprised many of the same bacteria, but were sufficiently dissimilar overall, that a reliable PMSI prediction for a decomposition event that took place in one location could not be made using a bacterial assemblage recovered from the other marine location. Such findings indicate that ecological factors unique to the specific body of water and the time of year in which a body is submerged – as well as the length of the PMSI – will affect the combination of microbial species found on the surface of the cadaver.

Aside from the studies conducted in New Zealand coastal waters [7, 8] and intertidal areas of Hawaii [15], other research efforts directed toward aquatic decomposition of human or animal remains that have also noted the activity of exogenous microorganisms during the decay process have made limited use of natural aquatic environments and have instead been carried out in artificial contexts – either in water-filled tanks [16] or in holes dug into the ground [17]. In such environments, the cadaver is exposed to a limited subset of variables that it may expect to encounter in a natural marine or freshwater environment, and they lack the inherent communities of bacteria and other microorganisms that reside in every natural body of water. Several studies [7, 8, 18] have provided evidence that the ecological context within which the submerged remains are found is extremely important as it can determine the types and relative abundances of colonising bacteria.

While the bacteriology of pig decomposition has been shown to closely resemble that of humans, which makes pigs acceptable models for bacteriological studies in terrestrial contexts, it remains to be seen whether marine bacterial succession data generated using pig carcasses are translatable to human cadavers. For logistical and ethical reasons, it may be currently impossible to systematically study human post-mortem bacteriology in natural bodies of water and this author knows of no study that has done so. As an alternative, however, it may be possible to generate sufficient data by sampling specific areas of submerged human bodies recovered from aquatic contexts before autopsy – provided as many details as possible regarding PMSI, the physical nature of the aquatic environment and of the body itself are also recorded for comparison.

In a preliminary analysis, Dickson [8] studied a series of five human cadavers that had been submerged in coastal marine or river environments, during different seasons, for intervals ranging from 12 hours to 15 days. Several cadavers exhibited visible microbial growth on the skin surface (Fig. 11.2) and, indeed, such findings are not uncommon on immersed remains. Multiple locations on each of the human bodies were sampled in order to elucidate which areas, if any, would be the most likely to return a positive bacterial sample, and thus would be the best areas for forensic practitioners to examine if the marine bacterial succession method was to be used to determine PMSI in future forensic casework. Figure 11.3 shows that the greatest sampling success rate was achieved with

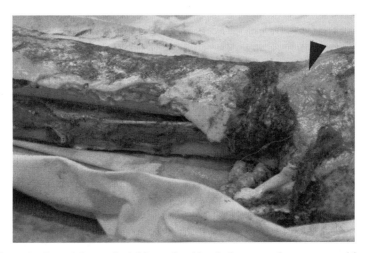

Fig. 11.2 Marine bacterial growth visible on the skin of a human cadaver recovered from coastal waters of New Zealand. (Photograph courtesy of G Dickson.) (*See insert for colour representation of the figure.*)

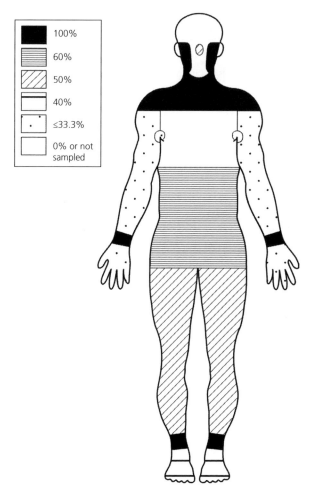

Fig. 11.3 Proportion of successful marine bacteria samples taken from different areas of the bodies of recovered human cadavers. (Courtesy of Dickson, 2012.)

samples taken from the face, neck and shoulder areas. Of the factors considered by Dickson [8] relating to cadaver treatment, both clothing and extensive scavenging appeared to have the greatest negative impact on the likelihood of obtaining a positive bacterial sample. A lack of clothing over the face and neck areas upon submersion may go some way toward explaining why these areas, in particular, produced a greater proportion of successful samples. Future cases in which human cadavers are sampled for aquatic bacteria should focus their sampling efforts on the face and neck region (or those areas of the body not covered by clothing) and areas where microbial growth is visible, but not parts of the body that have been visibly disturbed by scavenger activity. Most individuals enter the water at least partially clothed; therefore, future research using clothed and unclothed cadavers is necessary in order to understand the exact quantitative and qualitative effects that layers of clothing have on marine bacterial communities and colonisation patterns. Future studies might also wish to examine the little understood interplay between endogenous flora of the skin and invading saprophytic bacteria from the surrounding environment, and the factors that govern this interaction.

Understanding the process of decomposition of cadavers in aquatic environments is essential if predictions are to be made regarding their post-mortem fates. Recent studies of microbial marine decomposition of human and animal remains have provided unprecedented insight into the microorganisms involved and their unique temporal patterns. Exogenous aquatic bacteria are important agents of taphonomic change of immersed bodies, but their actions may be influenced by factors such as water temperature, season, interactions between microbial community members and factors relating to the body itself, such as whether it is clothed or unclothed. Aquatic bacteria are also an extremely promising group of microorganisms for PMSI estimation in forensic death investigations due to their abundance in nature, global distribution and capacity to colonise a body almost immediately following submersion in a reliable and predictable manner.

This novel concept has a distinct advantage with its applicability to partial remains as well as complete cadavers recovered from aquatic environments. Although it shows much promise, the use of a microbial colonisation and succession tool for PMSI estimation is still in its infancy and significant research and development is required, particularly in relation to the factors discussed in this chapter, in order to gain a more comprehensive understanding of local microbial aquatic taphonomic processes and to hone the method to the level of precision required for forensic casework.

The use of energy-dispersive spectroscopy in forensic investigations

The scope of this section is to give the forensic investigator an overview of the potential of energy-dispersive spectroscopy (EDS) while imaging a specimen using scanning electron microscopy (SEM). EDS, also known as energy-dispersive x-ray spectroscopy (EDX or XEDS) or energy-dispersive x-ray analysis (EDXA), is an adjunct technique to SEM where elemental analysis of the object being viewed can be carried out during the same viewing session. When a specimen is viewed in the SEM, characteristic x-rays are produced by each of the various elements that make up the specimen. These are detected and converted by the EDS software to give the elemental composition of the specimen [19]. EDS is one of many different analytical methods that can be used to identify chemical composition or changes that occurred to materials during an incident, and thereby help reconstruct a sequence of events. When these specimens are extremely limited in size, SEM/EDS is often the only suitable method available for their elemental characterisation. An investigator should seek the advice of an experienced SEM/EDS operator when preparing specimens, and ideally should request the operator to prepare, mount and carry out the EDS analysis.

When the atoms that make up the elements of a specimen are impacted by the microscope's electron beam, this excites them to emit a unique x-ray spectrum. An atom at rest within the specimen contains electrons in discrete energy levels/shells. The electron beam causes excitation of the electron shell, resulting in the ejection of an electron from the inner shell, leaving a hole and the atom in an unstable state. When an electron from a higher energy outer shell fills this hole while trying to re-establish stability, a loss of energy is required, which releases an x-ray unique to its atomic structure detected by EDS [19]. Most modern SEM/EDS systems allow for a range of measurements, from highly focused spots of nanometre scale, to line scans and elemental surface mapping.

The advantage of EDS is that it can be used to analyse the elemental composition of most solid materials, while at the same time imaging the surface morphology using SEM. Biological materials can also be imaged and analysed after appropriate treatment to make them conductive. Depending on the technique and settings of the EDS system, analysis can be quantitative or qualitative. Materials that are electrically conductive do not require carbon coating, while those materials that are non-conductive do. For non-biological materials the technique is considered non-destructive and the specimen can be re-examined and analysed multiple times. The size of the specimen is only limited by the size of the SEM chamber and mounting stage system. Typically, a modern microscope with a large chamber can accommodate a specimen of 40 × 40 cm with a height of ~40 mm. Elements with atomic numbers ranging from those of beryllium to uranium can be detected [19].

A SEM equipped with an EDS system is one of the most frequent applications used for particle analysis to determine the proximity of a discharging firearm based on gun shot residue (GSR) elemental analysis. The SEM/EDS system is able to detect particles containing antimony, barium and lead that originate from primers used in the manufacturing of most firearm ammunitions [20]. This can then be referenced back to the ammunition, cartridge cases and residue on the firearm used in a crime. For GSR analysis, a two-sided sticky carbon tape tab is stuck on an aluminium mount prior to being patted on the surface of the article in question. The specimen is then carbon coated prior to being inserted into the SEM and subsequently analysed by EDS. Ancillary materials that may be of interest can also be characterised. These techniques can be used in the analysis of glass chips, paint chips, inks, soils and any other materials where a specimen can be prepared and inserted into a SEM. In many countries, the results can be compared to national databases using sophisticated software systems [21]. Proprietary software is also available from SEM manufacturers that automate many time consuming functions. A major advantage of an automated process is the removal of bias by the human operator who subjectively selects the areas or spots to be analysed.

The following Case studies (11.1–11.3) illustrate the range of use of EDS in a forensic context.

Case study 11.1

A person claimed that they bit down on a dental amalgam filling that had been an inclusion in their hamburger patty while eating at a well-known franchised restaurant chain. The offending metallic object was recovered by the restaurant and sent for SEM/EDS analysis to establish what it was (Figs. 11.4 and 11.5). The franchise chain also wanted to know the geographical origin of the amalgam and whether there were any differences in dental techniques or amalgam compositions internationally.

Based on the SEM/EDS and visual analysis, the forensic analysis found that the image looked like a 'three-quarter' noble alloy crown that was used to restore a mandibular first molar (tooth 36). Part of the internal surface looked like contoured ripples, indicating that the working cast die was wax dipped to form the pattern for the 'lost wax' casting process. Looking at the EDS analysis, the alloy appeared to be a typical palladium/silver Type 3 or 4 crown-and-bridge casting alloy, which was silver in colour. It therefore was not an amalgam restoration, as that alloy would contain high levels of mercury and silver and there was no mercury present in the EDS analysis. The presence of cadmium and gold lead one to believe that this restoration was soldered with a cadmium containing gold solder during manufacture (the small yellow areas on the silver coloured surface). Cadmium containing dental solders has been banned for at least the last 30 years, as the release of cadmium through corrosion in the oral environment is potentially carcinogenic. The restoration was therefore very old or was manufactured outside of current first world countries. There are thousands of alloy manufacturers worldwide, and each one manufactures 30 to 40 alloys for the dental market, so precise identification was not possible.

In this case, the most likely scenario was that the complainant dislodged a crown while eating at the restaurant and falsely claimed compensation. The restaurant secured the metallic object and had it forensically analysed. This evidence will be used should the case go to court and the complainant's dental records show a match to the lost crown.

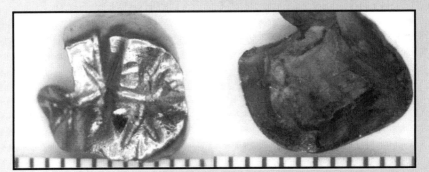

Fig. 11.4   A digital image of the occlusal surface (left side) and fitting surface (right side) of a cast all-metal dental three-quarter crown.

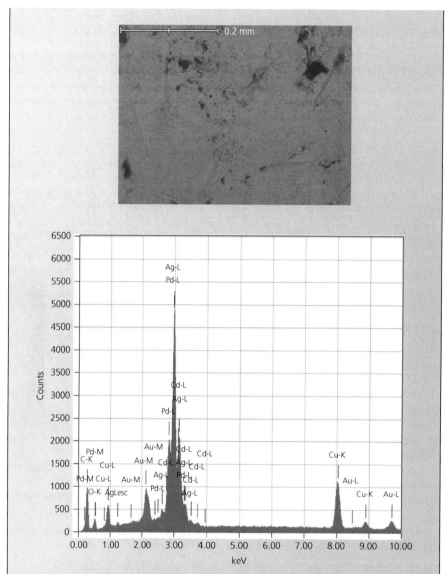

Fig. 11.5   The graph shows EDS analysis peaks indicating elements present based on a scan of the surface of the crown (top image).

Case study 11.2

A person claimed that they found a resin-like inclusion when they were eating a bar of hard dark chocolate (Figs. 11.6 and 11.7). Analysis showed ytterbium trifluoride, aluminium silicate and zinc sulphate/sulfite. The forensic analysis found the particle was from a Resin Modified Glass Ionomer Cement (RMGIC). This material can be used as a

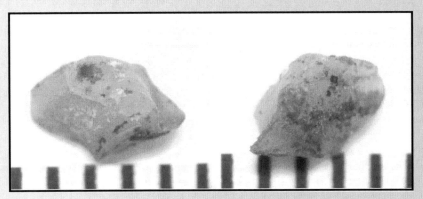

Fig. 11.6 The front and back views of a RMGIC particle. The discolouration is accumulated surface staining that occurred over time.

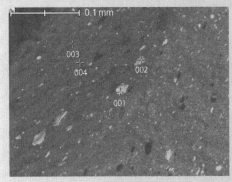

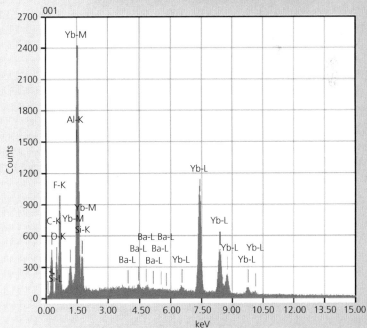

Fig. 11.7 Example of a graph showing EDS element peaks based on spot scans (crosses numbered 001 to 004 in top image).

tooth filling material or a cement for bonding various materials to tooth structure. A typical powder is an acid-soluble calcium fluoroaluminosilicate glass, similar to that of silicate. The fluoride portion acts as a ceramic flux. Lanthanum, strontium, barium or zinc oxide additives provide radio-opacity. The typical make-up of the raw materials of a RMGIC are: silica 41.9%; alumina 28.6%; aluminium fluoride 1.6%; calcium fluoride 15.7%; sodium fluoride 9.3% and aluminium phosphate 3.8%. Ytterbium (III) fluoride (YbF3) is used as an inert and non-toxic tooth filling because it continuously releases fluoride ions [22].

As in Case Study 11.1, the analysis could be matched to the complainant's dental records should the case go to court.

Case study 11.3

This dental study was based on the allegation that imported porcelain-fused-to-metal crowns manufactured in China contained toxic elements, namely lead in the veneer porcelain and arsenic in the dental alloy [23]. The SEM/EDS mapping analysis (Figs. 11.8 and 11.9) showed that the crowns contained no toxic elements and consisted of typical nickel chromium dental alloys and typical dental veneer porcelain.

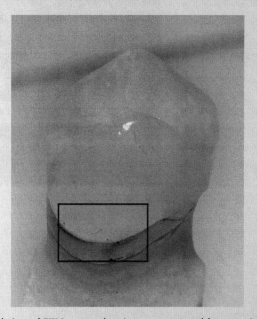

Fig. 11.8 Palatal view of PFM crown showing area prepared for scanning incorporating the palatal metal alloy collar, metal/porcelain junction and porcelain veneer. (Waddell et al. 2010. Reproduced with permission from *New Zealand Dental Journal*.)

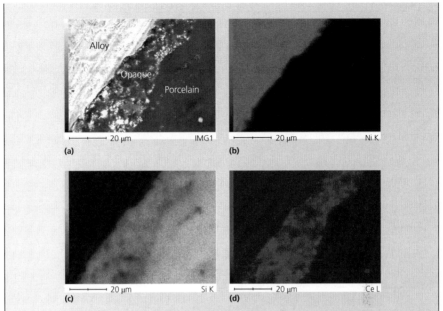

Fig. 11.9 Example of EDS mapping analysis of (a) the alloy, opaque and veneering porcelain regions; (b) alloy region scanned for nickel shown in grey; (c) opaque porcelain and veneering porcelain scanned for silica (the major component of veneering porcelain) shown in light grey; (d) opaque porcelain scanned for cerium (cerium oxide has high refractive index and is added to porcelain to make it more opaque) shown in light grey. (Waddell et al. 2010. Reproduced with permission from *New Zealand Dental Journal*.)

These three cases serve to illustrate a small example of how EDS spots, line scans and elemental surface mapping analysis can be of use to the forensic investigator. EDS should be regarded as an essential investigatory tool. Good-quality valid results are usually achieved by an experienced SEM/EDS microscopist.

References

1 Galton F. (1892) *Finger prints*. MacMillan and Co., London.
2 Goff ML. (2000) *A Fly for the Prosecution: How Insect Evidence Helps Solve Crimes*. Harvard University Press, Cambridge, Massachusetts.
3 Prichard JG, Kossoris PD, Leibovitch RA et al. (1986) Implications of trombiculid mite bites: report of a case and submission of evidence in a murder trial. *Journal of Forensic Sciences* **31**, 301–306.
4 Landmark Criminal Case: UC Davis Entomologist Links Insects in Car Radiator with Defendant's Whereabouts [Internet] (2007) May 30. Available from: http://169.237.77.3/news/kimseyinsecttestimony.html. Accessed August 2015.
5 Crosby TK, Watt JC, Kistemaker AC et al. (1986) Entomological identification of the origin of imported cannabis. *Journal of the Forensic Science Society* **26**, 35–44.

6 Gill-King H. (1997) Chemical and ultrastructural aspects of decomposition. In: Haglund WD, Sorg MH (eds) *Forensic Taphonomy: The Postmortem Fate of Human Remains*, CRC Press, Boca Raton, pp. 93–108.

7 Dickson GC, Poulter RTM, Maas EW et al. (2011) Marine bacterial succession as a potential indicator of postmortem submersion interval. *Forensic Science International* **209**, 1–10.

8 Dickson GC. (2012) Microbial marine decomposition of human and animal remains. Unpublished PhD Thesis, University of Otago, Dunedin, New Zealand.

9 Carter DO, Yellowlees D, Tibbett M. (2007) Cadaver decomposition in terrestrial ecosystems. *Naturwissenschaften* **94**, 12–24.

10 Saukko P, Knight B. (2004) *Knight's Forensic Pathology*. 3rd edn, Arnold, London.

11 Doberentz E, Madea B. (2010) Estimating the time of immersion of bodies found in water – an evaluation of a common method to estimate the minimum time interval of immersion. *Revista Española de Medicina Legal* **36**, 51–61.

12 Heaton V, Lagden A, Moffatt C et al. (2010) Predicting the postmortem submersion interval for human remains recovered from U.K. waterways. *Journal of Forensic Sciences* **55**, 302–307.

13 Haskell NH, McShaffrey DG, Hawley DA et al. (1989) Use of aquatic insects in determining submersion interval. *Journal of Forensic Sciences* **34**, 622–632.

14 Kirchman DL. (2002) The ecology of Cytophaga-Flavobacteria in aquatic environments. *FEMS Microbiology Ecology* **39**, 91–100.

15 Davis JB, Goff ML. (2000) Decomposition patterns in terrestrial and intertidal habitats on Oahu Island and Coconut Island, Hawaii. *Journal of Forensic Sciences* **45**, 836–842.

16 Payne JA, King EW. (1972) Insect succession and decomposition of pig carcasses in water. *Journal of the Georgia Entomological Society* **7**, 153–162.

17 O'Brian TG, Kuehner AC. (2007) Waxing grave about adipocere: soft tissue change in an aquatic context. *Journal of Forensic Sciences* **52**, 1–8.

18 Pakosh CM, Rogers TL. (2009) Soft tissue decomposition of submerged, dismembered pig limbs enclosed in plastic bags. *Journal of Forensic Sciences* **54**, 1223–1228.

19 Goldstein J, Newbury DE, Joy DC et al. (2003) *Scanning Electron Microscopy and X–ray Microanalysis*. 3rd edn, Springer, New York, pp. 297–353.

20 ASTM E1588–10e1 (2010) *Standard Guide for Gunshot Residue Analysis by Scanning Electron Microscopy/Energy Dispersive X–ray Spectrometry*. ASTM International, West Conshohocken, PA.

21 Ward DC. (2000) Use of an X-ray spectral database in forensic science, *Forensic Science Communication* **2**, 3.

22 Sakaguchi RL, Powers JM. (2012) *Craig's Restorative Dental Materials*. 13th edn, Elsevier Mosby, Philadelphia.

23 Waddell, JN, Girvan L, Aarts JM et al. (2010) Elemental composition of imported porcelain-fused-to-metal crowns – a pilot study. *New Zealand Dental Journal* **106**, 50–54.

CHAPTER 12

Odontology opinions

Denice Higgins and Helen James

Forensic Odontology Unit, University of Adelaide, Australia

Introduction

An opinion is the interpretation of facts, based on knowledge within a particular field (published literature) and experience of the practitioner giving the opinion. Giving an opinion is a privilege of expert status in a given field. Outside identification of human remains by the traditional comparison of dental records, a forensic odontologist may be asked to give an expert opinion on a number of other topics. This chapter will discuss the general principles involved in giving an opinion, situations where an opinion may be sought and the fundamentals of report writing. Accompanying the text is a series of case studies to highlight the range of opinions that may be given by the forensic odontologist.

General principles

The formation of an expert opinion requires management, examination, evaluation and presentation of relevant dental evidence. Provision of an expert opinion entails great responsibility, potentially affecting the lives of individuals. Experts are bound by a canon of ethics and have a duty of care when providing an opinion. Other forensic practitioners may need to be consulted to aid in an investigation and collaboration between various specialists is often important in forming accurate opinions. A forensic odontologist may consult with another dental specialist, pathologist or anthropologist to provide clarifying information necessary to the formation of an opinion. The principles discussed below are inter-related and therefore difficult to prioritise, but are all factors to consider when giving an opinion.

All opinions formed must have a solid scientific basis, based on current philosophy and methodology within the discipline. A valid opinion can only be formed if relevant knowledge is comprehensively understood and applied. The opinion should be formulated in a manner that is generally accepted by the

Forensic Odontology: Principles and Practice, First Edition. Edited by Jane A. Taylor and Jules A. Kieser.
© 2016 John Wiley & Sons, Ltd. Published 2016 by John Wiley & Sons, Ltd.

relevant scientific community. If the view formulated is outside mainstream acceptance then this should be stated in the opinion.

The role of the forensic odontologist is to give impartial advice to those seeking the opinion and, when necessary, to assist the courts by providing expert knowledge and interpretation of evidence to assist in the pursuit of the truth. Biased or inaccurate opinions can have widespread and potentially immutable ramifications. The forensic odontologist should not be an advocate for the party who requested the opinion, but should provide a detached, objective assessment.

It is important for any forensic practitioner when giving opinion evidence not to stray from their area of expertise. Definition of the area of expertise should take into account the individual practitioner's education and experience. As dental practitioners, forensic odontologists have an in-depth understanding of orofacial and dental anatomy, morphology and pathology. They are also aware of expected standards associated with provision of dental treatment, dental record keeping and dental practice management. This knowledge, along with a working knowledge of radiological and digital image production and analysis, forms the range of expertise for a forensic odontologist and are the likely areas in which opinion may be sought. Any opinion should consider the purpose for which the opinion was sought and should be restricted by the scope of the request and the area of expertise of the odontologist. All opinions should be substantially or wholly based within this area of expertise.

Limitations of the opinion should be freely acknowledged. These may include both technical areas of analysis methodology and personal training and experience. If a colleague has greater knowledge, then deferring to their opinion may be a wise option. The odontologist's reputation can, in fact, be enhanced if they indicate to investigators or courts when a second opinion may hold more weight.

Timely consideration and distribution of both oral and written opinions is a key concept. Investigators seeking information to attribute identity or preserve evidence do not want lengthy delays. It is also important to remember when speaking to police and lawyers, that nothing should be considered 'off the record'. The odontologist must assume anything said in discussion may be used in court. Similarly, an 'unofficial' conversation with a journalist may be reported in the news, with the potential to compromise an investigation or cause a mistrial.

Opinions for an opposing party should not be used as an opportunity to 'smokescreen' by attacking minor matters such as a typographical error. Neither should they be used to personally criticise a colleague. Review of another's opinion should always be fact based and should fall within the odontologist's area of expertise.

The opinion offered by an odontologist is not exempt from scrutiny outside of the legal proceeding for which it is requested. In many countries, experts are immune from litigation concerning opinions given in evidence provided that they are based on fact and the expert has not knowingly lied under oath. In other countries, if the opinion of the odontologist is considered to cause damage to a foreseeable victim, civil or criminal action can be brought against them.

Types of opinions

Scenarios where the opinion of a forensic odontologist may be sought, include, but are not limited to, the areas discussed below.

Identification of dental structures

Odontologists may be asked to comment on dental material found by crime scene officers, customs officials or members of the general public (Case study 12.1). Single teeth or tooth fragments and dislodged dental restorations may be used to identify individuals, and may also aid in the location of individuals. Odontologists can give opinion both at the scene and at the mortuary to recognise and identify dental materials or link such evidence to an individual (either the victim or the suspect) or to evidence found in another location (Case study 12.2). This will aid in the investigation of the crime. An opinion may also serve to conserve time and resources by determining whether recovered material is suspicious and requires further investigation. For example, in Australia ancient Aboriginal remains are

---

Case study 12.1

Background: Odontologists were asked to provide an opinion concerning the finding of a single tooth in a suburban backyard (Fig. 12.1).

Issues: Is the tooth human? What is a likely explanation for the find?

Opinion: The tooth is a human upper-left second deciduous molar (FDI designation 65), which has been previously restored and has caries extending to the pulp chamber. The disto-buccal root has been fractured. Based on the root status, the tooth would have come from a child in the age range of 6–8 years. It is likely that the tooth was extracted for clinical reasons subsequent to the deep restoration (breaking the root tip). It is not possible to say when the tooth was extracted (i.e. how long it had been buried).

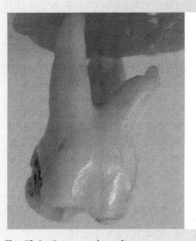 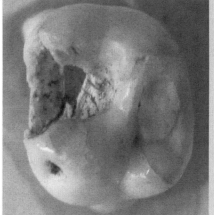

Fig. 12.1   Recovered tooth.

Case study 12.2

Background: A victim of an alleged assault claimed that she had been attacked in the suspect's house. The suspect denied that the woman had ever been inside his house. Police located a fragment of tooth at the house and odontologists were asked to give an opinion as to whether the fragment of tooth belonged to the victim.

Issues: DNA harvesting may damage the exhibit and may not yield a good result, as the fragment is predominantly enamel and will take time to process. An odontology examination can be performed in a relatively short time frame. The speed with which odontologists can associate scenes is a valuable tool to investigators.

Opinion: The tooth fragment shows anatomical correlation with the remaining portion of tooth and can be clearly shown to belong to the alleged victim (Fig. 12.2). The suspect must be mistaken or not truthful in his assertion that the victim has not been at the location, unless secondary transfer from clothing or footwear had occurred.

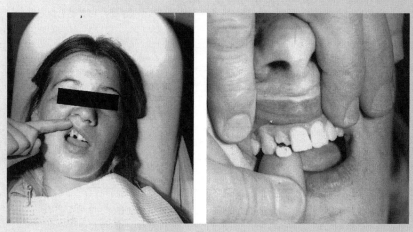

Fig. 12.2   Alleged victim, with fractured upper right lateral incisor (12) and associated tooth fragment.

---

commonly encountered. These need to be identified as such and repatriated, but further investigation by police is not required.

Opinions may also be sought on whether teeth are human or non-human. Teeth of some animals, such as pigs, can look remarkably similar to human teeth to the untrained eye, and fragments of teeth and bones can be difficult to discriminate between human and non-human (Case study 12.3). High-impact incidents, and those involving incineration of humans and pets, may result in commingling of remains. Odontologists work with anthropologists to separate material and can provide opinion on non-human teeth. Trading in ivory and other animal parts is prohibited in many countries and correct identification of non-human material may be required [1]. Ivory can be distinguished from tooth enamel and bone by the presence of cross-sectional criss-crossing line patterns

Case study 12.3

Background: Police attending a scene to locate a body excavated an area that displayed increased vegetation growth. They requested an opinion with regards to teeth that were located close to the surface during the excavation (Fig. 12.3).

Issues: Are the remains human? What features are used to differentiate dentitions?

Opinion: The dental formula of adult pigs (*Sus scrofa domestica*) is I3.C1.P4.M3 and the molars are, at first glance, quite similar to human teeth. However, careful study of the morphology, in particular the bell shape to the crown, identifies these teeth as being of non-human origin.

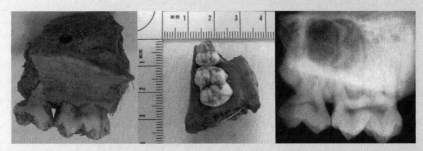

Fig. 12.3 Teeth and bone recovered from potential crime scene.

that create diamond-shaped areas. Museums may also seek the opinion of an odontologist with regards to which species teeth and skulls belong, so a comprehensive knowledge of dental comparative anatomy is required (Case study 12.4).

Allegations of objects found in foodstuffs may precipitate legal action and opinion may be sought from an odontologist as to the composition of the object if it is suspected to be of dental origin. The odontologist may be asked simply to identify the object, or to examine the complainant to ascertain if the dental matter has come from their mouth. This would negate the claim that the manufacturer or chef introduced the foreign body.

Where odontologists have niche knowledge in a particular field of research, opinions may be sought in that area. For instance, a dentist, dental specialist or a dental company representative may require assistance in identifying the type of implant present in an individual's dentition (Case study 12.5). This information may be needed where there is failure of an abutment, or the super-structure supported by an implant requires restoration, or if further implant treatment is required adjacent to a previously placed implant. Knowledge of the type of implant allows use of the correct driver to remove the abutment, as an incorrect driver may bur the fitting and the abutment may prove difficult to remove. Features such as tapering, threading, holes and apex shape are considered when trying to identify a brand [2]. As implants evolve there is constant changing of shapes, attachments and surface textures leading to new designs and the ceasing

Case study 12.4

Background: Odontologists were asked to assist museum staff to reconstruct the skull of an African elephant (*Loxodonta Africana*) and restore the broken teeth (Fig. 12.4).

Issues: What is the dental formula for an elephant? How are individual teeth identified by type and location? What materials are suitable for reconstruction?

Opinion: Elephants have bilateral single opposing molar teeth, replaced six times in a typical elephant's lifetime (polyphyodont) by horizontal migration from the rear of the jaw bones. The molars have loop-shaped dental ridges used to grind food. The tusks are modified incisors in the upper jaw. Tooth-coloured filling materials, and in particular glass ionomer materials, can be used to restore the teeth.

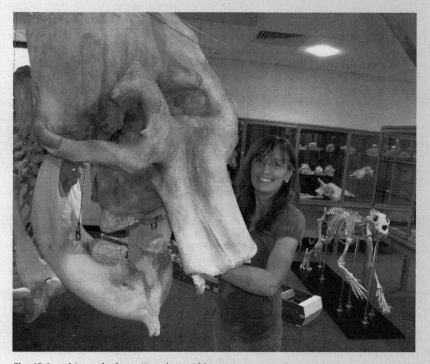

Fig. 12.4   African elephant (*Loxodonta Africana*).

of production of the older types. There are currently over 200 dental implant companies and the popularity of implants as a treatment option continues to grow. An implant placed 30 years ago may not be easily recognised by a recent dental graduate. Not all odontologists will be experienced in this capacity. Web-based recognition software may assist, but referring to a colleague with expertise in this particular area is recommended.

Case study 12.5

Background: Odontologists were asked to give an opinion concerning the type of implant, to determine what drivers were needed clinically to remove a failing implant. A South African dentist had placed the implant in England in 2000.

Issues: What features will allow recognition of the brand of implant? Will location data assist in identification?

Opinion: Dental endosseous implants may be placed in patients to support replacement of one or more missing teeth. Modern dental implants are designed to osseointegrate where the implant material, such as titanium, forms an intimate bond to bone. Various features of implants are seen on radiographic images that allow differentiation of the brand of implant. In this case the implant characteristics include a bell-shaped head; threading, non-tapering body; a rounded apex and no visible holes (Fig. 12.5). A number of possibilities should be considered, including Euroteknika, Osteocare®, Noble Biocare® and IDI System®. An early Zimmer Inc. implant has the best total fit of features. This type of implant was in common use in both the United Kingdom and South Africa at the relevant time and the dentist was likely to be familiar with the product. A Zimmer Inc. implant was, therefore, considered the most probable brand.

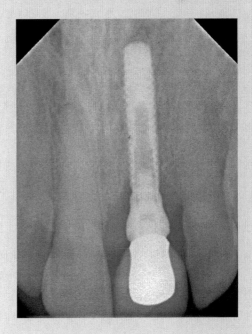

Fig. 12.5 Dental implant.

Injuries sustained to the teeth or other oral structures

An odontologist may be asked for an opinion with regard to an injury that has been sustained to the teeth and/or orofacial structures of an individual. Usually opinion is sought as to the likely cause of the injury, what force was required to

Case study 12.6

Background: Odontologists were asked to give an opinion about hard tissue injuries. The victim claimed he was hit once, but medical evidence shows two jaw fractures (Fig. 12.6).

Issues: What direction and degree of force was involved? How do the injuries relate to the statement of the victim?

Opinion: Deep tooth roots close to the border of the mandible make a weak point susceptible to fracture. This lessens the amount of force required to break the jaw from an oblique blow to the angle of the mandible. Such a blow will also be likely to fracture the contra-lateral TMJ (i.e. one blow, two breaks). Comment on the prognosis of the lower-left second molar could also be made by the odontologist but would have more weight from a clinical specialist such as an oral and maxillofacial surgeon.

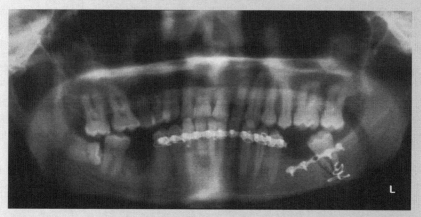

Fig. 12.6   Post-trauma OPG.

cause the injury and how much time had passed since the injury occurred. The odontologist may also be asked whether or not a given scenario is likely to have caused the injury (Case study 12.6).

Injuries may be sustained to the teeth, jawbones, oral and perioral soft tissues and the temporomandibular joints (TMJs). Injuries to the soft tissues can be in the form of contusions, abrasions and lacerations or even avulsion of sections of tissue. These injuries can occur as a result of an accident or assault, and in some instances are self-inflicted (intentional or otherwise). For example, a person may bite their own tongue or lips intentionally, as an act of self-harm, or involuntarily during the course of an assault or accident. Injuries to teeth may involve one or more teeth and can include total or partial avulsion, chips of varying severity and fractures involving the crown and/or roots as a result of impact trauma. The bones of the maxillofacial skeleton can also be involved in injury, sustaining fractures of varying severity. Most often an injury will involve more than one tissue and more than one type of wound.

Injuries can also be indirectly induced. For example, stress can induce bruxism, having a detrimental effect, not only on the teeth and dental restorations, but also on the TMJs [3]. The side effects of some medications, such as those used for pain relief, can cause damage to the teeth by decreasing saliva flow. Drug-induced xerostomia can have a debilitating effect on the dentition [4].

Ideally the forensic odontologist will undertake a careful examination and documentation of any injuries. In many cases, however, the odontologist is provided with the results of examinations, such as written records, photographs and radiographs, performed by other persons rather than directly examining the victim. It is important, regardless of who performs the examination, that injuries are documented as close as is practical to the time of the incident before the effects of healing or medical intervention occur. It is also important, where available, that the forensic odontologist is provided with an accurate timeline of events.

Dating the time of occurrence of any injury based on appearance alone is difficult for many injury types, especially contusions. If dating of an injury is key to the investigation then further examinations, such as histological or biochemical analyses, may be necessary. This may then fall outside the area of expertise of the odontologist. The odontologist may be limited to concluding that the injury is recent or not recent rather than a more accurate timescale. Other experts, such as the pathologist, clinical forensic medical officer or histologist, may also be asked to provide this opinion evidence.

When considering the extent of an injury to the teeth, it is important to consider the condition of the dentition prior to the alleged incident. Access to dental records describing the state of the dentition prior to the incident would help establish a baseline with which to compare the condition of the dentition after the incident. The previous state of health of the periodontal tissues and the level of bony attachment would be particularly important in the case of avulsed or loose teeth.

An injury report may be required for assistance in criminal investigation of an event, but may also be required for personal injury compensation claims that are not of a criminal nature (i.e. civil complaints). For example, an individual may sustain an injury in an accident that is covered by insurance or work cover and may require a report and financial estimates for treatment to repair the damage (Case study 12.7). Generally a report should not be prepared without permission from the patient or the patient's legal guardian, unless it is authorised by law as part of a legal proceeding.

When reports are requested with regards to treatment required to rectify an injury, both immediate and long-term requirements must be considered as well as consideration of complications that could result in the future as a result of the injury. For example, a tooth that sustains a fracture may, in the short term, require repair by provision of a direct restoration or a crown, but in the future could require endodontic therapy and post crown placement or extraction and implant placement. All treatment of a restorative nature has a finite lifespan so

Case study 12.7

Background: A report was requested by insurers about the diagnosis and prognosis of injuries to a cyclist who allegedly fell onto the road after being hit by an opening car door.

Issues: The insurer has asked if the injuries were caused by the collision, what treatment is required, as well as treatment costs.

Opinion: The upper central and lateral incisors have all sustained fractures of varying severity (Fig. 12.7). The upper-right central incisor (11) has a complex root fracture and is likely to require extraction and implant replacement. The upper-left central incisor (21) may require endodontic therapy and crown. Restoration of the lateral incisors may be by composite resin or porcelain onlay. The injuries sustained are consistent with the described incident but, unless an eye witness, the odontologist should be wary of attributing causation. Short- and long-term effects of the direct trauma and indirect consequences of the victim's inability to properly clean the teeth due to pain and discomfort must be considered.

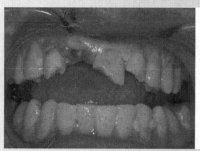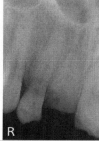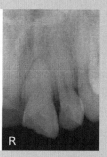

Fig. 12.7 Intra-oral and radiographic images of oral trauma.

will need replacement at given intervals; therefore provision for this is required in the treatment estimate. The life expectancy of dental restorations is generally five to ten years. It is also important to note in an estimate of treatment expenses that all figures quoted are based on current fees and do not make any provision for inflation.

Preparation of a report for a third party is subject to a number of statutory regulations including the Code of Conduct set down by the relevant professional Board, privacy and defamation laws and to common law. Privacy laws dictate the collection, use and disclosure of all personal information.

Injuries caused by teeth

The opinion of an odontologist is often requested regarding injuries that have potentially been caused by the biting action of teeth. Bite injuries inflicted by people on other people often occur during assault, sexual assault, child abuse, self-defence and consensual sexual activities. Biting injuries may also involve animals as well as humans. People can sustain injuries inflicted by the teeth of either domestic or wild animals. Opinion sought from the forensic odontologist may include insight into whether or not teeth caused the injury and, if so, whether or not the injury is consistent with human or animal teeth.

Most often bite injuries of interest are seen on the skin of a victim or suspect. The quality of the injury can be very variable, from a vague area of bruising or scratches to distinct indents, lacerations or areas of avulsed tissue. Other factors, such as the amount of force used, movement of the individuals involved and the time since the event occurred, will also play a role in the final appearance of the injury.

When assessing a potential bite mark the first matter to decide is whether or not the mark is likely caused by teeth (Case study 12.8). If the answer to this is

Case study 12.8

Background: Odontologists were asked to analyse a suspected bite mark. The request states that the victim alleges she was bitten and 'teeth ripped down the arm towards the wrist'.

Issues: Is the injury a bite mark? Can it be associated with a specific dentition?

Opinion: Repetitive abrasions to the forearm are seen (Fig. 12.8). The injury pattern displays few features to suggest dental origin. Healing skin tags suggest that the direction of inflicting is across the arm from outer (lateral) to inner (medial) aspect, not vertically down the arm. Parallel (repetitive) injuries to accessible areas, such as the arm or thigh, suggest self-infliction and should be regarded as such until shown to be otherwise. From the appearance, location and disposition of this injury, self-infliction using fingernails is likely. Self-inflicted injuries do not preclude a prior assault (sexual or otherwise) and may be a case of 'gilding the lily'.

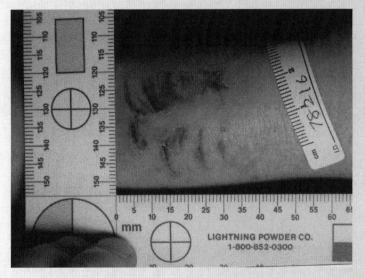

Fig. 12.8   Arm abrasions. (*See insert for colour representation of the figure.*)

negative then the odontologist may be asked as to the likely cause of the patterned injury. Objects such as bottle tops and belt buckles [5], defibrillator marks [6] and various dermatoses [7] can make patterns that, to the untrained eye, may appear as a bite mark. On some occasions injuries may be reported as bite marks when in fact they have a different aetiology.

Case study 12.9

Background: Odontologists were asked to give an opinion where a young boy was alleged to have had his 'mouth washed out with soap' as a disciplinary measure.

Issues: Is soap a stable medium for bite registration? Can the teeth of the alleged victim be correlated with the soap (Fig. 12.9)? If not, is this because the soap has not been in contact with the child's mouth or because changes have occurred due to growth of the child (e.g. exfoliation of deciduous teeth)? Is this child abused?

Opinion: Indentations in the soap remnants are consistent with human incisor teeth. In this case comparison of the teeth marks to the dentition of the child could be made that failed to exclude him as the source of the tooth marks. As an exhibit, the soap needs to be stored at a constant temperature. Child abuse implies intentional harm by the primary care giver(s); however, the incident may not proceed to court.

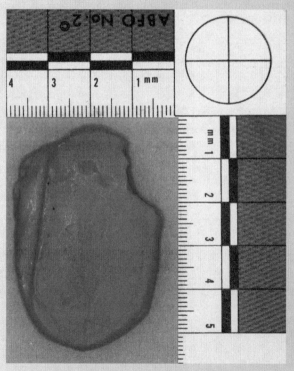

Fig. 12.9 Bite mark in soap.

Bite mark analysis can be considered as a form of tool-mark investigation. Bite marks have gross characteristics such as two semi-circular marks made of a series of smaller marks caused by teeth; class characteristics, which restrict the origin of the mark that is, distinguish between humans and different animal species; and individual characteristics that can be used to distinguish between individuals. In addition to visual and morphometric analysis of bite injuries other forms of analysis may be performed including histological, biochemical and immunological studies. All bite marks have the potential to yield DNA, analysis of which has a greater chance of isolating the individual who caused the injury; hence all suspicious marks should be swabbed for DNA before any other procedure is performed. Swabbing of wounds for DNA is, however, often overlooked in hospital emergency departments.

There are occasions where bite marks in foodstuffs or other inanimate objects may be of interest, particularly to link offenders to the scene of a crime. The clarity of the bite, and suitability for analysis, will depend on the substrate, with solid substrates yielding better results than porous objects [8]. The perishable nature of food means it should be examined as soon as possible and opinions should be tempered by the limitations of the evidence.

The most commonly investigated animal bites inflicted on humans occur during attacks by domestic dogs. The ability to link a given dog to an attack by morphological or metric comparison is limited, like human bites, by properties of the skin and lack of data to differentiate dog dentitions. DNA analysis can help distinguish between dog breeds as well as between individual dogs. Other animals that can cause bite injuries include other domesticated animals such as cats, rabbits and horses; wild animals such as dingoes; and marine animals such as sharks.

Examination of surfboards and scuba equipment where a body has not been located after a suspected shark attack may shed light on the presence of tooth marks. This could assist the coroner in finding the cause and manner of death despite the lack of human remains. The teeth of the great white shark (*Carcharodon carcharias*), in particular, produce characteristic striations in bitten objects [9].

Aside from assessment of bite mark injuries involving humans, a forensic odontologist may be consulted regarding biting injuries inflicted on one animal by another. Valuable livestock can be killed or injured by domestic or wild animals and opinion may be required in compensation claims or to identify the perpetrator in order to prevent further attack. Conservation efforts to protect protected species of animals are often hampered by feral animals such as cats and dogs, but also other non-domestic animals such as foxes and dingoes or even other protected species. An odontologist may be asked to give an opinion as to the likely species that has caused injury to another animal that is potentially at risk of extinction so that efforts can be made to protect the animal or species of interest (Case study 12.10). In these cases bite marks may be seen in skin, bone or other materials, such as collars and radio-tracking devices [10].

Case study 12.10

Background: Odontologists were asked to assist wild life investigators concerned with the death of a protected species of fairy penguins (*Eudyptula minor*) by assessing if the predators were human, a land-based domestic or a feral animal, or a marine animal.

Issues: What features can be used for comparative dental anatomy?

Opinion: Human intervention was considered unlikely due to the repetition, spatial arrangement and size of paired sets of puncture wounds on the penguins' skins. The injuries are consistent with the blunt trauma puncture wounds associated with animal bites. Arch shape, inter-canine distance and tooth size, shape and arrangement were considered for a number of species. *Canis familiaris* (dog), *Vulpes vulpes* (fox) and *Felis catus* (cat) were excluded on the basis of arch and tooth size. *Acrtocephalus pusillus doriferus* (Australian fur seal), *Acrtocephalus fosteri* (New Zealand fur seal) and *Neophoca cinerea* (Australian sea lion) could not be excluded (Fig. 12.10).

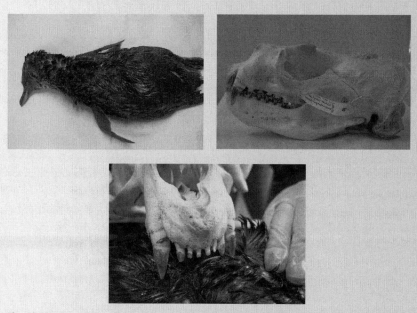

Fig. 12.10 Comparison of injuries to fairy penguins (*Eudyptula minor*) with dentition of New Zealand fur seal (*Acrtocephalus fosteri*).

Child abuse

Deliberate injuries to children may involve both damage to the oral tissues and bite injuries. Damage to the lips, frenula or gingivae of infants from fists or force applied to drinking bottles, pacifiers or other objects, may occur. When biting injuries are seen on children or babies it is not uncommon for the biter to blame other children, such as siblings or school classmates, or domestic animals, for the

Case study 12.11

Background: Child Protection Services investigating injuries to a child asked odontologists for an opinion about the child's oral health.

Issues: What is normal oral health in a child in a given region? Is significantly adverse oral health child neglect?

Opinion: The dentition of the child shows gross caries of the upper anterior teeth, with a draining sinus proximate to the upper-right deciduous central incisor (51) and residual inflammation at the site of the upper-left deciduous lateral incisor (62) (Fig. 12.11). This is due to prolonged and frequent exposure to sugar, combined with lack of good oral hygiene, and is not common in most communities. Neglect is failure to give proper care or attention to a child, and may include failure to modify diet or seek dental treatment.

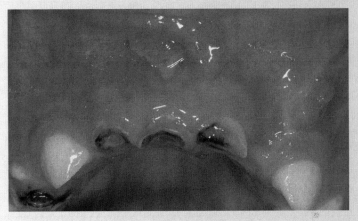

Fig. 12.11   Intra-oral image of widespread dental decay.

injury. Odontologists may be asked if such injuries are human, and whether they are consistent with adult dentition.

Opinion may also be sought concerning widespread decay of the teeth in a child. Prolonged exposure to sugar due to long-lasting sweets or inappropriate diet will cause extensive damage to the teeth. If parents or care givers have disregarded advice from a dentist or other healthcare professional to alter the child's diet or have not had the child's condition treated, this may be construed as neglect (Case study 12.11).

Anatomical/morphometric comparisons

To successfully undertake identification of an individual by dental comparison, dental records depicting individualising features are required. In some instances, however, sufficient dental records may not be available. If the individual did not have dental treatment or a treating dentist could not be located, then no dental records would be available. Alternatively any available dental records may be limited if the individual had good dental health, infrequently attended a dentist or the treating practitioner kept poor records. In these instances an odontologist may be asked to give an opinion on identity based on comparison of the dental, oral and facial features of an individual with features noted in photographic records. Available images can be in the form of family photographs or portraits, driver's licence/passport photographs or digital images. The increasing popularity of social media and the concurrent improvement in the photographic capabilities of mobile phones has greatly increased the availability of high-quality facial photographs available for such comparison.

Direct superimposition of ante-mortem and post-mortem images is problematic, as ante-mortem photographs rarely contain a scale with which the image can be resized to life size, and angles and distances from the camera are difficult to replicate. Comparisons of proportions (photo-anthropometry) and the quantitative analysis of form (morphometric analysis) are, however, possible to perform. If dental casts or impressions are available in ante-mortem records then geometric morphometric analysis, either directly or with the aid of 3D scanners and computer software, may also be possible.

Morphometric/anatomical comparison of dental and orofacial features may also be requested to aid in criminal investigation of living individuals suspected of being involved in crimes or other incidents that have been captured photographically or on Close Circuit Television (CCTV) footage. This involves the examination of two images to determine points of similarity or difference. Individual dental and facial features are compared and a subjective conclusion is reached. While irreconcilable differences can potentially exclude two images from the same individual, it is unlikely that the comparison will allow the odontologist to definitely conclude that the two images are of the same individual. Any conclusions formed are based on subjective observations and, as no database exists with regards to the rate of occurrence of specific features, no statistical weight can be given to this form of evidence. The number of features that can be compared and deemed to be similar will increase the weight of the evidence. Extreme caution should be exercised if image quality is poor. While the knowledge and understanding of the maxillofacial complex is well within the purview of the forensic odontologist, other forensic practitioners such as physical anthropologists and forensic artists may also perform this type of comparison extending to other body structures.

Odontologists may be asked to consider the change in appearance that occurs over time with growth of individuals. Changes to the maxillofacial complex during growth and development occur in a predictable sequence and are used by orthodontists for treatment planning. Families of children reported missing always retain hope that they will be found alive, even after many years, and may request opinion on the likely appearance of the child at time intervals for media release purposes. Opinion may also be sought about age changes in adults. This may occur to reunite families or, in cases of suspected war crimes, when photographs may be many years apart.

Age estimation

Age estimation of humans has a number of indications, largely as an aid to identification of unknown deceased persons, but also for those living person for whom there is no record or accurate record of their date of birth. They could be a refugee, an immigrant, an adopted child or a person facing criminal charges. Situations where the opinion of age may be sought from a forensic odontologist include: as an adjunct to identification in cases where identity is suggested, but little dental evidence is available to establish identity; to add to a profile in a case where identity is unknown so as to narrow down the number of possible individuals; to distinguish between two or more bodies when identity is known and for paleodemographic study of archaeological specimens. In the living, age estimation may be sought for the purpose of criminal proceedings to determine if the individual in question is to be charged as an adult or a minor, or for civil purposes including application for school entry, social welfare benefits, employment or other areas where age is a restriction (Case study 12.12).

It is not possible to accurately pinpoint an exact chronological age for an individual without knowledge of their date of birth. However, studying biological indicators can make an approximation of chronological age. Biological maturity can be grouped into four physiological divisions: somatic, skeletal, dental and

---

Case study 12.12

Background: Odontologists were asked to give an opinion on the age of a young man from a third-world country involved in a serious crime. If over 18 years of age, the individual would be tried in the adult court, with potential for the death sentence.

Issues: How accurate are age-estimation methods? What factors affect the age range? Would the serious consequences alter your scientific judgement?

Opinion: The scientific assessment of age is based on the recognition of certain biological changes known to take place at certain stages during growth and development and beyond. These changes occur gradually over periods of time and may vary significantly according to race, sex, genetic background, geographic location, socio-economic status and lifestyle, diet, condition of health and medical treatment. Biological age therefore cannot be expressed in precise terms of chronological age but, at best, within an age range derived from population studies. All permanent teeth, except the third molars, are fully erupted into the oral cavity and have reached the stage of root closure. The third molar teeth have commenced development. Dental age may also be considered in conjunction with skeletal development. Whilst recognising the potential for variation due to his ethnic background, the clinical and radiographic evidence indicates that this person, at the time of examination, has a chronological age consistent with that of a person aged 16 years with a range from 14 to 18 years (Fig. 12.12).

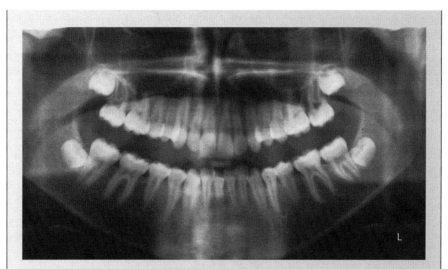

Fig. 12.12 OPG showing dental development.

sexual. Examination of the stage of biological maturity can give estimation of chronological age, but with varying degrees of certainty based on the maturity indicator used and the age of the individual. Dental age has been shown to correlate with chronological age with a higher degree of certainty than the other biological indicators and is less affected by extrinsic factors such as nutrition [11].

During development of the dentition a number of predictable changes occur that can be used to estimate age. These include formation, maturation and eruption of both the deciduous and adult dentition. Once development is finished, however, the prediction of age becomes more problematic with only structural and chemical changes evidencing the passing of time. There are numerous methods of age estimation discussed in the current literature, but no single method is likely to cover all possible situations. Often, several methods of age estimation will be utilised and the results combined to derive a final opinion. Any method used must be scientifically based and must have been validated. Any opinion formed must include a measure of error, and if a population database is used this must be relevant to the case at hand.

Tooth selection and sampling for DNA

When DNA identification of highly degraded human remains is required, teeth are often the tissue of choice for sampling [12]. The unique structure and location of teeth within the jawbones protects the DNA within tooth tissues from the degrading effects of environmental factors such as heat and water, but also from other insults such as fire. The very low porosity of teeth also helps protect the DNA from within and from environmental contamination and exogenous DNA.

However, the success rate of genetic analysis of teeth is highly variable due to the fact that teeth have a unique and complex structure, with DNA content and distribution being affected by many ante- and post-mortem factors [12]. Hence, the forensic odontologist is best qualified to determine how the evidence is examined and to direct the collection and sampling of these tissues.

A comprehensive understanding of tooth structure and the relationship between DNA and the mineralised tissues and the factors that impact this is critical for optimal sample selection. Each case is different and requires careful consideration of the available teeth. The forensic odontologist will determine the most appropriate tooth and specific tooth tissue to sample, and has the necessary skills and expertise to remove teeth from the jaws without compromise and to sample the individual tissues. In degraded teeth the DNA present is often fragmented and in limited quantity. It is important to select the most appropriate tooth and to sample it in a manner that targets the DNA-rich tissues while avoiding complicating compounds such as calcium and collagen, without causing further destruction to the DNA and while avoiding contamination [12].

Contamination of tooth samples with exogenous DNA can occur during initial collection and storage of teeth, so special precautions should be taken to minimise this risk. All personnel working on or near samples that will be used for DNA analysis should wear clean disposable gowns that fully cover the torso, neck and arms, facemasks, gloves and hair covers. If teeth have been handled in a manner that could potentially expose them to contamination, then decontamination procedures may be required. Forms of decontamination include washing with sodium hypochlorite, exposure to UV light and removal of the outer surface by grinding or sanding. Teeth that are firmly retained within the jawbone are unlikely to become contaminated.

As teeth possess value to the identification process beyond that of DNA analysis they should not be arbitrarily destroyed, but should be carefully examined and documented prior to sampling [12]. Adequate photographs and radiographs should be taken so that comparison with dental records is still possible should these records become available at a later date. Careful sampling can also retain sections of the tooth, for example the enamel, which has no DNA but may be useful for chemical analysis or morphometric comparison. Radiocarbon dating of tooth enamel can indicate not only the year of birth (post 1943), but also, in some instances, the year of death of an individual [13, 14]. Tooth enamel provides a more accurate measure of these dates than bone as, unlike bone, it does not undergo continual remodelling.

Once the appropriate tooth and tooth tissue have been selected then the method of DNA extraction needs to be decided. If pulp tissue is sampled then direct polymerase chain reaction (PCR) or an extraction protocol with a short lysis time will be sufficient to liberate the DNA from the cellular components of the pulp. If, however, dentine and/or cementum are sampled an extraction protocol with a much longer lysis time will be required to liberate sufficient DNA from the tissues. DNA contained within the dentine and cementum can be intimately associated with the hydroxyapatite mineral so removal of this mineral via a demineralisation step may also be required and involve an overnight incubation period, which then greatly increases the processing time [12].

Oral pathology

Oral microflora contributes both directly and indirectly to human physiology, nutrition and defence systems [15]. Resident organisms are usually in harmony with the host, but can change to opportunistic pathogens if they reach usually inaccessible sites or encounter changes to normal biology due to exogenous factors (for example, prolonged antibiotic treatment) or endogenous changes to host defences. Dental caries and periodontal disease are the most common expressions of imbalance in normal oral microflora.

Evidence suggests that the oral cavity can also allow pathogenic bacteria and their toxins to distribute systemically, leading to infections and inflammation in distant body sites. Selective subtypes of oral species have been associated with cardiovascular disease, adverse pregnancy outcomes, rheumatoid arthritis, inflammatory bowel disease, colorectal cancer and respiratory tract infections. Species such as *Fusobacterium nucleatum*, *Fusobacterium necrophorum*, *Porphyromonas gingivalis*, *Streptococcus mutans* and *Campylobacter rectus* have been linked to potentially fatal lung, liver, spleen and brain abscesses and meningitis [16]. The odontologist may be asked to provide opinion as to whether the cause of death or serious injury is related to an infection of dental or peri-oral origin (Case study 12.13).

Oral piercing as a cosmetic enhancement is a growing trend [17]. Life-threatening situations have been reported associated with such piercings and include the development of endocarditis [18], cerebral brain abscess [19] and Ludwig's angina [20]. Airway obstruction [21], air embolism during implant surgery with a faulty drill, allowing both air and water into the cavity being drilled [22], intra-operative or post-operative haemorrhage [23–27], and anaphylaxis associated with dental materials [28] have also been reported as oral events having fatal consequences.

Dental malpractice

Dental malpractice is considered as a failure to provide care of a reasonable standard. The standards are upheld by a governing body, such as a professional dental board, and are what a practitioner would have done using proper procedures and appropriate materials.

Dental malpractice claims are of concern to all dental practitioners. The prosecution or the defence (adversarial system), or the court (inquisitorial system) may require the opinion of a forensic odontologist. The odontologist's knowledge and expertise both as a dental and forensic practitioner, places them in the ideal situation to contribute to these cases. Due diligence and careful examination of the evidence, as in all opinions given, is required in these cases.

Case study 12.13

Background: The cause of death of a young man was determined to be organ failure with complicating septicaemia. Post-mortem culture showed the infection to be *Staphylococcus aureus*. Odontologists were asked if recent dental extraction of the upper-right permanent canine (FDI designation 13) was a) clinically justified and b) the source of the infection?

Issues: What is normal oral microflora? What conditions may alter the balance?

Opinion: Extra-oral radiography shows that the patient was in poor dental health, with a number of decayed teeth, retained roots and periapical pathologies (Fig. 12.13). Extraction of the upper-right canine tooth as a result of acute infection would be appropriate primary treatment. *S. aureus* is a Gram-positive bacterium. It is not normally resident in the oral cavity microflora, but is common in the upper respiratory tract, nasal cavity and skin, and may become an opportunistic pathogen. In this case entry to the systemic system may have been via the ethmoid plate, facial veins or the open socket following extraction, or have been unrelated to the oral condition, that is septicaemia may have been secondary to dental treatment or the result of an unrelated portal of entry.

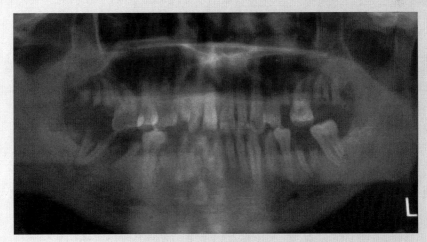

Fig. 12.13   OPG showing widespread dental decay.

Evidence requiring examination will predominantly be the treating practitioner's records, including details of treatment provided, radiographs, photographs, laboratory slips, medical history forms, financial records and any correspondence between the dentist and patient. Other evidence may include the treatment records of subsequent treating dentists, medical practitioners or pathologists (Case study 12.14). Original records are crucial to the review of these cases. Additions to case files after the event can be constituted as fraudulent and can nullify the defendant dentist's insurance and can also expose the dentist to criminal charges of perjury. Determination of whether an injury sustained is the cause of the plaintiff's symptoms or not and whether the treatment provided or not provided is the proximal cause of the symptoms are important to determine.

In some instances a malpractice suit can be brought about not because treatment was performed inappropriately or poorly resulting in injury, but because the practitioner failed to diagnose a condition, the patient was not adequately informed of the risks, alternate treatment options were not made available or the patient's expectations of the treatment were not met. In these cases attention will focus on how the disease would have progressed if correct diagnosis and treatment had been provided, and whether the treatment that was provided was required and whether or not the patient was adequately informed of the likely risks of the procedure and informed consent was obtained. In instances where compensation is claimed because the treatment provided did not meet the patient's expectations, a record of correspondence between the dentist and patient (including verbal communication) is vital.

Case study 12.14

Background: Odontologists were asked to give an opinion on whether a dental record met appropriate standards.

Issues: What legal standards determine appropriate record keeping? Could this record be used to defend a claim of malpractice?

Opinion: The record is largely illegible (Fig. 12.14). Dates and details of treatment could not be reliably established. The documentation does not comply with the Dental Board of Australia standards for record keeping, and is highly likely to be insufficient for any legal defence.

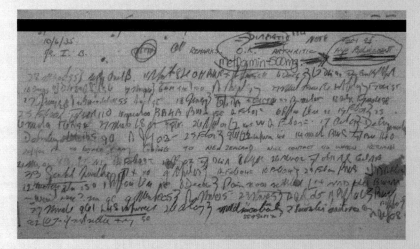

Fig. 12.14 Substandard dental records.

Oral and dental injury can also occur as a result of treatment from healthcare professionals other than dental and dental allied professionals. For example, claims can be brought against an anaesthetist for injury sustained during intubation. Opinion may be sought about the likelihood of such an injury, given the oral condition of the patient, and what steps the anaesthetist might have taken in pre-anaesthetic consultation and at the time of intubation.

The odontologist may also be asked to comment in cases of suspected fraud, where money has been received from the patient, health fund or government agency for work not actually performed. This may range from exaggeration of the number of tooth surfaces restored in order to maximise a benefit, to claims of expensive services that were never provided. Such cases may involve both the living and deceased. When identification by dental comparison is undertaken and the conclusion of exclude is reached, consideration must be given to whether it is a true exclusion (that is, not the person named in the records), the wrong records have been received (another person with the same name) or whether records have been inadvertently or deliberately falsified. Careful examination of dental records is required and substantiating proof of discrepancies should be documented.

Report writing

A forensic report is a formal means of communication between the forensic practitioner and other professionals. Currently, in Australia and New Zealand, there are no formal laws governing the specific format and content of a report of expert opinion, although jurisdictions may have Court Practices Directives as a guide. An expert report may be required to inform legal practitioners or lay persons involved in assessing compensation claims or to outline expert testimony in a court appearance. The content of the report may vary depending on the individual and jurisdiction from which the request for the report came. In all instances the report should address the ultimate questions of the case. Sometimes expert opinion may be required to identify errors or deficits in testimony provided by fact witnesses, while in other cases it may be required to meet the burden of proof in establishment of claim or defence.

Expert reports should start with a preamble, outlining the scope of forensic odontology and the qualification of the expert, to show that the analyses undertaken and opinions expressed are within the area of expertise of the individual practitioner. When reports are given on a regular basis over time, the recipient of the reports may become familiar with those writing them, to the point where they may suggest that, in the interests of brevity, the preamble can be dispensed with.

Chain of evidence details should include information about when and who has made the request for the opinion, and what was requested. A detailed description of material provided should be given and actions undertaken need to be stated. Opinions drawn must be based on the evidence and the information utilised, and basis and rationale for the opinion should be clearly stated. Facts and opinion need to be clearly defined and the reliability and relevance of the opinions given should be unambiguous. All technical and complex processes should be explained so that a layperson can understand the information provided. The basis of the opinions given should be objective and unbiased and the methods used to test the facts and form the opinion should be appropriate. If the report relies on information provided by others, this must be clearly stated in the report, as should any assumptions made. Limitations such as the quality of the evidence provided, methodology or technical difficulties and boundaries to the conclusions that can be reached should also be clearly stated. Many jurisdictions have directions for experts that require reports to contain a stipulation such as: I have considered all relevant materials and have made appropriate enquiries and no matters that I regard as significant have, to my knowledge, been withheld.

Reports should be written in a clear and concise manner, with language to match the understanding capacity of the reader of the report. Technical terms, such as tooth numbers and anatomical terms, need to be clearly explained. Above all reports should be succinct. Long, waffling reports are of little use to either investigators or courts. Ideally, all reports should be peer reviewed before they are issued. An independent review should examine the facts and conclusions that have been reached. If there is material disagreement then a frank reassessment is indicated. The peer review should also check for grammar and typographical errors, and that all evidence upon which the opinion was given is present in the case file.

Requests to change a report by third parties, such as police or lawyers, should be resisted. The report is legally binding and should not be modified unless fresh evidence has emerged or the odontologist is sure that they have made a mistake. All reports should contain a statement to the effect that the opinion given is based on the evidence available at the time of its completion. This allows that, if subsequent evidence becomes available, the opinion may be superseded.

References

1 Goonerathne I, Gunatilake PGL. (2010) A histological and a forensic odontological approach to identify ivory and ivory substitutes for forensic purposes: a case study. *Sri Lanka Journal of Forensic Medical Science and Law* **1**, 33–34.

2 Berketa J, Hirsch R, Higgins D et al. (2010) Implant recognition as an aid to identification. *Journal of Forensic Science* **55**, 66–70.

3 Craig P, Clement JG. (2012) The dentist's responsibility with respect to a no–fault motor accident compensation scheme. *Journal of Forensic Odontostomatology* **30**, 40–46.

4 Titsas A, Ferguson MM. (2002) Impact of opiod use on dentistry. *Australian Dental Journal* **47**, 94–98.

5 James H, Cirillo GN. (1989) Bite mark or bottle top? *Journal of Forensic Science* **49**, 119–121.

6 Grey TC. (1989) Defibrillator injury suggesting bite mark. *American Journal of Forensic Medicine and Pathology* **10**, 144–145.

7 Gold MH, Roenigk HH, Smith ES et al. (1989) Human bite marks. Differential diagnosis. *Clinical Pediatrics* **28**, 329–331.

8 Dorion RBJ. (2011) *Bitemark Evidence: A Color Atlas and Text*. CRC Press, Florida.

9 Cirillo GN, James H. (2004) Pattern association: a key to recognition of shark attacks. *Journal of Forensic Odontostomatology* **22**, 47–48.

10 James H, Acharya AB, Taylor JA et al. (2002) A case of bitten bettongs. *Journal of Forensic Odontostomatology* **20**, 10–12.

11 Demirjian A. (1978) Dentition. In: Falkner F, Tanner JM (eds) *Human Growth 2 Postnatal Growth*, Plenum Press, New York, pp. 413–444.

12 Higgins D, Austin JJ. (2013) Teeth as a source of DNA for forensic identification of human remains: A review. *Science and Justice* **53**, 433–441.

13 Ubelaker DH, Parra RC. (2011) Radiocarbon analysis of dental enamel and bone to evaluate date of birth and death: perspective from the southern hemisphere. *Forensic Science International* **208**, 103–107.

14 Spalding KL, Buchholz BA, Bergman LE et al. (2005) Forensics: age written in teeth by nuclear tests. *Nature* **437**, 333–334.

15 Marsh PD, Martin MD. (2009) *Oral Microbiology*. 5th edn, Elsevier, Edinburgh, pp. 1–7.

16 Han YW, Wang X. (2013) Mobile microbiome: Oral bacteria in extra-oral infections and inflammation. *Journal of Dental Research* **92**, 485–491.

17 Plastargias I, Sakellari D. (2014) The consequences of tongue piercing on oral and periodontal tissues. *ISRN Dentistry* **2014**, Article ID 876510, 6 pages.

18 Friedel JM, Steblik J, Desai M et al. (2003) Infective endocarditis after oral body piercing. *Cardiology in Review* **11**, 252–255.

19 Martinello JRA, Cooney EL. (2003) Cerebellar brain abscess associated with tongue piercing. *Clinical Infectious Diseases* **36**, e32–34.

20 Perkins CS, Meisner J, Harrison JM. (1997) A complication of tongue piercing. *British Dental Journal* **182**, 147–148.

21 Costain N, Marrie T. (2011) Ludwig's angina. *American Journal of Medicine* **124**, 115–117.

22 Messier DY. (1978) Coroner's report: circumstances of a death related to implant surgery procedures. *International Journal of Oral Implantology* **6**, 50–63.

23 Green AW, Flower EA, New NE. (2001) Mortality associated with odontogenic infection. *British Dental Journal* **190**, 529–530.

24 Moghadam HG, Caminti MF. (2002) Life-threatening hemorrhage after extraction of third molars: case report and management protocol. *Journal of the Canadian Dental Association* **68**, 670.

25 Funayama M, Kumagai T, Saito K et al. (1994) Asphyxial death caused by post–extraction hematoma. *American Journal of Forensic Medicine and Pathology* **15**, 87–90.

26 Lifschultz BD, Kenney JP, Sturgis CD et al. (1995) Fatal intercranial hemorrhage following pediatric oral surgical procedure. *Journal of Forensic Science* **40**, 131–133.

27 Okada Y, Suzuki H, Ishiyama I. (1989) Fatal subarachnoid haemorrhage associated with dental local anaesthesia. *Australian Dental Journal* **34**, 323–325.

28 Gangemi SI, Spagnolo EV, Cardia G et al. (2009) Fatal anaphylactic shock due to a dental impression material *International Journal of Prosthodontics* **22**, 33–34.

CHAPTER 13

Forensic odontology management

Helen James and Denice Higgins

Forensic Odontology Unit, University of Adelaide, Australia

Introduction

Management considerations in forensic odontology can be categorised into the domains of administration, education and research. This chapter provides an overview of issues to be considered in these areas. Once likened to herding cats, management of a group of odontologists can be a challenging and stimulating experience. It is, however, a necessary task: police, forensic scientists and lawyers need both a contact point to arrange services and an end point of responsibility ('the buck stops here' concept originally suggested by US President Harry Truman). The traits that characterise a good forensic odontologist, such as knowledge currency, attention to detail, solution seeking and team approach, should translate to good management skills.

Administration

Administrative tasks include the management of funding, personnel and resources; the development and maintenance of procedures and protocols (including formulation of standard operating procedures and operational health safety and welfare considerations); Disaster Victim Identification (DVI) planning; and media management.

Most developed countries have a forensic odontology component to their forensic response capability because it has been demonstrated that odontology can provide a rapid, reliable and cost-effective means of identification of deceased persons. Attempts to dispense with odontology services have usually been quickly reversed. The most likely funding source for forensic odontology services is through regional government. Government agencies that may provide funding for coronial identifications and legal opinions include justice, law enforcement and health departments.

Although forensic odontology is a recognised, and in some countries a registered speciality, it is rarely a full-time employment option. Most odontologists

---

Forensic Odontology: Principles and Practice, First Edition. Edited by Jane A. Taylor and Jules A. Kieser.
© 2016 John Wiley & Sons, Ltd. Published 2016 by John Wiley & Sons, Ltd.

work in other areas of public or private dentistry and, in reality, often personally subsidise the forensic component of their practice as a service to the community. Co-funding through university teaching and postgraduate training programs is a model that has advantages. The academic environment gives added resources to forensic groups and promotes a culture of teaching and evidence-based research.

Forensic odontologists are a rare group within the dental community, contributing only a small fraction to the total dental workforce. Dental Board of Australia statistics for 2014 [1] show 18,243 registered dentists and 27 specialist forensic odontologists (approximately 0.15% of the workforce). Even allowing for general dental practitioners without formal qualification but with interest and/or experience in the field, those dentists working in the discipline still equate to less than 1% of the registered dentists in Australia. It is likely that these numbers are mirrored in other countries. There may be a number of reasons for this, including the fact that training is expensive, jobs are scarce and it has been described as a 'ghoulish' occupation that many feel they could not undertake. It is often a secondary career option for dentists who have financial security but wish to expand their professional life or contribute to the community.

It is important that personnel are managed with care to encourage both retention of trained odontologists and the involvement of newcomers. Senior odontologists need to organise ongoing training for other staff and allow them the time and resources to pursue development opportunities. This may include development and delivery of educational material, attendance at conferences and involvement in research. It is also important for a group's senior odontologist to consider succession planning for their retirement and to assist colleagues to achieve a range of case experience and skills, in order to ensure a smooth transition of leadership.

As well as trained personnel, many other resources are required for all aspects of odontology services including equipment (for example, computer hardware and software; and imaging devices such as x-ray machines and cameras) and consumables (for example, office stationery, personal protective equipment and staff amenities). Funding for major and minor equipment may be provided as part of an employment contract or secured via application for grants from national and local funding bodies such as the National Health and Medical Research Council (NHMRC), and the Australian Research Council (ARC).

The equipment required to perform forensic odontology tasks is dependent on the particular task at hand, but all areas require some basic office equipment. Minimum office equipment could be considered to comprise a desk and chair with phone and computer (including software such as: Microsoft® Office™, Adobe Acrobat®, Adobe Photoshop® and Internet, virus and security programs), printer and scanner. If the odontologist is expected to maintain records and exhibits then a secure storage capacity is also essential. Court cases, with appeals, may take many years to finalise, meaning that such storage needs to be long-term, with

Table 13.1 Journals of professional interest to forensic odontologists.

- *Journal of Forensic Odontostomatology*
- *Journal of Forensic Sciences*
- *Forensic Science International*
- *Forensic Science, Medicine and Pathology*
- *Journal of Forensic and Legal Medicine*
- *Journal of Comparative Human Biology*
- *Journal of Emergency Management*
- *Journal of Contingencies and Crisis Management*
- *Science and Justice*

high-level security. To protect against loss of data due to computer failure, fire, flood or theft, off-site backup of electronic data should also be considered.

Another important resource is access to standard reference books in forensic odontology and related fields, such as forensic pathology, genetics and anthropology, forensic science, imaging and law. In addition, access to current and past scientific literature is vital, requiring subscription to those journals that do not have free public access and the availability of Internet services for those that do. Potentially relevant journals are listed in Table 13.1.

Specific odontology tasks have their own equipment requirements although some pieces of equipment may be utilised over several different tasks (for example, camera equipment and a calibrated scale for use in imagery). The primary task undertaken by the odontologist is identification of deceased persons, which involves examination of both ante-mortem records and post-mortem remains. Examination of ante-mortem records requires relatively little extra equipment on top of the standard office equipment discussed previously. Additional equipment requirements may include an x-ray viewer and magnifying glass for the examination of radiographs and a ruler and set of callipers for measuring features on casts and dental appliances. Standardised ante-mortem and post-mortem dental description forms, such as the Interpol DVI forms can be used to record dental findings, in either paper or electronic format. Alternatively, computer software such as DVI System International® [2] or WinID® [3] may be utilised. Standardised recording format, achieved by a pre-determined local code guide for common dental conditions and treatment options, allows uniform reconciliation and reporting.

Considerably more equipment is required for the examination of post-mortem remains. This equipment may belong to the local forensic service or may be the property of the forensic odontologists. It may be housed at the mortuary or brought with the odontologist to each case. Consumables, such as personal protective clothing, masks and gloves, can usually be sourced at the mortuary. Equipment required to perform a post-mortem examination includes standard dental examination instruments, such as mirror, probe and tweezers.

Additionally, jaw spreaders and mouth props may be needed to allow access to the dentition, and extraction instruments, such as elevators and forceps, will be needed if tooth sampling for DNA is requested. If dental casts are required then disposable impression trays will also be needed. Instruments used on deceased persons cannot be subsequently cleaned and reused on the living so dedicated post-mortem equipment is essential.

In most developed countries dental radiography as a diagnostic tool is routinely undertaken, and consequently establishing identification by dental means relies heavily on the comparison of ante-mortem and post-mortem radiographic images. Post-mortem dental radiography requires a dedicated radiation source for plain dental radiography. The x-ray unit may be wall mounted, attached to a floor stand or hand held. If capture of radiographic images outside of the mortuary setting is required then the unit needs to be portable and battery operated. Images may be captured digitally or on film. Digital imagery is preferable as it decreases the required radiation dose, avoids chemicals required for development of film and allows immediate access to the images. Immediate access to imagery allows for correction of sensor placement and tube angulations to facilitate capture of ideal images for comparison. If film is utilised it is important to consider that film has a shelf life that should not be exceeded for best quality images. Extra-oral fluoroscopy or computer tomography (CT) may also be available for use in the mortuary. Odontologists should know how to interpret these images and may request them if views will assist identification. Situations where such views may be helpful include when bone plates and screws are present, or if sinus views or medical films depicting oral structures are available for comparison.

Extra-oral and intra-oral cameras can be used to record features of the face and teeth for comparison with ante-mortem photographs to assist in identification. High-resolution images can potentially be used for superimposition, if angulations and perspectives of ante-mortem images can be replicated.

A scene case is a self-contained unit that is stocked and quickly available if an odontologist is asked to attend the scene of an incident or event. This may be to assist recovery of remains or to examine an injury. The case may contain a folder with journal pages, dental identification forms, template forms for pattern injury examination of alleged victim and alleged biter; camera, ABFO No 2 ruler; multi-colour pen; gloves; and impression trays, materials and mixers (Fig. 13.1). Crime scene over-clothing, stout boots, hat, sunscreen and drinking water may also be considered. Similarly, a pre-packed equipment case can be kept on standby for DVI deployment.

All equipment requires some level of maintenance; from simple cleaning to more involved regimes such as software upgrades and electrical testing. Equipment such as cameras and hand-held x-ray machines are battery operated and the batteries need regular charging. A schedule should be established to ensure that charged batteries are always available. The frequency of charging

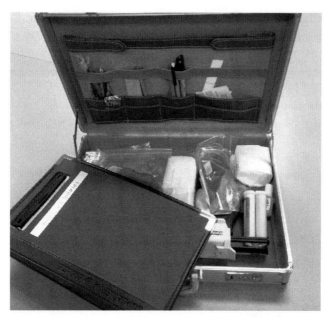

Fig. 13.1 Scene case.

will depend on the type of batteries, the appliance and the amount of use. A log should be kept to record maintenance processes, such as the date and time of battery charging. As an occupational safety measure only trained personnel should test electrical appliances to ensure that they are fit for use. Similarly, radiation testing of x-ray machines and lead aprons is required annually or in accordance with any local legalisation.

Equipment such as printers and scanners should be calibrated and colour balanced when acquired. A validation study should be undertaken to assess accuracy and precision of scanned images and to determine the limitations of the system. Well-maintained good-quality equipment and a validated protocol will allow high accuracy and high precision, as well as results that are repeatable (same operator) and reproducible (different operator).

All equipment deteriorates with time. A program of planned obsolescence should be considered to ensure optimal function of equipment and to accommodate new technologies. Knowing when equipment is due for replacement assists with budget planning.

It is vital to have a quality management ethos in forensic odontology, and to develop and implement protocols to maximise and correctly interpret dental data to achieve the successful, scientifically sound and rapid outcomes expected by instructing authorities, impacted parties and the forensic odontology specialist community [4].

Development of procedures should be based on current, scientifically valid methods taking into consideration the resources available. This requires a wide and detailed knowledge of the current literature that meets the best-practice global standards of forensic odontology. Critical areas to consider include collection and transportation of evidence, examination and recording techniques, interpretation of data, reporting, presentation of findings and preservation of evidence in a secure environment.

Protocols to manage and store both physical and electronic data are crucial. Loss of data can occur by physical misplacement, mixing with another dataset, incorrect file type (lossy files) or corruption of storage media. Data need to be indexed, isolated from other case material, and retained until no longer required for legal purposes. This may, in some cases, be many years through court cases and appeal processes.

Odontologists do not work in isolation. It is important for protocols to incorporate interdisciplinary interactions and to demonstrate understanding of the roles of police, pathologists and other forensic scientists. Care needs to be taken that odontologists do not disturb scene evidence or allow biological contamination to occur from one case to another. Odontologists may be asked to have their DNA profiles uploaded to a DNA database for exclusionary purposes.

Reporting templates can be useful tools to standardise format and language and ensure that all relevant evidence is collected, documented and presented. Facts should always be separated from opinions. Technical terms need to be defined and jargon should be avoided. Mechanisms for audits and peer review of opinions need to be clearly established.

Standard Operating Procedures (SOPs) are documented, detailed, prescribed operational practices, which are created to ensure that operations are carried out optimally and always in the same manner. The principle of having SOPs in place is to provide a working and tested set of rules that can be implemented to maintain appropriate quality levels [4]. SOPs need to be written, tested in controlled circumstances to ensure anticipated results are achieved, distributed and implemented. Most procedures in forensic odontology can be performed using a number of different methodologies with varying degrees of skill required. Selection of a particular methodology must be based on a detailed review of the scientific literature, tests performed in practical situations and error levels established where possible [4]. SOPs should be regularly revised and updated to encompass changing circumstances and in the face of emerging technologies. Group discussion and feedback mechanisms are recommended to formulate and update SOPs [5].

Educational emphasis and work practices differ between regions. Odontologists must understand and implement SOPs as formulated, but equally must have defined mechanisms to initiate discussion about review of SOPs. Communication clarity, both written and spoken, is crucial. As a specialised discipline within dentistry, forensic odontology standards are mandatory. They afford legal protection, if questioned about methodology, and allow quality management when training newcomers to the discipline. Odontologists must commit to remaining professionally current in their knowledge, be willing to accept peer review and to change their practices if necessary, recognise their limitations and not go beyond those boundaries. It should also be their manager's responsibility to recognise, record and allow for those limitations when allocating areas for their employment.

Occupational health, safety and welfare (OHSW) is concerned with protecting the safety, health and welfare of people engaged in work. Most developed countries have legislation to ensure worker safety and organisations have policies and procedures relating to the safety of employees and visitors, based around the relevant regional legislation. These laws set out the general requirements for protecting health and safety in the workplace and give powers to government inspectors to scrutinise workplaces and investigate health and safety issues. In many countries inspectors may not need an appointment to make a visit to a workplace, and may call at any workplace at any time to carry out an inspection, investigate an injury or incident that has occurred, or audit health and safety systems. Prosecutions, resulting in penalties and fines, may follow breaches of OHSW regulations.

Odontologists' roles in OHSW are often not clearly defined because of differing conditions of employment that may apply. Odontologists may be employed by forensic service providers, universities or regional health services; they may also be classed as contractors or, in some case, as volunteers. Consequently they may be involved in OHSW as a coordinator, employee, contractor or volunteer. It is also possible to have more than one site of employment – for example, some work is done on university campus and some at the local mortuary. Both areas may require odontology OHSW input into management systems. If defined as a contractor then a complete policy may need to be developed. Odontologists acting in a management, coordinator or contractor role must ensure OHSW policies and procedures are in place and are followed; identifying and assessing risk in areas specific to odontology and proposing risk minimisation strategies.

Many organisations use a management system to implement OHSW measures. Occupational Health and Safety Management Systems (OHSMS) have been defined as "a combination of the planning and review, the management organisational arrangements, the consultative arrangements, and the specific program elements that work together in an integrated way to improve health and safety performance" [6]. The use of OHSMS has become common in workplaces both in Australia and other developed economies as a response to defective protocols exposed by disasters such as the Piper Alpha oilrig fire [7]. OHSMS involve the deliberate linking and sequencing of processes to achieve specific objectives and to create a repeatable and identifiable way of managing OHSW and apply corrective actions where necessary [8]. The elements of an OHSMS are displayed in Table 13.2. AS/NZS 4801 is an Australian and New Zealand standard, which outlines requirements related to Health and Safety Management Systems and provides a self-assessment checklist [9].

Table 13.2 Elements of an Occupational Health and Safety Management System.

- Commitment to a Safe Workplace (framing a policy)
- Recognising and Removing Hazards (using a hazard identification checklist)
- Maintaining a Safe Workplace (including safety checks, maintenance, reporting hazards, information and training, supervision, accident investigation and emergency planning)
- Safety Records and Information (including records and standards required to be kept by law)

		Consequences				
		Negligible	Minor	Moderate	Major	Severe
Likelihood	Almost certain	Medium	High	Very high	Very high	Very high
	Likely	Medium	Medium	High	Very high	Very high
	Possible	Low	Medium	High	High	Very high
	Unlikely	Low	Low	Medium	Medium	High
	Rare	Low	Low	Low	Medium	Medium

Fig. 13.2 Risk assessment matrix.

The OHSW policy is a written statement of commitment to OHSW and, in many countries, is a legal requirement. The policy should indicate the responsibilities and accountabilities of both management and workers. Procedures should be developed to outline how the requirements of the policy will be met for specific areas of concern. Planning should set goals, objectives and priorities. For each goal the steps or actions needed to achieve it should be identified and for each action, responsibility, timeframe and date for review of progress should be assigned.

OHSW training for odontology coordinators should include roles and responsibilities under the prevailing legislation; hazard identification and management; conducting audits; incident investigation and injury management. They, in turn, need to ensure that odontologists working with them have the knowledge and skills necessary to work safely, and that mechanisms for hazard and incident reporting are clearly defined. Odontology coordinators may be asked to sit on a Health and Safety Committee to contribute knowledge related to general office and mortuary issues and also to those specific to odontology working conditions.

A hazard is something that has the potential to cause injury or illness. Effective hazard management involves identifying the hazard, assessing risk based on likelihood and consequences (Fig. 13.2), and formulating mechanisms to minimise risk and evaluate outcomes. Hazards in forensic odontology are summarised in Table 13.3.

The nature of forensic odontology casework means it can be extremely stressful. Psychological ill health may result from ongoing work-related stress, where odontologists may be subjected to demands and expectations that are out of keeping with their abilities, skills or coping strategies. Factors that may

Table 13.3 Hazards in forensic odontology.

- Psychological
- Chemical agents
- Sharps
- Biological pathogens
- Radiation
- Ergonomic

contribute to psychological injury include demanding workloads; unrealistic timeframes for completion of work; lack of skills and training; inability to discuss issues or problems; poor relationships with supervisors and/or other workers; and real or perceived lack of counselling and support. Risk can be minimised by providing workers with a job description statement and making them aware of their roles, responsibilities and rights; holding regular staff meetings to provide opportunity for debriefing and problem solving; providing training in procedures to ensure workers are competent to perform their roles; reducing opportunities for fatigue related to work; providing counselling avenues; and encouraging group social interaction.

Stress for odontologists may be due to accumulative interactions or following a critical incident. Disaster stress is a complex interaction between environmental and task stressors; job competency; perceptual and emotional defences; and management and follow-up support. A Critical Incident Stress Management (CISM) program, with appropriate counselling services, should be identified by the odontology coordinator. Critical Incident Stress Debriefing (CISD) should be linked and blended with crisis support services, including individual crisis intervention, family support services, referrals for professional care, if necessary, and post incident education programs [10]. This may be most appropriately sourced in conjunction with police and other emergency services.

Disaster workers are also at risk of both acute and chronic post-traumatic stress disorder (PTSD). Experienced personnel may experience low levels of problems [11]; however, exposure to a disaster setting can also have both short- and long-term mental and physical consequences on some professionals [12]. The prevalence of PTSD in rescue/recovery occupations has been reported as ranging from 5% to 32%, with the highest rate reported in workers with no prior training in disaster work [13]. Studies also suggest an increase in physical health problems and health care utilisation associated with exposure to traumatic events and disaster work. Health problems may include fatigue, musculoskeletal complaints, and cardiac, respiratory and gastric symptoms. A study by Swygard and Stafford found exposures to different types of hazards, including insect bites, skin lesions, diarrhoea and other gastrointestinal complaints, during or soon after deployment [14]. Thormar et al. also reported that PTSD has been associated with increased smoking, alcohol and drug abuse [15]. Post-traumatic Stress Management is complex, and appropriate specialist services need to be identified as part of an OHSW plan.

It is essential for odontologists to have good team dynamics, with managerial protocols to minimise potential problems and a work culture of management and team support. Team members must take care of themselves and also be mindful of the stress levels in colleagues. The results of a study of emergency workers suggested that support from supervisors reduces the severity of PTSD symptoms; and spirituality and support from co-workers promotes professional growth after trauma [16].

Aside from disaster work, respiratory and skin disorders have both been reported in forensic personnel associated with identification of deceased personnel [17]. Methacrylates, rubber latex proteins, and glutaraldehyde are the predominant allergens in dentistry. Reactions from cell-mediated contact allergy may include urticaria and occupational asthma [18]. Spray disinfectants may be used in mortuaries and may cause respiratory problems. Formalin and formaldehyde from preserved bodies may present a hazard if subsequent autopsy or odontology examination is required. Nausea, headaches and respiratory irritation have been noted. Risk minimisation includes use of non-latex gloves where needed and wiping rather than spraying surfaces. Breathing apparatus may be considered for cases involving re-examination of preserved or partially preserved bodies. Odontologists with latex allergy should take with them a supply of their preferred gloves if deployed to a location other than their usual work environment.

Sharps injuries are one of the most common types of injury incurred by healthcare workers [19] and are a potential hazard in forensic odontology when examining deceased persons. Risks include injury from scalpels and dental probes as well as fractured bones, and are compounded by biological pathogens. Risk minimisations include care in tissue dissection; correct disposal of single-use scalpels into a sharps container; and correct cleaning techniques for dental examination instruments.

In many mortuaries it is presumed that all deceased persons carry some infectious disease. Occupational blood-borne virus (BBV) transmission, including human immunodeficiency virus (HIV), hepatitis B and hepatitis C, has been reported for health workers but assessment of transmission incidence and absolute risk of infection has rarely been published. Incidences in forensic odontology are uncertain, most likely due to under-reporting. Common routes of administration of infection include absorption (through open cuts or scratches on the skin or eye); direct inoculation (needles, scalpels, etc. providing a direct means of injection of an infection into the bloodstream); oral ingestion (smoking, eating or drinking prior to hand washing) and aerosol inhalation. Risk control includes personal protective equipment, including protective clothing, gloves, safety glasses or a full-face shield; personal hygiene; designated clean and dirty areas within the mortuary (with appropriate SOP); and correct disposal of linen and waste materials. Working surfaces must be disinfected routinely by swabbing with a suitable disinfectant and instruments must be correctly cleaned and autoclaved.

Forensic odontology radiology comprises the performance, interpretation and reporting of diagnostic radiological procedures that pertain to the law. A number of special features must be considered in developing protocols to meet the varying operational situations the forensic odontologist might face. Material may be fragmented, decomposed, incinerated, fragile, not readily movable or handling might cause contamination of, or damage to, evidence. The site where the x-rays need to be taken is not generally dedicated to dental treatment or radiography. Casework can involve moving between multiple locations, local or distant; having to remove x-ray equipment from a site immediately after use; not having a solid support footprint or operating space available for conventional equipment; or working in areas where use of equipment could create a danger to the operators or destroy vital evidence.

The odontology coordinator must ensure that ionising radiation is managed safely, in accordance with regional laws, and exposure to radiation is at a level as low as reasonably achievable by using appropriate control measures. Lower doses will be achieved using digital x-ray sensors. Monitoring of the radiation dose of all registered workers can be achieved by personal dosimeters. In many countries all staff and postgraduate students using sealed sources x-ray diagnostic apparatus (plain and fluoro) require a license. The law may require that the machine is locked when not in use; a radiation warning sign 'Danger – Radiation Area' is displayed; personal protection by use of lead apron and correct exposure technique is followed; and that a transport log for moving a hand-held machine is maintained.

Portable radiation sources, such as the Nomad™ Hand-held X-ray Unit (Aribex, Inc., Oram, USA) are now commonplace in forensic odontology. They allow for flexibility in scene and mortuary work but can lead to poor radiation hygiene if operators become careless. Compliance with local legislation with respect to use of such units is mandatory. A radiation plan, including safety manual and SOP for operating equipment, needs to be developed. Likewise, a schedule for maintaining equipment is required. Radiation safety testing of the x-ray unit and lead apron, and electrical testing of battery chargers should occur annually. Lead aprons need to be hung, rather than folded, to minimise cracking.

Chemical, Biological, Radiation or Nuclear (CBRN) incidents are a potential risk for odontologists deployed for DVI. While planning, training exercises and recent operations have honed skills in many areas of DVI, odontologists in general have little experience with CBNR. In the event of an unintentional incident or terrorist attack involving CBNR, decontamination procedures may require the expertise of hazardous materials (HazMat) technicians. The process may impact on evidence collection for DVI both at the scene and in the mortuary phase [20]. The levels of personal protective equipment (PPE) required for all odontology examinations may be escalated to full body suit and gloves that are resistant to both chemical and biological agents, and a self-contained breathing unit. Many odontologists will have had no training with such apparatus and should avoid entering Hot or Warm Zones without full guidance in the use of the equipment.

While many of the hazards described above are more obvious, and potentially more harmful, it should not be forgotten that a large part of the odontologist's work is office orientated. Occupational Overuse Syndrome (OOS) related to the use of computers is a potential hazard that should not be overlooked. Australian Standard AS 3590 – 1990 recommends arrangement of computer workstations in such a way so that the risk of OOS injuries is reduced [21]. Work surface height; chair height and backrest support; screen and keyboard placement; type and position of the mouse; and lighting for monitors to reduce glare and reflection need to be considered. Correct desk set up should include: a swivel chair with stable base, adjustable seat height and back support; sufficient legroom under the desk; and similar distance from screen to keyboard. It is important to change posture regularly and take frequent short breaks to minimise fatigue.

Incidents and near misses need to be reported to the site OHSW manager to allow investigation of cause and remedial action. For example, a knife rack placed too close to a light switch may result in a sharps injury. In addition, in some jurisdictions mandatory reporting is required to a government regulatory body for incidents that result in, or could potentially result in, death of a worker. An example for odontology would be electrical shock from faulty equipment. Incidents are documented and investigated to identify cause and prevent similar issues recurring. Incident reports need to be kept and may be audited.

In many countries there are legal requirements to maintain a range of OHSW records, including injury/incident reports and investigations; workers rehabilitation and compensation records; first aid records; training records; certificates and licences; and hazard report forms (including actions taken). A plan for foreseeable emergencies, including natural events such as fire or earthquake, biosecurity breaches or medical emergencies may also be required. The OHSW plan, as a whole, should be reviewed regularly to ensure currency.

Regional pre-event planning by odontologists for identification of victims of a mass casualty event is crucial. This needs to involve close liaison with the person designated to command operations in the region if a disaster should occur and, preferably, input into the regional DVI committee. Administrative tasks for senior odontologists will include appointing, equipping and training a first-response odontology team; identifying equipment needs and sources; designating experienced odontology team leaders for each phase of the disaster; identifying personnel with appropriate expertise to augment local team members if indicated by the scope of the disaster; and writing SOPs to be implemented. Such tasks are encompassed by an Odontology Disaster Response Plan.

Senior odontologists may be asked to comment for a 'human interest' or media fill-in story, or on a particular event. Employment conditions for odontologists may specify no media interviews, or not without organisational media training. The media may be interested as a matter of general interest or current controversy, and some are adept at misquoting for sensational effect. Queries regarding current investigations, matters before the courts (*sub judice*) and DVI operations should be referred to the police media office for comment.

Education

Identification by means of the teeth has been described in the literature for a considerable period of time [22], but such work has not always been confined to the dental profession. Historical accounts tell us that a wife of an Emperor of Rome and valet to a Duke of Burgundy were involved in early identification work, along with doctors and relatives of deceased people. Silversmith Paul Revere, who supplemented his income by part-time dentistry, is credited with the first professional identification when he recognised his handiwork in the form of a crafted silver wire bridge [23]. Many dentists have subsequently given time and expertise on an informal basis. The first educational courses in forensic odontology were established in Scandinavia in the mid 20th century [22] and programs have since been established in many countries.

Training can range from single-issue courses for interested dentists through to specialist registration programs. Regardless of the intended outcome, training needs to be comprehensive, objective and creative so that participants reflect the learning outcomes and graduate attributes of the training provider. A good training program will have a reputation that will attract future students to the discipline.

Trainees have expectations of currency in knowledge and methodology and acquisition of skills to allow them to practise in the discipline. Successful students and graduates will demonstrate visible improvements in knowledge, methodology, critical judgements, and problem-solving skills, and a team focus. They should be encouraged to provide critical review of the training program content and delivery during and after graduation.

A primary focus of training programs should be to have graduates involved in the discipline on completion of their studies. This should include, where possible, casework, teaching and research. Coughlin (2009) suggested adaptation of the traditional format for acquiring medical skills ('see one, do one, teach one') could be successfully applied to other disciplines [24]. Teaching and presenting on the many aspects of forensic odontology has the advantage of improving communication skills and boosting expertise in the eye of the courts.

Odontologists may be invited to speak to many different groups (Table 13.4). It is important to tailor presentations to the knowledge level and expectations of the target audience, and to provide both information and entertainment. The

Table 13.4 Presentations.

- Dental practitioners
- Dentists
- Hygienists
- Therapists
- Prosthetists
- Dental assistants
- Dental students
- Associated and related fields
- Forensic scientists
- Medical practitioners
- Legal
- Police
- Coroner
- Legal fraternity
- Government
- Community

focus of each presentation may change: for example, to increase the profile of odontologists; to inform allied forensic practitioners of our expertise; or to initiate improvement in dental standards. Odontologists must hone their skills in oral presentation and take every opportunity to promote the discipline. Being 'flashy with fright' at the thought of public speaking is no excuse. Measures of successful presentations may include obvious interest of the audience; implementation of change in a target audience; and repeat invitation.

Many countries require professionals to adopt a life-long learning approach. Australian dental professionals are required to complete a minimum of 60 hours of continuing professional development (CPD) over a three-year period to maintain registration with the Dental Board of Australia. Odontology Fellows of the Royal College of Pathologists of Australasia (RCPA) are expected to complete 500 hours, in a range of categories, over five years. The format of CPD undertaken by odontologists is a matter for individual preference. Books, journals and web-based tutorials on forensic issues are readily available. Conferences, offering block hours of education and a social mix for those with similar interests, are an excellent way of gaining knowledge and seeing the world. Regional working groups provide focus on local issues. Many countries have a forensic odontology society, which may accept national and international members.

Research

Research involves investigation undertaken to gain knowledge, understanding and insight. The goal of research is to contribute to a scientific body of knowledge of a profession. It is understood by researchers that the term encompasses both intellectual honesty and integrity, and scholarly and scientific rigour. Research may be used to develop theories, test questions or validate new techniques; moving from empirical statements to those based on evidence [25]. Many countries have an assessment system that evaluates the quality of research conducted against national and international benchmarks. Excellence in research for Australia (ERA), which is administered by the Australian Research Council (ARC), strives to identify and promote excellence in research in Australian higher education institutes [26].

Research related to forensic odontology may utilise both human and animal models. Human research may include case studies or group comparisons, surveys, observation and experimentation. Animal research may include use of tissues or body parts; or functional experiments. All research requires the overview of approval from an ethical committee. The purpose of ethics approval is to assess risks and benefits to protect human subjects and their records; to warrant that animal use is justified by the projected scientific benefits; and to ensure safety and confidentiality are incorporated into the design of each study [27].

Research is not without a monetary cost, which must be met by the researcher or institute with whom they are associated. Grants are a way to fund research projects and may be awarded by governments or private enterprises. A grant application is intended to convince reviewers and the agency to fund the project. The type of information and the level of detail in the grant proposal will vary depending on the guidelines provided by the funding agency. In general the elements of a grant proposal include: objectives, background and significance, design, target and sampled populations, outcomes, intervention, anticipated results and conclusion, and schedule and personnel [27]. Many agencies, like journals, have specific instructions and may return incomplete or non-conforming proposals. Criteria for funding will include: relevance to the agency; scientific soundness (research question and hypotheses, and the research design and sample size); capability of the researchers; and cost of the project.

Publication of research results in the scientific literature provides the basis for evolving knowledge in the discipline. Peer review is the appraisal of theories, methodologies and conclusions by other experts in the field in order to uphold credibility in the scientific process. Screening of submitted manuscripts and funding applications commits authors to accepted standards within the discipline and reduces publication of irrelevant findings and unwarranted interpretations.

Conclusion

As well as coordinating casework, management in forensic odontology should encompass nurturing staff and resources; developing standards and protocols; teaching and training; and contributing to knowledge in the discipline. Although forensic odontologists are primarily 'tradespeople' providing opinions on a range of services, coordinators should maintain links with the academic world and encourage active participation by staff in teaching and research.

References

1 Dental Practitioner Registration Data (2014) Available from: http://www.dentalboard.gov. au/About-the-Board/Statistics.aspx. Accessed August 2015.

2 Andersen TL. (2005) DVI System International: software assisting in the Thai tsunami victim identification process. *Journal of Forensic Odontostomatology* **23**, 19–25.

3 McGivney J. (2013) WinID3. Available from: http://www.winid.com. Accessed August 2015.

4 Lake AW, James H, Berketa JW. (2012) Disaster Victim Identification: quality management from an odontology perspective. *Forensic Science, Medicine and Pathology* **8**, 157–163.

5 Taylor J. (2009) Development of the Australian Society of Forensic Odontology Disaster Victim Identification Guide. *Journal of Forensic Odontostomatology* **27**, 56–63.

6 Gallagher C. (2000) Occupational health and safety management system types and effectiveness. Deakin University, Melbourne.

7 Cullen WD. (1990) *The Public Enquiry into the Piper Alpha Disaster*. London, H.M. Stationery Office.

8 Bottomley B. (1999) Occupational health and safety management systems: Strategic issues report, Sydney.

9 Occupational health and safety management systems – Specification with guidance for use. Self assessment checklist: NCSI Publication. (2001)

10 Mitchell JT. (1983) When disaster strikes.... The critical incident stress debriefing process. *Journal of Emergency Medical Services* **13**, 49–52.

11 Marmar CR, Weiss DS, Metzler TJ et al. (1996) Characteristics of emergency services personnel related to peritraumatic dissociation during critical incident exposure. *American Journal of Psychiatry* **157**, (suppl 7) 94–102.

12 Fullerton CS, Ursano RJ, Wang L. (2004) Acute stress disorder, posttraumatic stress disorder and depression in disaster or rescue workers. *American Journal of Psychiatry* **161**, 1370–1376.

13 Javidi H, Yadollahie M. (2012) Post-traumatic stress disorder. *International Journal of Occupational and Environmental Medicine* **3**, 2–9.

14 Swygard H, Stafford RE. (2009) Effects on health of volunteers deployed during a disaster. *American Journal of Surgery* **75**, 747–752.

15 Thormar SB, Gersons BP, Juen B et al. (2010) The mental health impact of volunteering in a disaster setting: a review. *Journal of Nervous and Mental Disease* **198**, 529–538.

16 Ogińska-Bulik N. (2013) Negative and positive effects of traumatic experience in a group of emergency service workers – the role of personal and social resources. *Medycyna Pracy* **64**, 463–472.

17 Huusom AJ, Agner T, Backer V et al. (2012) Skin and respiratory disorders following the identification of disaster victims in Thailand. *Forensic Science, Medicine and Pathololology* **8**, 114–117.

18 Hamann CP, Rodgers PA, Sullivan KM. (2004) Occupational allergens in dentistry. *Current Opinion in Allergy and Clinical Immunology* **4**, 403–409.

19 Elder A, Paterson C. (2006) Sharps injuries in UK health care: A review of injury rates, viral transmission and potential efficacy of safety devices. *Occupational Medicine* **56**, 566–574.

20 Hanzlick R, Nolte K, de Jong J. (2009) The Medical Examiner/Coroner's Guide for Contaminated Deceased Body Management. *American Journal of Forensic Medicine and Pathology* **30**, 327–338.

21 Screen-based workstation [cited AS 3590]. Available from: http://www.standards.org.au. Accessed August 2015.

22 Hill IR. (1984) *Forensic Odontology: Its Scope and History*. Alan Clift Assoc., Solihull, pp. 35–94, 132, 185, 209.

23 Luntz LL. (1977) History of forensic dentistry. *Dental Clinics of North America* **21**, 7–17.

24 Coughlin CN. (2009) See one, do one, teach one: Dissecting the use of medical education's signature pedagogy in the law school curriculum. *Georgia State University Law Review* **26**, Article 4.

25 DePoy E, Gitlin LN. (1994) *Introduction to Research Multiple Strategies for Health and Human Services*. Elsevier, Mosby, pp. 16–27.

26 Excellence in Research for Australia. Available from: http://www.arc.gov.au/excellence-research-australia. Accessed August 2015.

27 Bordage G, Dawson B. (2003) Experimental study design and grant writing in 8 steps and 28 questions. *Medical Education* **37**, 376–385.

CHAPTER 14

Application of post-mortem computed tomography to forensic odontology

Richard Bassed[1] and Eleanor Bott[2]

[1] Victorian Institute of Forensic Medicine, Victoria; and Monash University, Australia
[2] Healthscope Pathology, Australia

Introduction

Advanced medical imaging, including computed tomography (CT), has in many ways revolutionised the practice of clinical medicine and dentistry. This revolution has occurred over the last three decades, and further advancements and new applications for imaging are consistently being discovered. CT technology enables direct imaging and differentiation of soft tissue structures, such as liver, lung, brain, blood vessels (with contrast media) and fat. It is especially useful in searching for space-occupying lesions, tumours and metastases, revealing their presence and size, spatial location and extent. CT imaging provides excellent tissue contrast (although differentiating soft tissue organs without contrast media can be challenging), as well as high spatial resolution. This enables the use of CT in dentistry for detailed examination of the facial skeleton and the teeth. The image post-processing capabilities of CT, creating both multi-planar reconstructions and three-dimensional (3D) displays, further enhances the value of CT imaging for dentists and maxillofacial surgeons. For instance, 3D CT is an invaluable tool for surgical reconstruction following facial trauma. It can be said that it would be quite rare today to find in clinical practice a dentist planning complex implant or third molar surgery without first consulting detailed CT imaging of the area of interest. The voxel based nature of CT data – a voxel being the 3D version of a pixel – allows for accurate measurement of distance in all directions, and high-resolution imaging (numerous voxels in a small space) allows good assessment of bone density and alerts clinicians to the presence of anomalies and anatomical variation.

Before discussing the application of CT imaging to forensic odontology, it is appropriate to briefly outline what exactly CT imaging is, and how it has evolved into a useful tool in forensic practice.

Forensic Odontology: Principles and Practice, First Edition. Edited by Jane A. Taylor and Jules A. Kieser.
© 2016 John Wiley & Sons, Ltd. Published 2016 by John Wiley & Sons, Ltd.

The essence of CT imaging involves a radiation source emitting a finely collimated fan-shaped x-ray beam rotating rapidly about a patient. A series of detectors also rotate about the patient opposite the radiation source, both detectors and radiation source being located in a large ring shaped 'doughnut'. The patient moves through the x-ray beam on a sliding gantry at a prescribed rate, and the result is a volume of data that can be manipulated in order to demonstrate different bodily structures of differing densities based on their varied ability to attenuate the x-ray beam (differential density is expressed as Hounsfield Units (Hu) where water is 0 Hu, air is –1000 Hu, bone will be from +700 Hu upwards depending on density, and tooth enamel will be anywhere from 2000 Hu to over 3000 Hu).

The first commercially viable CT scanner was invented in 1971 by Sir Godfrey Hounsfield, at the EMI Central Research Laboratories in the UK. The first patient brain-scan, performed on 1 October 1971, revealed a brain tumour in a 41-year-old female patient. These early clinical CT scanners provided slice thicknesses of between 8–13 mm, and scan times of up to 20 minutes. Since then technology has improved in quantum leaps in a relatively short period of time. Enhancements in image quality and speed of acquisition, and significant reductions in slice thickness, have been the major foci of development. Scanners now produce images with ever greater speed and higher resolution, enabling increasing accuracy in diagnoses and enhanced precision in the performance of medical procedures. The applications for CT imaging in clinical medical practice, and more recently in dental practice are numerous, ranging from diagnosis and treatment planning, to involvement in image-guided surgical procedures (biopsy) including the use of robotics.

Although, historically, the images generated were in the axial or transverse plane and perpendicular to the long axis of the body, modern scanners allow this volume of data to be reformatted in various planes or even as volumetric (3D) representations of individual structures. Multi-detector computed tomography (MDCT) helical imaging utilises an array of detectors at one time, which results in a shorter scan time than single detector units and higher resolution images, down to slice thicknesses of less than 0.5 mm. The latest generation of scanners incorporates a 'dual energy' function. Dual Source CT (DSCT) is a relatively new technique used for diagnostic medical imaging that uses two different x-ray tubes in a single CT unit. With the additional tube comes the advantage of exposing the patient to two different energy spectrums. The advantage of DSCT is that by employing two energy settings tissues and materials can be better differentiated based on their attenuation characteristics, allowing for example, the possibility of differentiating between various dental restoration materials using imaging alone.

MDCT scanners and increasingly DSCT scanners are the current standard for clinical medical and dental practice, and while imaging of living individuals is limited by the health risks associated with radiation exposure, no such limits apply to imaging of the deceased. In forensic practice radiation dose is unimportant and therefore the deceased are able to undergo total body CT imaging at the highest resolution without consequence. The lack of heartbeat, respiration and general body movement also acts to maximise the quality and diagnostic value of the images.

Computed tomography and medico-legal death investigation

Forensic odontologists, pathologists and anthropologists all saw the potential for this imaging modality in the forensic setting early on, but the high cost and lack of available scanners meant that forensic practice lagged clinical practice in adopting this technology. The first documented forensic use of CT was by Schimacher and associates in 1977 where they described a gunshot wound to the head [1]. There is anecdotal evidence of the use of post-mortem CT imaging in Japan in the mid 1980s, but articles describing the utility of post-mortem computed tomography (PMCT) did not really begin to appear until the mid 1990s [2–5].

PMCT imaging is now well established in forensic medical practice in many jurisdictions and research has demonstrated the many ways this imaging modality can assist the forensic pathologist, odontologist and anthropologist [6–12]. The advantages of PMCT in the forensic setting include assistance in determination of the appropriate death investigation procedures, autopsy planning, provision of information leading to identification of the deceased and in research. As a general protocol guide the CT scanner in use at the Victorian Institute of Forensic Medicine (VIFM) in Melbourne captures 0.5–1 mm thick slices of the head and neck and 1–2 mm slices of the remainder of the body, although higher resolution images can be acquired if needed for particular cases (paediatric cases, angiography). These datasets are then viewed using proprietary software packages on individual workstations. Reconstruction algorithms are applied to the dataset and these can be configured in various ways to highlight different anatomical features – for example either soft tissue or bone – in both 3D volumetric reconstructions and/or 2D multi-planar reformations.

This technology significantly aids the death investigation process, allowing the instigation of a 'triage' procedure during which questions surrounding identity, trauma, presence of foreign bodies and certain disease processes can be rapidly and easily addressed without the need for invasive procedures. This triage process has been formalised in some institutes whereby a duty pathologist will conduct a series of preliminary investigations with the aim of determining whether or not a full autopsy is required [13]. These investigations comprise an external examination, perusal of any relevant medical records, perusal of the circumstances surrounding the death, some initial toxicology testing, and examination of the post-mortem MDCT images. The integration of PMCT imaging has enabled forensic pathologists, in certain types of cases, to determine a reasonable cause of death without the need for a traditional autopsy. In the event that an autopsy is required, the scans can be examined prior to the autopsy and can serve to aid autopsy planning, to anticipate hazards and to view areas of the body that would normally be difficult to access during the autopsy procedure.

There has been considerable discussion in the popular press, and among some forensic practitioners, arguing that PMCT imaging would be able to replace the autopsy entirely; the so-called 'virtopsy' approach [14]. Almost 10 years of experience with this imaging technique in forensic practice in Australia and elsewhere has shown that this is not yet the case. Whilst post-mortem MDCT offers the pathologist and odontologist an unparalleled ability to look inside a deceased individual and to examine internal structures in both two and three dimensions (Fig. 14.1), there are still many medical and/or forensic issues that can only be resolved with the performance of a traditional autopsy. There is, however, considerable thought being devoted to proposals that aim to utilise imaging in conjunction with partial or 'targeted' autopsy procedures, including the use of angiography, which may serve to reduce the degree of dissection undertaken in certain cases [15].

As technology develops over time and new scanners displaying internal structure in ever greater detail and resolution come into clinical use, it is anticipated that the range of forensic applications for post-mortem radiology will expand. An example of this relevant to forensic odontology practice is the introduction of DSCT scanners. These may, once the requisite research is complete, enable practitioners to differentiate between different dental restorative materials by means of their radiation absorption characteristics (see later). This opens the possibility of eventually being able to accurately describe the dental condition of a deceased

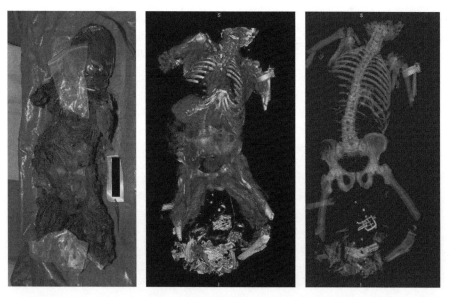

Fig. 14.1 Example of CT 'dissection'. (Reproduced with permission of the Victorian Institute of Forensic Medicine.) (*See insert for colour representation of the figure.*)

individual via imaging alone, without any requirement to physically examine the body. Another example, of relevance to forensic pathology, is the emerging sub-speciality of post-mortem angiography whereby techniques are being developed to inject contrast media into the circulation of deceased individuals in order to better visualise pathology related to the cause of death [16].

Another forensic discipline with an interest in post-mortem CT imaging is forensic anthropology. Active research is now being conducted in this field to discover whether it is possible to determine the biological profile (sex, stature, age, ancestry) of a set of decomposed remains using imaging alone [17–19]. Several studies have been conducted to determine the dimensional accuracy of CT imaging for measuring skeletal elements, and for examining growth centres for age-estimation purposes [20,21].

From a medico-legal viewpoint, full body CT scans are kept indefinitely, there-fore forming a permanent digital record of each case, and can thus be examined at any time if issues surrounding death should arise after the body has been interred or cremated. The images may also be used to provide a pictorial representation of complex injury patterns for use in court (Fig. 14.2). These images are often clearer for juries to understand, and are far less confronting when compared to images of the deceased. Thought is now being given to the production of 3D models, printed from CT volumetric datasets in a variety of materials, which may be used for teaching and court presentation purposes [22,23].

Application of PMCT to odontology

MDCT imaging is particularly useful for the examination of hard tissues within the body: the teeth and skeleton, where fine details of dental structure and the delicate facial skeleton can be visualised in exquisite detail. Research concerning the use of CT imaging for identification, trauma analysis and age estimation has been conducted for several years now with promising early results [24–32]. The ability to reconstruct CT data in three dimensions and to manipulate these in 3D space on a computer screen provides what is in effect a three-dimensional radio-graph of the hard tissues. These images are dimensionally accurate representa-tions of reality. As such, they are much easier to interpret than conventional radiographs, which are two-dimensional views of three-dimensional objects, and are thus prone to interpretative error, especially when very accurate descrip-tion and measurement of complex craniofacial injuries is required.

Prior to the implementation of PMCT, analysis of skeletal injury to the head and face often required complex dissection, a difficult and time-consuming proce-dure with obvious stressful implications for the family of the deceased. The act of dissection itself may also alter the relationship between fractured skeletal ele-ments, further complicating the situation with regards to accurate reporting. The ability to look inside the body with 3D imaging facilitates visualisation of those

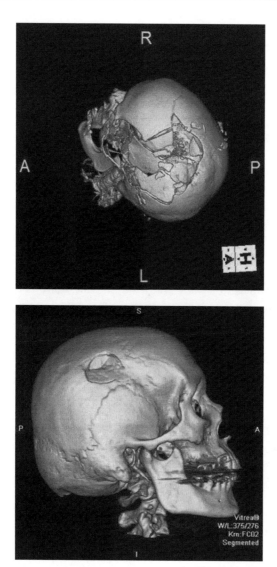

Fig. 14.2 Pictorial representation of injuries – useful for evidence presentation in court. (Reproduced with permission of the Victorian Institute of Forensic Medicine.)

parts of the skeleton that are difficult to access and describe via conventional dissection, such as the internal bones of the facial skeleton. Accurate description of the injuries to deep facial structures can have forensic significance in cases where degree of force may be an important consideration. The diagnostic quality of these images means that facial dissection can be avoided in many instances (Fig. 14.3).

The majority of the workload of a forensic odontologist involves the identification of unknown human remains. This is conducted by comparing ante-mortem dental information relating to a known individual with post-mortem information gleaned from the deceased. The vast majority of dental identifications are

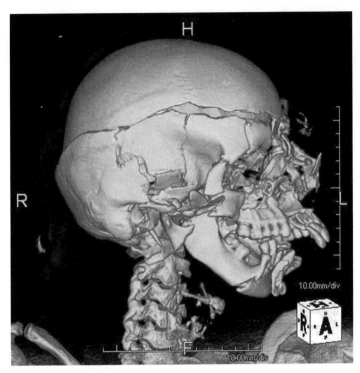

Fig. 14.3 Description and analysis of complex facial fractures facilitated using MDCT. (Reproduced with permission of the Victorian Institute of Forensic Medicine.)

confirmed by comparison of dental restorations via their description within dental charts and by comparison of ante-mortem and post-mortem radiographs. This is one area where the limitations inherent in post-mortem CT imaging become apparent. Although it is possible to see that there are restorations within teeth in CT images, it is often difficult and sometimes impossible to properly visualise the shape and size of these in many instances. Metal flaring artifact, or beam hardening (Fig. 14.4), will act to obscure the necessary fine detail in metallic restorations, and can also obscure restorations in adjacent teeth, and composite resin/glass ionomer cements/porcelain restorations can be difficult to distinguish from sound tooth structure. Some of these issues are being addressed by the use of dual-energy scanners, and it is now becoming possible to accurately visualise tooth-coloured dental restorations, and even amalgam restorations, particularly in individuals where there are only a few restorations. This is especially helpful in the visualisation of the various types of tooth-coloured restorations (Fig.14.5). Metal artifact is also much reduced with the use of DSCT, although it is still not often possible to achieve complete clarity regarding the morphology of most amalgam restorations. With further research and technological advancement, it will soon be possible to differentiate between restoration types [11,33–35], with the Holy Grail being to be able to replicate with PMCT the quality and clarity of conventional ante-mortem radiographs.

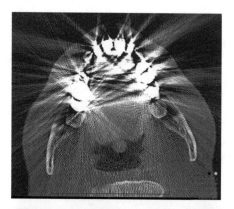

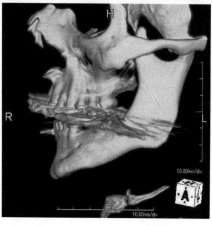

Fig. 14.4 Metal flare from amalgam restorations obscuring anatomical structure. (Reproduced with permission of the Victorian Institute of Forensic Medicine.)

One area of odontology practice that is particularly amenable to CT analysis is age estimation, using both the developing dentition and the skeleton (Fig. 14.6). The ability to determine a scientifically based age range for an unknown deceased individual aids investigators in the search for identity by eliminating a large number of possible matches due to age. In disaster victim identification, for example (see below), age estimation has been used to discriminate between, and thus identify, individuals when other means of identification were not possible (Fig. 14.7) [28].

Determining the legal status of unknown age living individuals – adult or child – is also an active area of research, with efforts currently underway to construct age estimation formulae for modern populations of interest to legal systems across the world [25]. Of course there are a multitude of issues that are yet to be overcome, including the ethical questions involved in exposing living individuals to ionising radiation with no definite medical need, and the considerable logistical and financial problems associated with getting this imaging technology to the populations of interest – inevitably from developing countries with limited resources. MDCT imaging is nevertheless beginning to play a major

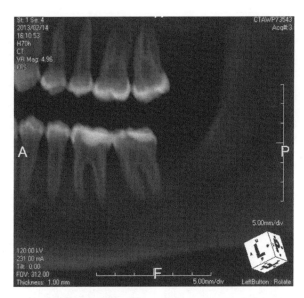

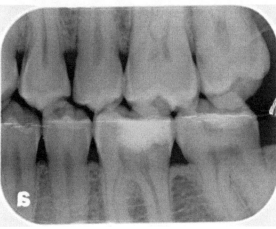

Fig. 14.5 Image on the top is a 3D DECT reconstruction using the bone algorithm and shows the detailed morphology of composite resin restorations in the lower molar teeth. The image on the bottom is a conventional ante-mortem bite-wing radiograph of the same person. (Reproduced with permission of the Victorian Institute of Forensic Medicine.)

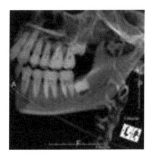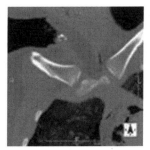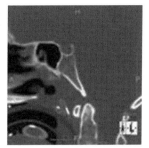

Fig. 14.6 CT images displaying development of the third molar tooth, the medial clavicular epiphysis and the spheno-occipital synchondrosis. All are useful in estimating the age of individuals in the middle to late teenage years. (Reproduced with permission of the Victorian Institute of Forensic Medicine.)

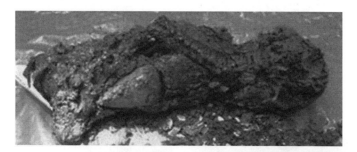

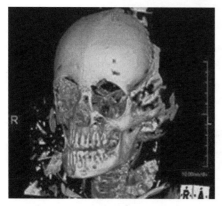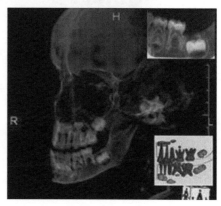

Fig. 14.7 Age estimation using CT images can identify an individual if no other people in that age range died in the incident. It also serves as an elimination tool – therefore saving investigation resources. (Reproduced with permission of the Victorian Institute of Forensic Medicine.) (*See insert for colour representation of the figure.*)

role in age estimation research, and as more institutions around the world are beginning to adopt this technology for forensic purposes, this will only increase. (For a fuller discussion of age estimation and the input of CT imaging please see Chapter 7.)

Computed tomography and Disaster Victim Identification (DVI)

The Victorian bushfire disaster of February 2009 represented the first time a CT scanner was utilised in an organised way in a major DVI operation [35,36]. It is clear from this operation that CT imaging had a profound impact on mortuary operations (DVI phase two). For the first time in a DVI setting it became possible to discover identifying information within a deceased person that would otherwise require extensive and time consuming dissection to find. Prior to any physical examination of a body in the mortuary it is now possible in many cases to discern various features within a deceased person that can greatly aid the identification process. This allows practitioners to target specific areas within a body without having to conduct a complete autopsy. Some of the identifying features discovered on CT would never have been found even with a full autopsy, as some prostheses/medical conditions are located in areas not normally examined in the course of a standard autopsy procedure. And in many DVI operations there is no place for full autopsies, with the medical examination being limited to a dissection for identification purposes only – for example, a laparotomy to assess presence/absence of uterus and gall bladder. In this scenario many internal cardiac and joint prostheses would possibly be missed without the application of full body imaging technology.

Triage of multiple deceased in DVI

Of particular relevance to DVI mortuary operations is the potential ability to triage cases based on full body CT imaging. This triaging benefits the identification process in several ways and informs case progression through the mortuary. Body admission procedures during DVI operations at the VIFM in Melbourne begin with full body CT scanning of all victims as soon as they are admitted and have been appropriately numbered. No attempts are made to open body bags or to reposition the deceased. A team of practitioners consisting of a radiologist, radiographer and an odontologist examine the CT scans. Anthropological expertise for image analysis is sought when required.

The task of the radiographer is to reconstruct the raw CT data using various algorithms so as to provide the clearest and most diagnostic images possible (both 2D and 3D) for the radiologist. The radiographer can also assist the odontologist in providing dental images with reduced artifact and enhanced detail in cases of interest to the dental team. The radiologist will analyse the images of all deceased persons involved in the incident and will be able to draw broad conclusions based on the following criteria:

1 human/non-human;
2 gender;
3 age – adult or child;
4 commingling of remains – human/non-human/multiple deceased in one body bag;
5 specific identifying features – dental work/medical prostheses/disease processes.

The radiologist and odontologist will then construct a brief report detailing findings for every case. This report will be provided to the mortuary teams at the beginning of the examination and will guide pathologists and odontologists in their investigations (Fig. 14.8).

In certain situations, especially where disruption and incineration are prevalent, the radiology examination may not be able to answer some of the above questions, but in many instances CT imaging will input into almost every case.

Figures 14.9–14.13 illustrate examples of CT imaging produced in various DVI scenarios. All of these individuals have suffered damage to a greater or lesser degree, making the discovery of most of these features a difficult proposition without the use of PMCT capability.

VIFM CT DVI screening proforma

VIFM #: _____   DVI #: _____

Date: _____   Reported by: _____

CT Technical issues: _____

State of body (circle appropriate):   Intact   Severely burnt   Remains   Individual parts

Details: _____

Type of remains (circle appropriate):   Human   Non-human   Co-mingled   not able to be determined

Details _____

Gender (circle appropriate):   M   F   not able to be determined

Based on _____

Growths plates (circle appropriate):   Y   N   not able to be determined

Location _____

Disease (circle appropriate):

Coronary artery calcification   Y   N   not able to be determined

Systemic vascular calcification   Y   N   not able to be determined

    (if so where) _____

Osteoarthritis   Y   N   not able to be determined

    (if so where) _____

Other _____

Identification:

Teeth (details) _____

Medical devices (details) _____

Other _____

Summary (circle):

Gender: Male   Female   not able to be determined

Estimated age: <12 months   1-5y   5-13y   13-20y   20-40y   40-60y   >60y   Don't know

ID features: Teeth   Medical devices   Other _____

Fig. 14.8 Report format used by radiologists at the VIFM for assessment of PMCT imaging delivered to mortuary teams to assist with DVI operations. (Reproduced with permission of the Victorian Institute of Forensic Medicine.)

Recent research coming out of the Swiss virtual autopsy (VIRTOPSY) project demonstrates personal identification via the comparison of normal anatomy and disease processes using post-mortem CT imaging. The practitioners involved in this study compared ante-mortem images of various anatomical structures with the post-mortem CT imaging. Comparisons were made between structures including

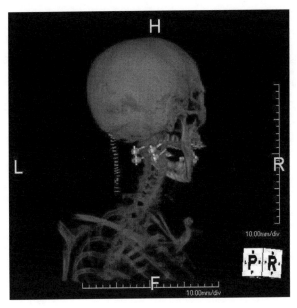

Fig. 14.9 A series of four titanium fixtures placed in the posterior cervical region. These may not be found during the course of a normal DVI pathology examination, especially considering the burned nature of the remains. This represents a most useful identifier, especially when this information can be compared to ante-mortem imaging and surgical notes. (Reproduced with permission of the Victorian Institute of Forensic Medicine.)

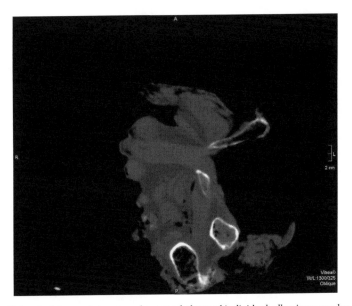

Fig. 14.10 CT detail of the genital region of a severely burned individual, allowing a gender determination to be made (male). Given the nature of the remains determining gender may be problematic with normal physical examination methods, and although not in itself identifying, this fact immediately eliminates half of the population, thus narrowing the possibilities for identification. (Reproduced with permission of the Victorian Institute of Forensic Medicine.)

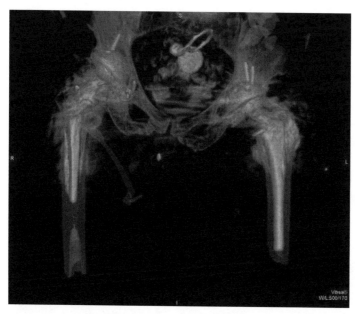

Fig. 14.11 Bilateral prosthetic hip replacements in burned remains. As this area is not routinely dissected in the normal DVI autopsy protocol, these could easily be missed. The degree of burning means that any external signs of past surgery will have been obliterated. These prostheses have on them serial numbers that can be related back to medical records, thus providing a positive identification. (Reproduced with permission of the Victorian Institute of Forensic Medicine.)

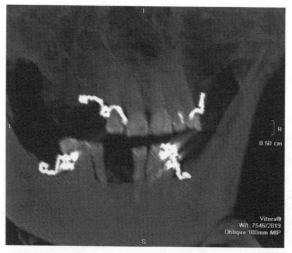

Fig. 14.12 Detail of dental restorative work that can be visualised when appropriate algorithms are applied to the raw CT data. Even though the shape detail of restorations is unclear due to metal artefact, it is possible to see the clasps of upper and lower acrylic partial dentures, a pin in an upper lateral incisor and metallic restorations in lower premolar teeth. (Reproduced with permission of the Victorian Institute of Forensic Medicine.)

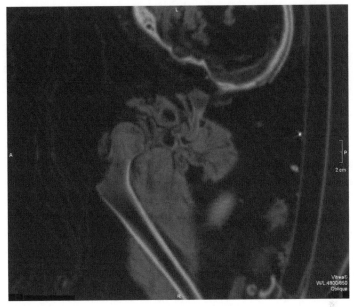

Fig. 14.13 A small section of a larger set of commingled and fragmented remains. This image shows the head of a femur with separate diaphysis and epiphysis clearly visible, indicating a child. Other bones in this set of remains were diagnosed by the radiologist as adult, thus confirming a commingled situation of at least two individuals requiring very careful examination to separate them. (Reproduced with permission of the Victorian Institute of Forensic Medicine.)

sinuses within the skull, the appearance of natural disease, bony trabeculae in long bones and dental features [37]. All of these techniques can now be applied in any DVI scenario, thus facilitating the identification process and resulting in faster completion times.

CT and dental identification in DVI

Until very recently the value of CT imaging to forensic odontology and identification has been realised in being able to recognise the presence of dental treatment in a deceased person prior to performing an examination. In DVI operations this has proven invaluable in that it allows a rapid triage and targeting of cases that are likely to provide quick and easy identifications, allowing more time for complex cases. This approach saves time and means that for many victims, identification and release can occur relatively rapidly. Dental pathology can be diagnosed fairly clearly and the presence of obvious treatment such as root canal therapy, crown work, recent extractions, orthodontic and prosthetic appliances and titanium implants can be readily seen. However, while restorations (especially metallic) can be seen and attributed to a particular tooth, it is not possible in most instances to determine the exact morphology of that restoration due to the presence of metal artifact. In mouths with large numbers of amalgam restorations it can be difficult determining which teeth are filled, let alone which tooth surfaces are included in each restoration (Fig. 14.4). This means that for many cases an accurate dental chart cannot be constructed using CT imaging alone, and conventional dental examination and radiography will be required. There is, however, hope that future advances in PMCT imaging will allow construction of accurate dental charts that will minimise the necessity for physical examination and dissection in a large number of cases. As discussed previously, the latest generation DSCT scanners are offering new opportunities for forensic odontology, in that it is now possible to resolve restoration morphology to a level of clarity not previously seen (Fig. 14.5).

One area where CT imaging is of immense value in DVI is in age estimation of individuals who are still developing their dentition. Imaging of the dentition is clear and precise with regards to tooth development, and as long as the appropriate reference data table/formulae are available, useful age estimates can be made that can considerably narrow the investigation as to identity. This is particularly useful in incidents where there may be a number of children, all of different ages, who are unable to be separated on the basis of visual examination due to trauma or incineration but who can be readily separated according to age based on dental development [28].

If CT scanning is to be employed in a DVI operation it is essential that the appropriate expertise is available to reconstruct raw data with appropriate algorithms, and that practitioners are able to correctly interpret the images. Dentists need to be familiar with the type of scanner used and the imaging software that is being employed, as well as possessing a significant level of experience in reading and interpreting CT images.

Logistics and infrastructure

Advanced medical imaging technology is expensive. Hence the vast majority of scanners used in the world are dedicated to the diagnosis and treatment of the living. Very few forensic institutes can afford the luxury of a dedicated CT scanner and, of those, many rely on older superseded technology. Some forensic institutes have an arrangement with a local hospital that will allow them to scan certain cases if a particular need arises, but only after hours and very rarely at that.

Not only is CT imaging prohibitively expensive for many jurisdictions, it is also resource hungry in terms of the infrastructure and space required to house the scanner, image storage capacity, the power supply, the expertise required to run and repair the machine and the medical expertise needed to interpret the images. In general, the only time a CT scanner will be employed in a DVI scenario is if the disaster occurs in a jurisdiction that possesses a dedicated forensic CT capability. The exceptions to this are the military of countries such as the USA, who have mobile CT scanners that are deployable to operational theatres.

The other notable exception is the British Forensic Identification Imaging System (FIMAG), which has a number of mobile CT scanners dedicated to forensic purposes [38,39]. The FIMAG system is based on developing capability to scan multiple victims of a mass fatality event at the scene, or as close to the scene as possible, thus avoiding the pitfalls associated with body transport and storage (body numbering errors, further damage or degradation of remains due to rough handling). This system will also ease the demand placed on local forensic facilities, which will have their regular caseloads to deal with and thus may not be in a position to cater for a large number of deceased at one time. Once the scans have been completed, the images can be viewed remotely from anywhere in the world. There is no need for the radiologist to be actually present on site. This also applies to the odontologists who perform the initial CT assessment of the dentitions of the victims. They can be located at their home office and can construct reports to be sent to the on-site mortuary team.

Conclusion

Computed tomography has already been, and will increasingly continue to be, a revolution for forensic practice. MDCT has enhanced our ability to assess the deceased in terms of identity and cause and manner of death, and has fostered many areas of research, the results of which are now beginning to inform new ways this imaging modality can be used in the forensic setting. In some ways it has not been quite the revolution that some had hoped for – in terms of it not being able to replace entirely the need for autopsy and physical examination. The aims of the VIRTOPSY project are yet to be fully realised, and no doubt there will always be a need for dissection in the medico-legal death investigation process. For forensic odontology, some cases are now amenable to positive identification without the necessity of directly examining the oral cavity of the deceased. For most cases, and until imaging techniques are refined (especially in terms of metal artifact and restoration type differentiation), conventional examination methods still apply. For DVI, a case can be made for saying that PMCT has had a profound impact, especially in terms of the triage of multiple deceased persons, the rapid recognition of identifying features and forensic evidence and the increasing ability to perform scientifically robust identifications using imaging alone. It remains to be seen whether the technology can be made economically viable so as to become a standard part of any DVI operation, no matter where it may occur.

It behooves all of us as practitioners to familiarise ourselves with the possibilities and limitations of this technology, and to conduct research into new applications that will add to the current body of knowledge concerning the use of advanced imaging in medico-legal death investigation.

References

1   Wullenweber R, Schneider V, Gremme T. (1977) A computer-tomographical examination of cranial bullet wounds. *Zeitschrift fur Rechtsmedizin – Journal of Legal Medicine* **80**, 227–246.
2   Haglund WD, Fligner CL. (1993) Confirmation of human identification using computerized tomography. *Journal of Forensic Sciences* **38**, 708–712.

3 Riepert T, Rittner C, Ulmcke D et al. (1995) Identification of an unknown corpse by means of computed tomography (CT) of the lumber spine. *Journal of Forensic Sciences* **40**, 126–127.

4 Rouge D, Telmon N, Arrue P et al. (1993) Radiographic identification of human remains through deformities and anomalies of post-cranial bones: a report of two cases. *Journal of Forensic Sciences* **38**, 997–1007.

5 Oliver WR, Chancellor AS, Soltys M et al. (1995) Three dimensional reconstruction of a bullet path: Validation by computed tomography. *Journal of Forensic Sciences* **40**, 321.

6 O'Donnell C, Rotman A, Collett S et al. (2007) Current status of routine post-mortem CT in Melbourne, Australia. *Forensic Science, Medicine and Pathology* **3**, 226–232.

7 Thali MJ, Dirnhofer R, Vock P. (2009) *The Virtopsy Approach. 3D Optical and Radiological Scanning and Reconstruction in Forensic Medicine.* CRC Press, Florida, pp. 169–185.

8 Burke MP. (2012) *Forensic Pathology of Fractures and Mechanisms of Injury.* CRC Press, Florida, pp. 75–107.

9 Levy AD, Theodore Harcke H. (2011) *Essentials of Forensic Imaging.* CRC Press, Florida, pp. 11–29.

10 Murphy M, Drage N, Carabott R et al. (2012) Accuracy and reliability of cone beam computed tomography of the jaws for comparative forensic identification: a preliminary study. *Journal of Forensic Sciences* **57**, 964–968.

11 Jackowski C, Wyss M, Persson A et al. (2008) Ultra-high-resolution dual-source CT for forensic dental visualization–discrimination of ceramic and composite fillings. *International Journal of Legal Medicine* **122**, 301–307.

12 O'Donnell C, Woodford N. (2008) Post-mortem radiology – a new sub-speciality? *Clinical Radiology* **63**, 1189–1194.

13 O'Donnell CJ, Woodford N. (2010) Imaging the dead. Can supplement but not replace autopsy in medicolegal death investigation. *British Medical Journal (online)* **341**, c7415.

14 Thali MJ, Jackowski C, Oesterhelweg L et al. (2007) VIRTOPSY – the Swiss virtual autopsy approach. *Legal Medicine (Tokyo)* **9**, 100–104.

15 Pollanen MS, Woodford N. (2013) Virtual autopsy: time for a clinical trial. *Forensic Science, Medicine and Pathology* **9**, 427–428.

16 Grabherr S, Doenz F, Steger B et al. (2011) Multi-phase post-mortem CT angiography: development of a standardized protocol. *International Journal of Legal Medicine* **125**, 791–802.

17 Stull KE, Tise ML, Ali Z et al. (2014) Accuracy and reliability of measurements obtained from computed tomography 3D volume rendered images. *Forensic Science International* **238**, 133–140.

18 Brough AL, Morgan B, Robinson C et al. (2014) A minimum data set approach to post-mortem computed tomography reporting for anthropological biological profiling. *Forensic Science and Medical Pathology* **10**, 504–512.

19 Morgan J, Lynnerup JN, Hoppa RD. (2013) The lateral angle revisited: a validation study of the reliability of the lateral angle method for sex determination using computed tomography (CT). *Journal of Forensic Sciences* **58**, 443–447.

20 Brough AL, Rutty GN, Black S et al. (2012) Post-mortem computed tomography and 3D imaging: anthropological applications for juvenile remains. *Forensic Science, Medicine and Pathololopy* **8**, 270–279.

21 Sakurai T, Michiue T, Ishikawa T et al. (2012) Postmortem CT investigation of skeletal and dental maturation of the fetuses and newborn infants: a serial case study. *Forensic Science, Medicine and Pathology* **8**, 351–357.

22 Brennan J. (2010) Production of anatomical models from CT scan data. Masters Dissertation, De Montfort University, Leicester, United Kingdom.

23 Negi S, Dhiman S, Sharma RK. (2014) Basics and applications of rapid prototyping medical models. *Rapid Prototyping Journal* **20**, 256–267.

24 Bassed RB, Briggs C, Olaf H et al. (2011) Age estimation and the developing third molar tooth: an analysis of an Australian population using computed tomography. *Journal of Forensic Sciences* **56**, 1185–1191.

25 Bassed RB, Briggs C, Drummer OH. (2011) Age estimation using CT imaging of the third molar tooth, the medial clavicular epiphysis, and the spheno-occipital synchondrosis: A multifactorial approach. *Forensic Science International* **212**, 273.

26 Graham JP, O'Donnell CJ, Craig PJG et al. (2010) The application of computerized tomography (CT) to the dental ageing of children and adolescents. *Forensic Science International* **195**, 58–62.

27 Bassed RB. (2011) Advances in forensic age estimation. *Forensic Science Medicine and Pathology* (online) doi: 10.1007/s12024–011–9280–3

28 Bassed RB, Hill AJ. (2011) The use of computed tomography (CT) to estimate age in the 2009 Victorian Bushfire Victims: A case report. *Forensic Science International* **205**, 48–51.

29 Wang JJ, Wang JL, Chen YL et al. (2012) A post–processing technique for cranial CT image identification. *Forensic Science International* **221**, 23–28.

30 Bassed RB, Ranson D. (2012) Age determination of asylum seekers and alleged people smugglers. *Journal of Law and Medicine* **20**, 261–265.

31 Buitrago–Téllez CH, Schilli W, Bohnert M et al. (2002) A comprehensive classification of craniofacial fractures: postmortem and clinical studies with two- and three-dimensional computed tomography. *Injury* **33**, 651–668.

32 Ruder TD, Kraehenbuehl M, Gotsmy WF et al. (2011) Radiologic identification of disaster victims: A simple and reliable method using CT of the paranasal sinuses. *European Journal of Radiology* **81**, e132–e138, doi:10.1016/j.ejrad.2011.01.060.

33 Persson A, Jackowski C, Engström et al. (2008) Advances of dual source, dual-energy imaging in postmortem CT. *European Journal of Radiology* **68**, 446–455.

34 Stolzmann P, Winklhofer S, Schwendener N et al. (2013) Monoenergetic computed tomography reconstructions reduce beam hardening artifacts from dental restorations. *Forensic Science, Medicine and Pathology* **9**, 327–332.

35 O'Donnell C, Iino M, Mansharan K et al. (2011) Contribution of postmortem multidetector CT scanning to identification of the deceased in a mass disaster: Experience gained from the 2009 Victorian bushfires. *Forensic Science International* **205**, 15–28.

36 Cordner SM, Woodford N, Bassed R et al. (2011) Forensic aspects of the 2009 Victorian Bushfires Disaster. *Forensic Science International* **205**, 2–7.

37 Hatch GM, Dedouit F, Christensen AM et al. (2014) RADid: A pictorial review of radiologic identification using postmortem CT. *Journal of Forensic Radiology and Imaging* **2**, 52–59.

38 Rutty GN, Robinson C, Morgan B et al. (2009) Fimag: the United Kingdom disaster victim/forensic identification imaging system. *Journal of Forensic Sciences* **54**, 1438–1442.

39 Rutty GN, Robinson CE, BouHaidar R et al. (2007) The role of mobile computed tomography in mass fatality incidents. *Journal of Forensic Sciences* **52**, 1343–1349.

Index

Note: Page numbers in *italics* refer to Figures; those in **bold** to Tables.

Forensic Odontology: Principles and Practice, First Edition. Edited by Jane A. Taylor and Jules A. Kieser.
© 2016 John Wiley & Sons, Ltd. Published 2016 by John Wiley & Sons, Ltd.